# Psychiatry Morning Report

**Volume Editors:**

*I would like to dedicate this book to Carolyn Tamas, Emily Tamas, Ken Luther, Dr. Amy Holthouser, and all of my wonderful family and friends. And I would like to thank all of my former teachers.*
**-Rebecca L. Tamas**

*We dedicate this book to our partners, pets, friends, and all of the teachers we had along the way.*

*We'd like to acknowledge Deborah Meisel, MS who is about to become an excellent psychiatrist. Her infectious intellectual curiosity helped shape this book.*

*A very special thank and acknowledgment to Jack Krasuki, MD whose board-review courses made psychiatry easy to understand, and took us to the next step in our careers.*
**-Tammy Duong and Peter Ureste**

**Series Editors:**

*Michelle and I would like to dedicate this book to our amazing children, Mina and Aiden. They give us endless amounts of joy and happiness. We love hugging both of you every chance we get. We also would like to dedicate this book to our newborn baby girl, Sadie Hope who now completes the Dasgupta family.*

# Psychiatry Morning Report: Beyond the Pearls

**Series Editors**

## RAJ DASGUPTA, MD, FACP, FCCP, FAASM

Assistant Professor of Clinical Medicine
Division of Pulmonary/Critical Care/Sleep
  Medicine
Associate Program Director of the Sleep
  Medicine Fellowship
Assistant Program Director of the Internal
  Medicine Residency
Keck School of Medicine of the University
  of Southern California
Los Angeles, California

## R. MICHELLE KOOLAEE, DO

Rheumatologist, Presbyterian
  Intercommunity Hospital (PIH)
Assistant Professor of Medicine
Division of Rheumatology
University of Southern California
Los Angeles, California

**Volume Editors**

## TAMMY DUONG, MD

Assistant Professor of Clinical Psychiatry
Associate Program Director of the
  Psychiatry Residency Program
Department of Psychiatry
University of California San Francisco
San Francisco, California

## REBECCA L. TAMAS, MD

Division Medical Director, PsychBC
Assistant Clinical Professor
Department of Psychiatry and Behavioral
  Sciences
University of Louisville School of Medicine
Louisville, Kentucky

## PETER URESTE, MD

Assistant Professor of Clinical Psychiatry
Department of Psychiatry
University of California San Francisco
San Francisco, California

ELSEVIER

Elsevier
3251 Riverport Lane
St. Louis, Missouri 63043

*Content Strategist:* James Merritt
*Content Development Specialist:* Kevin Travers
*Publishing Services Manager:* Shereen Jameel
*Project Manager:* Manikandan Chandrasekaran
*Design Direction:* Bridget Hoette

Printed in China

Last digit is the print number: 9 8 7 6 5 4 3 2 1

Working together
to grow libraries in
developing countries

www.elsevier.com • www.bookaid.org

# LIST OF CONTRIBUTORS

**Elie G. Aoun, MD**
Forensic Psychiatry Research Fellow
Department of Psychiatry
Columbia University
New York, New York

**Lama Bazzi, MD, MRO, FAPA**
Clinical Assistant Professor
Department of Psychiatry
Maimonide Medical Center
New York, New York

**Amy Bischoff, MD**
Resident Physician
Department of Psychiatry and Behavioral
   Neuroscience
University of Cincinnati Medical Center
Cincinnati, Ohio

**Jeffrey Michael Bonenfant, DO**
Fellow
Department of Pulmonary, Critical Care,
   Hyperbaric and Sleep Medicine
Loma Linda University
Loma Linda, California

**Eugenia Brikker, MD**
Assistant Professor
Department of Psychiatry
University of Louisville
Louisville, Kentucky

**Sean Butterbaugh, MD, MBA**
Resident
Department of Psychiatry
Carolinas Medical Center, Atrium Health
Charlotte, North Carolina

**Peter Chung, MD**
Fellow
Department of Pulmonary Critical Care
   and Sleep Medicine
University of Southern California, Los Angeles
Los Angeles, California

**Lucas Cruz, MD**
Fellow
Department of Pulmonary and
   Critical Care
University of Southern California,
   Los Angeles
Los Angeles, California

**Raj Dasgupta, MD, FACP, FCCP, FAASM**
Assistant Professor of Clinical Medicine
Division of Pulmonary/Critical Care/Sleep
   Medicine
Associate Program Director of the Sleep
   Medicine Fellowship
Assistant Program Director of the Internal
   Medicine Residency
Keck School of Medicine of the University of
   Southern California
Los Angeles, California

**Earl Andrew B. De Guzman, MD**
Psychiatrist
Private Practice
Los Angeles, California

**Zachary Clayborne Dietrich, PsyD**
Clinical Psychologist
Psychological and Behavioral
   Consultants
Louisville, Kentucky

**Jessica Dotson, DO**
Resident Physician
Department of Psychiatry
University of Kentucky
Lexington, Kentucky

**Alison Duncan, MD**
Associate Medical Director for Psychiatric
   Emergency Services
Department of Psychiatry
Boston Medical Center
Boston, Massachusetts

**Tammy Duong, MD**
Assistant Professor of Clinical Psychiatry
Associate Program Director of the Psychiatry
   Residency Program
Department of Psychiatry
University of California San Francisco
San Francisco, California

**Courtney Eaves, DO, MBA**
Assistant Professor
Department of Psychiatry
University of Louisville
Louisville, Kentucky

**Rif S. El-Mallakh, MD**
Director, Mood Disorders Research Program
Department of Psychiatry and Behavioral
   Sciences
University of Louisville School of Medicine
Louisville, Kentucky

**Kelly Fan, MD**
Pulmonary and Critical Care Medicine Fellow
University of Southern California, Los Angeles
Los Angeles, California

**Julie Flygare, JD**
President & CEO
Project Sleep
Los Angeles, California

**Christian Gerwe, MD**
Resident Physician
Department of Psychiatry
University of Kentucky
Lexington, Kentucky

**Derek William Gilbert, MD**
Resident Physician
Department of Psychiatry
University of Kentucky
Lexington, Kentucky

**Terese C. Hammond, MD**
Pulmonary Critical Care Sleep Medicine
   Fellowship
Medical Director
Providence St John's Health Center ICU/
   Intensivist Program
Associate Professor of Clinical Surgery
University of Southern California, Los Angeles
Los Angeles, California

**Meredith E. Harewood, MD**
Child, Adolescent, and Adult Psychiatrist
Pacific Coast Psychiatric Associates
Los Angeles, California

**Tiya Johnson, MD**
Assistant Clinical Professor
Department of Pediatrics, University of
   Louisville
Louisville, Kentucky

**Kurtis S. Kaminishi, MD, MBA**
Geriatric Psychiatrist
Department of Psychiatry
University of California, San Francisco
San Francisco, California

**Walter Klein, MD**
Attending Physician, Pulmonary/Critical
   Care Medicine
Riverside University Health System Medical
   Center
Moreno Valley, California
Health Sciences Assistant Clinical Professor
   of Internal Medicine
University of California, Riverside
Riverside, California
Assistant Professor of Medicine
Loma Linda University
Loma Linda, California

**Jack Krasuski, MD**
Executive Director
American Physician Institute for Advanced
   Professional Studies LLC
Westmont, Illinois

**Lauren H. Marasa, MD**
General and Forensic Psychiatrist
Private Practice
Sacramento, California

**Daniel Martinez, MD**
Assistant Professor of Clinical Medicine
Keck School of Medicine of the University
  of Southern California
Los Angeles, California

**Tiffany Martinez, MA**
Phoenix, Arizona

**Charlene McAndrews, PMHNP-BC, ARNP**
Psychiatric-Mental Health Nurse Practitioner
PsychBC
Louisville, Kentucky

**Aarti Chawla Mittal, DO**
Associate Program Director
Pulmonary and Critical Care Medicine
  Fellowship
Loma Linda University School of Medicine
Loma Linda, California
Assistant Professor of Medicine
Department of Pulmonary and Critical Care
  Medicine
University of California, Riverside School
  of Medicine
Riverside, California

**Stefana Morgan, MD**
Geriatric Psychiatry Fellow
Department of Psychiatry
University of California, San Francisco
San Francisco, California

**Susie Morris, MD**
Chief, Consultation-Liaison Services
Department of Psychiatry
University of Southern California, Los Angeles
Los Angeles, California

**Roya Noorishad, MD**
Resident
Keck Medicine of the University of
  Southern California
Los Angeles, California

**Mitesh Patel, MD**
Psychiatrist
Stress Center
St. Vincent's Hospital
Indianapolis, Indiana

**Olesya Pokorna, MD**
Adult Psychiatrist
Department of Psychiatry
University of California, San Francisco
San Francisco, California

**Jessica Reis, MD**
Assistant Professor
Department of Psychiatry
University of Louisville
Louisville, Kentucky

**Reza Safavi, MD**
Assistant Professor of Psychiatry
Department of Psychiatry
Baylor College of Medicine
Houston, Texas

**Kimberly Shain, BA**
Medical Student
University of Kentucky College of Medicine
Lexington, Kentucky

**Emily Sykes, MD**
Resident Physician
Department of Psychiatry and Behavioral
  Neuroscience
University of Cincinnati
Cincinnati, Ohio

**Rebecca L. Tamas, MD**
Division Medical Director, PsychBC
Assistant Clinical Professor
Department of Psychiatry and Behavioral
  Sciences
University of Louisville School of Medicine
Louisville, Kentucky

**Peter Ureste, MD**
Assistant Professor of Clinical Psychiatry
Department of Psychiatry
University of California, San Francisco
San Francisco, California

**Edwin Valladares, MS**
Adjunct Professor
Sleep Disorders Center
Keck Hospital of University of Southern
    California
Los Angeles, California

**Destry Washburn, DO**
Assistant Professor
Department of Internal Medicine
Riverside University Health System Medical
    Center
Moreno Valley, California

**Haley Wehder, MD**
Medical Student
University of Kentucky College of Medicine
Lexington, Kentucky

**Lawson Wulsin, MD**
Professor Emeritus
Department of Psychiatry and Behavioral
    Neuroscience
University of Cincinnati
Cincinnati, Ohio

**Timothy Yff, MD**
Resident Physician
Department of Psychiatry and Behavioral
    Sciences
University of Louisville
Louisville, Kentucky

**William H. Zhu, MD, MS**
Resident
Department of Psychiatry
University of California, San Francisco
San Francisco, California

Drs. Dasgupta and Koolaee are to be congratulated for developing the new and much-needed series of case-based books for in-training and practicing medical professionals, *Morning Report: Beyond the Pearls*. With psychiatry volume editors—Drs. Tammy Duong, Rebecca Tamas, and Peter Ureste—the team has succeeded in delivering what every psychiatrist can use: in-depth, user-friendly clinical cases with practical take-home facts. Whether for the medical student, the resident, or the clinician in practice, *Psychiatry Morning Report* will keep us fresh, current, and sharp. I first met "Dr. Raj" on the set of the TV show *The Doctors*, where he was the go-to sleep medicine and pulmonary specialist for the past 6 seasons. "Dr. Raj" always has a smile on his face and brings positive energy to the show and truly personifies the core elements of a great teacher—engaging personality, great work ethic, and amazing knowledge of medicine. It is always a pleasure to work with Dr. Raj, and I am confident that this book is as enthusiastic, passionate, and informative as his segments on the show.

*Judy Ho, PhD, ABPP, ABPdN*
Licensed clinical and forensic neuropsychologist, media personality, and published author
Associate Professor of Psychology
Pepperdine University Graduate School of Education and Psychology

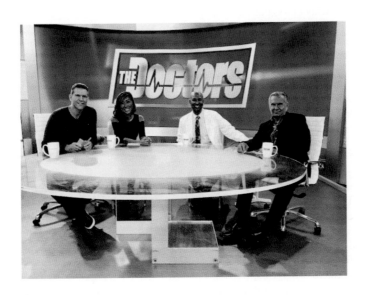

# Editorial by Hayley Gripp

At twenty-six years old, I look like my life is well put together. But what people don't see is a woman with Tourette syndrome, holding in her tics and managing her comorbid disorders—attention deficit disorder, obsessive-compulsive disorder, depression, and mild social anxiety. Imagine one hundred thoughts and emotions going through your head, feeling a tic come—like an urge to sneeze—and fighting to suppress it. Imagine straining to focus on one subject and forcing oneself to think positive thoughts while looking at the clock to see how soon you can decompress on your own. Yet despite these daily battles, I have no complaints. I have an incredible life. I realize that every struggle I have battled has not only made me stronger but also helped me give a voice to the voiceless.

Having an invisible disability like Tourette, I have always been an incredibly compassionate and nonjudgmental person. For those who don't know what Tourette syndrome is, it's a bioneurologic brain disorder that causes the body to make movements and sounds that it cannot control. Over 80% of people with Tourette are also afflicted by many other comorbid disorders. One in one hundred children have Tourette syndrome, but only one in every few thousand are diagnosed by a doctor. People who are not educated often discriminate or accuse me of making it up; it doesn't help that I am physically attractive and have a bubbly, outgoing personality when I am around people with whom I feel comfortable. Just a year ago I was discriminated against by another customer in Whole Foods Market for having tics, but these types of situations push me forward to continue educating others on my disability and the acceptance of those with disabilities.

Tics come and go, but the comorbid disorders are always there. Growing up, I experienced depression on and off as different forms of trauma or adversity developed in my life; however, through every difficult situation, I hung onto that tiny thread of hope—I chose to focus on the good. In middle school I was bullied so badly by a teacher for my disability (there were no laws to protect me at the time) that, at age sixteen, I went to Washington, DC, and lobbied to have the IDEA Act reinstated to include those with disabilities. The IDEA Act is a law that helps children with disabilities obtain proper accommodations in the education system to become successful students. It also protects students with disabilities from being bullied or abused by teachers. Right before I went to lobby to have the law updated, my mom asked me if I wanted to press charges against the teacher who bullied me. I told her, "No. I simply want to end the cycle of hate and make sure this doesn't ever happen to anyone else." I believe when we try to combat depression, anger, or frustration with other negative feelings, we are simply creating more negativity. I have learned that the more negative my thoughts, the worse my tics and comorbid disorders become.

A year after the law was reinstated and updated, my father died very suddenly. At this point, I could have fallen deeper into depression, but I chose life. Thinking positive thoughts helped me have more control over my tics. You may wonder how I am able to focus on the good. Well it's because I am so much more than my Tourette or other disabilities. On a daily basis, Tourette is probably one of the last things on my mind (unless I have a horrid flare-up of tics that day). Six months after my dad passed, I had a full ride to a private university for writing, but after a year I left so I could properly grieve my dad. Eighteen months later I started acting, and within 13 months had shot multiple commercials and a few small theatrical parts. On May 22, 2014, I was hit by a crazed driver. I was physically injured and also developed posttraumatic stress disorder, which in turn triggered my Tourette to become the worst it had ever been. In a heartbeat, I thought I lost everything. But I now know it was that day that I actually gained everything. I learned my calling in life is not acting but helping others. I began to speak nationally on Tourette syndrome and soon helped pass the CARE Bill, which granted funding for neurologic research to the Centers for Disease Control and Prevention (CDC). I also started learning about the education system and how I could use my experiences to help others. A few years passed, and I decided to progress from public speaking to mentoring teens with disabilities. I was trained to become a

COPAA-certified advocate, so I can be hands-on when helping fight for kids with disabilities who are denied proper accommodations in the education system. These days I still endure highs and lows. I will always deal with chronic depression, and if I become physically ill with a cold, my brain is psychologically tricked into thinking a sick cough is a tic. Depending on the severity, I can become bedridden, and it can be quite debilitating. In the past 2 years I have used social media as a platform to uplift others by sharing videos and other content of my highs and lows on Instagram, breaking the stigma that social media is only for the glamorous. On a weekly basis I receive about 40 direct messages from people experiencing depression, people facing disabilities, or people being bullied, and I do my best to answer every single one. Sometimes all it takes is one person to listen and provide words of affirmation to pull someone out of a difficult mentality. If my journey inspires people, how could I not help them find their strength when they reach out? I take things day by day, but no matter what I am faced with in life, I find solace in knowing that, by sharing my experiences, I am making a difference.

*Hayley Gripp*
Social Activist & Marketing Director
Lobbied to pass IDEA Act + CARE Bill
Educated over 300k on disabilities, diversity, and discrimination
COPAA-Certified Advocate
Founder of #PostWithintegrity movement
Cofounder of Inside/Out Wellness Weekend
Featured on: "Fox & Friends," "Buzzfeed," and "Yahoo News"

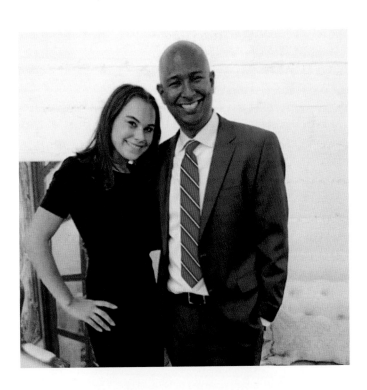

# PREFACE

It is with great pleasure once again that we present to you our fifth book in the *Morning Report: Beyond the Pearls* series, *Psychiatry Morning Report: Beyond the Pearls*. Writing the "perfect" review text has been a dream of mine ever since I was a first-year medical student. Dr. Koolaee and I envisioned a text that incorporates a focus on the United States Medical Licensing Examination (USMLE) Steps 1, 2, and 3, with up-to-date, evidence-based clinical medicine. We wanted the platform of the text to be drawn from a traditional theme that many of us are familiar with from residency, the "morning report" format. This book is geared toward a wide audience, from medical students to attending physicians practicing psychiatry. Each case has been carefully chosen and covers scenarios and questions frequently encountered on the psychiatry boards, shelf examinations, and wards, integrating both basic science and clinical pearls.

We would like to sincerely thank all of the many contributors who have helped create this text. Their insightful work will be a valuable tool for medical students and physicians to gain an in-depth understanding of psychiatry. It should be noted that although a variety of clinical cases in psychiatry were selected for this book, it is not meant to substitute a comprehensive psychiatry reference.

Dr. Koolaee and I would like to thank our volume editors, Dr. Duong, Dr. Tamas, and Dr. Ureste, for all of their hard work and dedication to this book. It was truly a pleasure to work with everyone associated with this book, and we look forward to our next project together.

# CONTENTS

# A Primer into Psychiatry

Tammy Duong ■ Peter Ureste ■ Jack Krasuski

## Introduction

Welcome to psychiatry! Whether you have chosen this path as a life-long career or are just visiting for a rotation, I hope your experience in psychiatry enhances your life in some way. This book is designed to walk through various psychiatric cases in a question–answer format to build the medical knowledge needed to become a successful psychiatrist. Each chapter is a stand-alone case and can be read in any order. This chapter, however, will guide you into practical skills for daily functioning, including taking a history, presenting and writing a note, briefly reviewing psychopharmacology, and considering ethical concerns. Along the way, we will discuss how psychiatry is similar and dissimilar to many other specialties within medicine.

## Psychiatric Interview

Initially, taking a psychiatric history can be intimidating for both the patient and a newly minted physician. Patients new to psychiatric visits can often be anxious and worried that they are being judged, "psychoanalyzed," or will be hospitalized against their will. New physicians often worry about what questions to ask or about offending the patient. It is important for both parties to be oriented to the psychiatric interview, including the goals of the encounter, which may be different according to the setting. For example, the goal of the encounter in the emergency department may be centered around safety, versus a psychotherapy visit that might focus on understanding the patient's patterns of behavior.

Similar to any other medical interview, the goal of the psychiatric interview is to collect information on symptomatology in order to come to a diagnosis and formulate a treatment plan. It often starts with an inquiry of the chief complaint and proceeds in a parallel fashion to other medical interviews. Table 0.1 illustrates the components of the psychiatric interview. A key component of the interview is the psychosocial context in which symptoms occur. For example, a patient may explain that their depressive symptoms began within the context of losing a job, relationship, or other major life transition. These details may help the clinician better understand the patient. A common mistake, however, is to solely focus on psychosocial context and not elicit details about symptomology. For each symptom, it is important to elicit the time of onset, symptom characterization, timing, alleviating and aggravating factors, associated symptoms, and its impact on functioning. These clues will help the psychiatrist build a differential diagnosis and explore the degree of impairment. For example, "anxiety" is a common chief complaint and on its own can yield little diagnostic information. However, a history of abrupt onset of anxiety that lasts 10 to 30 minutes, characterized by palpitations, sweating, chest discomfort, trembling, and fear of dying (panic attack), is different than the patient who is experiencing fear and worry

**TABLE 0.1 ■ Components of the Psychiatric Interview and Assessment**

| Identifying Patient Information | |
| --- | --- |
| History of presenting illness | Includes psychiatric review of systems (psychosis, depression, mania, anxiety) |
| Past psychiatric history | Onset |
| | Hospitalizations |
| | Outpatient/therapy |
| | Self-injurious behaviors/suicide attempts |
| | Medication trials |
| Past medical and surgical history | |
| Current medications | |
| Allergies | |
| Family medical and psychiatric history | |
| Social history | Family and relationship |
| | Dependent-care issues |
| | Current living arrangement and social support systems |
| | Education |
| | Employment history |
| | Legal history |
| | Trauma (verbal, physical, sexual) |
| | Substance use history (alcohol, tobacco, illicit drugs including cannabis) |
| Mental status examination | Appearance |
| | Behavior (includes psychomotor activity and abnormal movements) |
| | Speech |
| | Mood |
| | Affect |
| | Thought process |
| | Thought content |
| | Cognition |
| | Judgment |
| | Insight |
| | Impulse control |
| Vital signs and labs | CMP, CBC, TSH/FT4, RPR, HIV |
| Assessment | Includes diagnosis |
| Plan | #Problem 1 |
| | #Problem 2 |

*CBC,* Complete blood count; *CMP,* complete metabolic panel; *FT4,* free thyroxine; *HIV,* human immunodeficiency virus; *RPR,* rapid plasma regain; *TSH,* thyroid-stimulating hormone.

about social interactions, meeting unfamiliar people, and being scrutinized by others (social anxiety). Reviewing the cases contained within this book will help the learner select appropriate questions for the interview.

Most medical disciplines have a review of systems, and psychiatry is no exception. Outside of psychiatry, typical review of systems is organized by organ systems. Within psychiatry, the review of systems is often organized according to syndromic categories, such as depressive disorders, anxiety disorders, psychotic disorders, bipolar spectrum disorders, eating disorders, and more. Although it is not feasible to screen for every psychiatric disorder, the review of systems can be tailored to be pertinent for the patient. For example, a patient who presents with trichotillomania might also be screened for other obsessive-compulsive disorders.

In addition to past medical history, past psychiatric history is also a salient component of the interview. Important details to consider are prior episodes of psychiatric disease, psychiatric hospitalizations, suicide attempts, and/or self-injurious behaviors. This portion of the interview also covers prior psychiatric medication trials, including dosage, length of time of each trial, effectiveness of the medication, side effects, and reason for discontinuation.

A social history in the psychiatric interview often yields many clues to how the patient views, interacts, and copes with his or her surroundings. This portion of the interview focuses on topics such as where the patient grew up and relationships with parents, siblings, significant others, children, and friendships. Whether or not a patient can independently perform instrumental and basic activities of daily living is also in this section. Educational history becomes important if one is assessing cognitive status or neurodevelopmental disease. This section also assesses trauma history, such as verbal, physical, and sexual abuse, and legal history, such as probation, parole, arrests, or history of driving under the influence citations. Table 0.1 lists components of the social history pertinent to psychiatry.

## Mental Status Examination

The mental status examination is the psychiatrist's physical examination. Patients often convey unspoken information, which can serve as a window into the patient's inner workings. Just as costovertebral angle tenderness can be a sign of pyelonephritis, an inappropriately euphoric affect can be a sign of mania. Mental status examination is so important to the psychiatrist that there is an entire chapter devoted to it in this book! The examination often starts by describing the patient's appearance, behavior, and speech. For example, a female patient with mania may appear with bright-colored make-up, wear colorful clothes, yell incessantly and laugh intermittently, using hyperverbal speech that is pressured and rapid, making it difficult for the evaluator to ask their next question. In contrast, a patient with depressive symptoms may appear sad and poorly groomed with messy hair, often staring at the ground, crying, and exhibiting psychomotor retardation and speech that is slow and soft in tone. Other domains within in the psychiatric interview include mood (how the patient describes their emotional state), affect (how you observe their emotional state), thought process (linear, circumstantial, tangential, loose, word salad, for example), thought content (whether the patient has suicidal or homicidal ideations), perceptual disturbances (hallucinations or delusions), and cognition (whether the patient is alert and oriented, their short-term memory is intact, if they can pay attention and think abstractly, for example). The examination often concludes with an assessment of the patient's insight and judgment.

## Presenting the Case and Writing a Note

Presenting a patient case and writing a note are similar in that they both describe the just-gathered history as a cogent argument for or against a diagnosis. The information is presented in an organized fashion so that an experienced listener can follow along and come to an appropriate differential diagnosis.

Standard medical presentations start with an identifying sentence about the patient. It should include the patient's age, relevant past medical or psychiatric diagnoses, how the patient came into care, and the chief complaint. This immediately primes the listener on what to expect for the remainder of the presentation. The following are examples of an identifying sentence.

"Ms. McNeil is an 85-year-old woman with history of diabetes mellitus, hypertension, a right middle cerebral artery stroke in 2018, and no prior psychiatric history, who is presenting today as an outpatient as a referral from Dr. Kumar for memory problems."

"Mr. Johnson is a 20-year-old male with a history of methamphetamine use disorder, bipolar disorder, and one prior psychiatric hospitalization 1 year ago after a suicide attempt, who is brought in the emergency department today by police for disrobing in a grocery store and declaring he was the mayor."

Immediately, both identifying sentences provide high-yield information that helps the listener immediately form a preliminary differential diagnosis. In Ms. McNeil's case, she is a geriatric

TABLE 0.2 ■ **Common Biopsychosocial Factors That Influence Psychiatric Pathology**

| Biological | Genetic factors (family history) |
| --- | --- |
| | Epigenetic factors |
| | Developmental disorders |
| | Comorbid medical illness (neurodegenerative disease, traumatic brain injury, toxins) |
| | Prior episodes of psychiatric illness |
| | History of illicit drug use |
| | Response to medications |
| Psychological | Maladaptive behaviors and coping strategies |
| | Cognitive distortions |
| | Defense mechanisms |
| Social | Access to social support (spouse, friends, community) |
| | Religiosity |
| | Financial resources |
| | Access to safe housing |
| | History of violence/domestic violence |
| | Cultural influences |

patient, has a number of cardiovascular risk factors, and whose chief complaint is memory problems. The listener may start thinking about the differential diagnosis for neurocognitive disorders and will listen more carefully for symptoms consistent with these disorders. In Mr. Johnson's case, hearing about prior history of methamphetamine use, bipolar disorder, and a suicide attempt in the setting of disinhibited behaviors may have the listener wondering if the patient has relapsed in either of these disorders. Being called to medical attention by police is often a sign of significant impairment and clues the clinician on the severity of symptoms.

Many learners initially have trouble presenting the history of present illness. Patients, especially those whose thinking is impaired, often will not present their symptoms in a linear narrative. It is up to the clinician to consider the information and synthesize it into an orderly format understandable to the listener. Think of a presentation as presenting an argument; for example, if one were considering a diagnosis of generalized anxiety disorder, then the presentation would include pertinent positives and negatives related to this diagnosis. A well-presented case lays out a road map for the listener to reach the same destination and conclusions as the presenter.

The assessment is the opportunity for the learner to explain their clinical reasoning and hypothesis regarding a differential diagnosis. This is the time to pull together information from the history, mental status examination, and laboratory examination in order to draw conclusions. Psychiatric assessments often mention both protective and risk factors that influence the presentation and identify areas to work on in the plan. These factors are commonly divided into biological, psychological, and social factors (together referred to as the *biopsychosocial model*). Table 0.2 lists several common biopsychosocial factors that influence psychiatric pathology.

# Safety

All branches of medicine encourage a safe environment for the patient, physician, and staff. In addition to striving for a culture of being free from medical errors, psychiatrists also consider the suicide and violence risk within the clinical encounter. Psychiatrists often see patients during crisis or during the lowest points in their life. This book will discuss suicide and its risk assessment in depth in a later chapter.

On occasion, patients may be irritable, upset, or disinhibited from substances. Psychiatrists can use several techniques to deescalate tense situations, such as speaking in a calm voice, avoiding arguments, validating a patient's feelings, distracting them (such as offering the patient something to drink), or giving a patient appropriate space. Psychiatrists use their own feelings to inform them of the clinical situation; for example, if it feels uncomfortable/unsafe then it most likely is an unsafe situation! Trainees early in their careers often make the mistake of ignoring these feelings, as most new experiences in medicine are uncomfortable, and proceed anyway. However, it is always okay and permissible to ask for additional help, be accompanied by staff, or interview a patient in a more open room to avoid any party feeling trapped. If there is ever a question of potential violence, please leave the area and proceed to ask for help!

## Diagnostic and Statistical Manual of Mental Disorders, Fifth Edition (DSM-5)

DSM-5 is the standard reference book that psychiatrists use to diagnose psychiatric disorders. It is divided into 21 syndrome-based sections and contains the diagnostic criteria for specific disorders. For example, within the chapter for depressive disorders, you can find the diagnostic criteria for disruptive mood dysregulation disorder, major depressive disorder, persistent depressive disorder, premenstrual dysphoric disorder, substance/medication-induced depressive disorder, and depressive disorder due to another medical condition. Knowing the diagnostic criteria for each of these disorders will help guide which questions you ask during your interview.

DSM-5 is a useful tool for the psychiatrist, but it is far from perfect. There have been many revisions since its conception. As society and science change, so does the understanding of mental illness. Several disorders have been added, removed, or reorganized throughout time. Another major folly is that it is impossible to capture all the complex emotional, behavioral, cognitive, and physiologic processes that occur with each disease. There is no replacement for a thoughtful, empathic clinician!

The cases in this book use DSM-5 as a point of reference. Reading each case will help familiarize you with diagnostic criteria of mental disorders and help you learn what questions to ask during the psychiatric interview, but also offer insights into the field of psychiatry.

## Psychopharmacology

Being familiar with psychopharmacology is essential to understanding modern psychiatry. Although the topic is beyond the scope of this chapter, it is worth briefly mentioning a few highlights of neurotransmitters that affect the central nervous system (CNS) so that you will be able to follow along like a pro during rounds.

Drugs that affect the CNS do so by changing nerve ion flow to induce cell signaling. This can be done via voltage or ligand coupled channels. Neurotransmitters are chemicals that act as ligands to induce or inhibit downstream cell signaling. Common neurotransmitters relevant in psychiatry include acetylcholine, dopamine, serotonin, norepinephrine, glutamic acid, and gamma-aminobutyric acid (GABA). The drugs used in psychiatry will commonly target the receptors for one or more of these neurotransmitters, plus others. In order to introduce you to commonly used antidepressants, mood stabilizers, and antipsychotics, the end of this chapter contains a series of tables of these medications and dosage ranges (see Table 0.3).

## Psychotherapy

Psychotherapy training is one of the unique aspects of psychiatry training, but it can seem the most foreign to medical students at times. There are many different types of psychotherapies, but

**TABLE 0.3 ■ Commonly Used Psychotropic Medications and Dosage Ranges**

|  | Medication | Dosage Range |
|---|---|---|
| ***Antidepressants*** | | |
| Tricyclic antidepressants | amitriptyline | 25–300 mg/day |
| | clomipramine | 50–250 mg/day |
| | desipramine | 25–150 mg/day |
| | doxepin | 15–300 mg/day |
| | imipramine | 25–300 mg/day |
| | nortriptyline | 25–150 mg/day |
| Monoamine oxidase inhibitors | phenelzine | 7.5–90 mg/day |
| | selegiline | 6–12 mg/day |
| | tranylcypromine | 5–60 mg/day |
| Selective serotonin reuptake inhibitors | citalopram | 10–40 mg/day |
| | escitalopram | 5–20 mg/day |
| | fluoxetine | 5–80 mg/day |
| | fluvoxamine | 25–300 mg/day |
| | paroxetine | 5–40 mg/day |
| | sertraline | 25–200 mg |
| Serotonin norepinephrine reuptake inhibitors | duloxetine | 20–120 mg/day |
| | desvenlafaxine | 25–50 mg/day |
| | levomilnacipran | 40–120 mg/day |
| | venlafaxine | 75–225 mg/day |
| Atypical antidepressants | bupropion | 75–450 mg/day |
| | mirtazapine | 7.5–45 mg/day |
| | trazodone | 25–600 mg/day |
| ***Antimanic medication*** | | |
| Mood stabilizer | lithium carbonate | 300–1200 mg/day |
| Anticonvulsants | carbamazepine | 600–1200 mg/day |
| | lamotrigine | 25–200 mg/day |
| | oxcarbazepine | 600–2400 mg/day |
| | valproic acid/divalproex | 500–2500 mg/day |
| ***Antipsychotics*** | | |
| Typicals (first generation) | chlorpromazine | 50–800 mg/day |
| | fluphenazine | 3–45 mg/day |
| | haloperidol | 2–40 mg/day |
| | loxapine | 50–250 mg/day |
| | perphenazine | 8–60 mg/day |
| Atypicals (second generation) | aripiprazole | 15–30 mg/day |
| | clozapine | 300–900 mg/day |
| | lurasidone | 40–80 mg/day |
| | olanzapine | 5–20 mg/day |
| | paliperidone | 3–12 mg/day |
| | risperidone | 4–6 mg/day |
| | quetiapine | 150–600 mg/day |
| | ziprasidone | 60–160 mg/day |

at the basis they all aim to discover the patient's patterns of thinking and behaviors in order to reduce symptom severity and improve functioning. One way of doing this is exploring the defenses patients use to cope with unpleasant feelings. Defenses are further explained later in this book. Most residency training programs focus on supportive, psychodynamic, and cognitive behavioral therapy. Supportive psychotherapy aims to encourage a patient's adaptive behaviors and steer the patient away from maladaptive ones. Psychodynamic therapy focuses on examining how prior relationships affect current relationships. Cognitive behavioral therapy assumes that thoughts, feelings, and behaviors are interconnected and influence each other. This therapeutic modality aims to modify inaccurate thoughts and behaviors in order to alleviate symptoms. Other therapeutic modalities include family therapy, interpersonal psychotherapy, problem-solving therapy, and dialectical behavioral therapy.

## Ethics

Like all medical specialties, psychiatry must balance the tensions between doing good for the patient (beneficence); avoiding harm (nonmaleficence); honoring their autonomy; and equitably distributing risks, benefits, and resources (justice). One or more of these ethical principles may be in conflict with one another, and the psychiatrist must carefully consider these ethical principles. For example, for a case involving an actively suicidal patient who is involuntary hospitalized, the psychiatric treatment team must carefully balance beneficence with patient autonomy.

## Conclusion

Although brief, I hope this chapter gave you an overview and insight into the daily mechanics of operating as a psychiatrist. The structure of psychiatry is similar to many other formats you may have seen in other specialties but has a few very special qualities as well. Now that you can take an organized history, write a note, and speak the language like a pro, are you ready to learn more? Time to start!

### References

American Psychiatric Association. (2013). *Diagnostic and statistical manual of mental disorders* (5th ed.). Washington, DC: Author.

American Physician Institute. (2019). Dynamically structured psychiatric assessment & treatment: Free online course for mental health clinicians. Retrieved from www.masterpsych.com.

Katzung, B. G. (2018). *Basic & clinical pharmacology* (14th ed.). New York, NY: McGraw-Hill.

Stahl, S. M., & Grady, M. M. (2017). *Stahl's essential psychopharmacology: Prescriber's guide* (6th ed.). New York, NY: Cambridge University Press.

# CHAPTER 1

# Mental Status Examination

Zachary Clayborne Dietrich ■ Rebecca L. Tamas

---

A 61-year-old male arrives at the emergency department by ambulance after being in a three-vehicle collision resulting in two fatalities. After the event he is openly joking about the accident, appears apathetic to the loss of life, and has urinary incontinence while speaking to the police. Field sobriety tests are conducted by the police in response to his behavior. The test is quickly suspended when the patient takes more than the instructed nine steps forward on three attempts. A breathalyzer test shows negative for alcohol. He denies having any discomfort and tries to leave the hospital (requiring redirection by staff). He does not ask why he was brought to the hospital. His only visible injuries are minor chest contusions, likely from impact with the steering wheel. When asked how he's feeling, he repeatedly (and at times inappropriately) responds, "Right as rain." His wife has been contacted and is on her way to the hospital.

---

*What are your initial thoughts, and what do you want to know to help determine a diagnosis?*
When a patient presents with abnormal behavior (marked by deviations from social norms and difficulty with decision-making) the context of observed symptoms should be considered to establish an etiology. He has an alteration in affect, difficulty in making decisions, and urinary incontinence. The persistence of his presentation suggests that this is more than an acute psychological reaction to trauma. Mild traumatic brain injury (TBI) is also unlikely due to the lack of observable physical findings, although it cannot be entirely ruled out. Obtaining a reliable history about symptom onset, course, and duration is crucial for further diagnostic considerations.

Difficulty in planning during the field sobriety test, joking about the accident, and apathy to loss of life suggest a deficit in executive functioning. This type of deficit could occur due to psychological factors, frontal lobe injuries, or toxin exposure. Thorough history-taking and documentation of a mental status examination (MSE) can assist in diagnostic clarity and appropriate consultation. With the hypothesis that his behavior is due to executive functioning deficits the MSE can be tailored to highlight and identify the suspected dysfunction.

*What is being evaluated by conducting an MSE?*
The MSE is only one part of a complete medical workup that helps guide diagnosis and treatment planning. When performing the MSE, clinicians should record what they see and hear. They should observe how the person engages in the interview and notice any abnormalities in cognitive, perceptual, or motor skills. Table 1.1 shows the different parts of the MSE.

*How do you conduct a bedside MSE with challenging patients?*
Sometimes, as in this case, a complete MSE can be difficult to obtain. The clinician will need to have a more focused approach and try to gather as much information as possible. Generally, the examination starts before even speaking to the person. How the person is dressed, his or her

TABLE 1.1 ■ Components of the MSE

| Component | Example |
| --- | --- |
| Alertness, Attention | Alert, lethargic, obtunded, stuporous |
| Appearance | Good posture, increased psychomotor activity, malodorous |
| Behavior | Cooperative, uncooperative, agitated, good eye contact |
| Orientation | Awareness of person, place, time, situation |
| Speech | Fluent, pressured, rapid, poverty of speech |
| Language | Spontaneous, writing, reading, naming of objects |
| Thought Process | Organized, circumstantial (overly detailed and nonlinear), tangential (off topic), flight of ideas, looseness of association, perseverative |
| Thought Content | Delusions, hallucinations, obsessions, ideas of reference, illusions, suicidal ideations, homicidal ideations |
| Mood | Depressed, euthymic, anxious, manic |
| Affect | Congruent with mood, labile, full range of affect |
| Memory | Recent, remote, immediate |
| Insight | Good, limited, poor |
| Judgment | Good, limited, impaired, poor |

MSE, Mental status examination.

TABLE 1.2 ■ Levels of Alertness

| Level of Alertness | Description |
| --- | --- |
| Alert | Fully aware |
| Clouding of consciousness | Mild decrease in attention, tired |
| Confusion | More profound decrease in mental processing (e.g., disoriented) |
| Lethargy | Severely sedated |
| Obtunded | Mumbles, requires constant stimulation, decreased response to stimulation |
| Stupor | Requires vigorous stimulation to arouse |
| Coma | Unarousable, unresponsive to stimuli |

hygiene, posture, and level of consciousness are all information that can be assessed the moment the clinician walks into the room. Alertness and arousal are addressed by documenting abnormalities in the patient's response to stimuli (Table 1.2).

Thoroughly assessing attention and concentration requires more than passive observation by the clinician. Common ways to assess these include asking the person to spell a word forward and backward (or use a series of numbers or the months of the year). Using a five-letter word is often used, the most common being *world*. For those clinicians with English as a second language the word *planet* can be easier to use because *world* can sound like the words *war* and *wore*. Another commonly used task is serial 7s. The patient is asked to subtract 7 from 100 and keep subtracting 7 until told to stop. Using serial 7s measures attention, working memory, and concentration, and it requires the ability to do simple calculations. Determining the person's level of education is useful in assessing which of these methods would be the most appropriate. If a person has a very low level of education, then asking the months of the year (or spelling his or her own name forward and backward) may be easier.

Thought process can be organized, circumstantial (overly detailed), or tangential (off topic). The person may also have flight of ideas (thoughts that are loosely connected and jump from topic to topic; e.g., "fire engines are red, and books are read, there's a redhead in my class"), looseness of association (thoughts that are not well connected; e.g., "a cow was holding the phone for me in Iowa"), and perseveration (repetitive).

Thought content can include delusions (false beliefs that are unwavering), hallucinations (false sensory perceptions: auditory, visual, tactile, gustatory, olfactory), obsessions (intrusive and recurring thoughts), ideas of reference (e.g., thinking the radio is speaking directly to you or about you), illusions (false perceptions based in reality, such as thinking a coat is a person), suicidal ideations, and homicidal ideations.

---

When you enter his room you notice the patient had not buttoned his shirt correctly. He smiles at you and asks how your day is going, then laughs. You smell urine and notice that his pants are wet. You ask him what brought him in, and he tells you that he has been trying to leave because there is no reason for him to be there. When you inquire further about this he changes the subject and asks if you know what the score of the game is. You are not sure what game he is referring to so you try to move on to more questioning. He then gets up and tries to walk out of the room, requiring redirection.

---

Orientation is commonly established by obtaining and confirming the patient's name, location, date, and the reason the person is seeking treatment. Asking appropriate details and follow-up questions may provide clues to orientation. For instance, if this patient were brought by ambulance he may realize he is in the hospital but not know the name of the hospital or city. Efforts should be made to inquire further when given partial responses. It is recommended to ask the date separately and note detailed discrepancies. Also ask the year, document his response, then follow with "What month is it?" If the patient cannot recall the calendar date but correctly responds with year, month, and day of the week, that should be noted. Sometimes patients will try to convince the clinician that they know the answer when they do not. They may say, "You really gotta ask me that?" or "You think I don't know the date?" This can sometimes happen when people are embarrassed and are trying to cover up their deficits. When neurologic or psychiatric abnormalities are suspected, it is crucial to ask the person to explain the *situation*. This patient may know he is in the hospital but may not know why. When documenting, it is often possible to adapt to time constraints by using the abbreviation A&Ox4 (meaning "alert and oriented times 4") when all responses are accurate. The shortened A&Ox3 is used when the person's situation is omitted. When the patient may have a compromised mental state it is important to assess if the person knows the situation. It is never acceptable to use A&Ox2 without specifying to which two items the person is oriented.

Memory can be assessed briefly or in great detail, depending on the situation. Usually immediate, recent, and remote memory are assessed. Recent memory can be tested by telling the patient that he will be given three words to remember and that he will be asked to recite them back in a few minutes (usually 3–5 minutes later). The words chosen should not be items in the examination room; should be unrelated to each other (e.g., plate, cup, bowl); should not easily flow together (e.g., flying, red, balloon); and should be words that the clinician will remember. It is important to note that immediate recall is not a true measure of memory, but rather a measure of attention and focus; delayed recall is a more accurate measure of memory. Evaluating remote memory is more straightforward. Ask the patient to recall historical *and* verifiable personal events, and ask the patient the name of the current president, previous presidents, or other historical events. (Again, education level should be taken into consideration.)

Language is assessed through many different domains of communication. The attentive clinician can obtain much of this information during the assessment. Spontaneous speech is assessed throughout the interview by paying attention to fluency, frequency, and abnormalities (such as paraphasic errors or neologisms).

---

**CLINICAL PEARL**                                                              **STEP 2/3**

Paraphasic errors commonly are associated with aphasia (the inability to comprehend or formulate language). These errors are characterized by unintended syllables, phrases, or words. The three types of paraphasia are **literal/phonological** (e.g., saying "indotruction" instead of "introduction"), **neologistic** (creating new words like "perfectaration"), and **verbal** (in which another word is substituted for the word that was intended). Neologisms are sometimes observed in schizophrenia.

---

The patient's wife arrives and reports the changes in her husband appeared approximately 3 years before the accident. He was a partner at a corporate law firm and was forced into early retirement because of a decline in strategic abilities. He also made a series of inappropriate comments to female coworkers and had multiple unexplained absences. In addition, he shoplifted affordable items, gained weight due to binge eating, and did not appear concerned when she told him she may have cancer. He attended a few sessions of psychotherapy, and the therapist thought his behavior was due to grief from his forced retirement. There is no history of surgery, traumatic brain injury, stroke, or seizure. His wife shows you a medication list that does not provide any explanation for his presentation. His toxicology screen shows no illicit drug use. Lastly, his wife reports the patient had an aunt and grandparent who both had unspecified dementias.

---

Sometimes psychological factors (such as loss of a job) cause behavior changes. Other times the changes may be due to a medical condition. Social withdrawal and depression often precede short-term memory impairment in Alzheimer disease by 2 to 3 years. Manic-like symptoms often can precede motor dysfunction and cognitive impairment in Huntington disease by more than 10 years. When assessing mood, psychiatric symptoms should be noted but not used to completely rule out other physical or neurologic etiologies.

---

**CLINICAL PEARL**                                                            **STEP 1/2/3**

Mood and affect are often confused. Mood is pervasive and does not change moment to moment, whereas affect can fluctuate quickly. Patients will sometimes report having "mood swings," but they are really describing affect lability (also called affective instability).

Upon further evaluation of the patient, you note that he is oriented to time, person (first and last name), and place ("hospital"), but not to situation. Remote memory is intact, and recent memory for three words (apple, penny, table) is intact after 5 minutes. His mood appears euthymic. His affect is overexpressive and somewhat labile (e.g., laughing inappropriately at times). Speech is fluent and not pressured. He denies having any hallucinations or delusions, or suicidal or homicidal thoughts. He has poor insight and limited judgment. His urinary incontinence, lack of awareness to situation, and the collateral report from his wife warrant referral to neurology.

Subsequent neuropsychological assessment shows executive functioning to be moderately to severely impaired, with other domains relatively intact, including attention and memory. Results from neuroimaging reveal significant dorsolateral, orbitofrontal, and perisylvian atrophy of the frontal lobes (and some atrophy in the right medial temporal lobe). He is diagnosed with behavioral variant frontotemporal dementia.

---

**CLINICAL PEARL**                                                    **STEP 1/2/3**

Frontotemporal dementia is described in the *Diagnostic and Statistical Manual of Mental Disorders*, fifth edition, *(DSM-5)* as mild or major neurocognitive dysfunction with insidious onset of symptoms and gradual progression. Behavioral findings include three or more of the following: behavioral disinhibition, apathy or inertia, loss of sympathy or empathy, perseveration, stereotyped or compulsive behavior, hyperorality, and changes in eating habits. The language variant shows prominent decline in language ability (the form of speech production, word finding, object naming, grammar, or word comprehension). Memory loss is relatively spared in frontotemporal dementia compared with other cognitive domains and is less pronounced than in other dementias.

---

**BEYOND THE PEARLS:**

- There are standardized screening tests to assist in dementia-related diagnoses. The simplicity of these tests can mislead one to believe they are comprehensive. Often referred to as the "gold-standard" is the Mini-Mental State Examination (MMSE). However, in the example mentioned earlier the MMSE may yield a normal score (which would delay referral to neurology). Because Alzheimer disease was the primary consideration during creation of the MMSE, the examination does not test executive functioning as a primary function in any subtest, which may lead to a false negative in frontotemporal dementia (FTD).
- The Montreal Cognitive Assessment (MoCA) has increased sensitivity for FTD compared with the MMSE because of the additional executive-functioning tasks. However, both tests can be difficult to administer when impulsivity in the patient is a prominent factor.

## References

American Psychiatric Association. (2013). *Diagnostic and statistical manual of mental disorders* (5th ed.). Washington, DC: American Psychiatric Association.

Folstein, M. F., Folstein, S. E., & McHugh, P. R. (1975). Mini-mental state. A practical method for grading the cognitive state of patients for the clinician. *Journal of Psychiatric Research, 12*(3), 189–198.

Goodglass, H., & Kaplan, E. (1983). *The Assessment of aphasia and related disorders*. Baltimore, MD: Williams & Wilkins.

Julien, C. L., Thompson, J. C., Wild, S., Yardumian, P., Snowden, J. S., Turner, G., & Crauford, D. (2006). Psychiatric disorders in preclinical Huntington's disease. *Journal of Neurology, Neurosurgery, and Psychiatry, 78*(9), 939–943.

Lezak Muriel, D., Howieson, D. B., & Loring, D. W. (2004). *Neuropsychological assessment* (4th ed.). New York, NY: Oxford University Press.

Nasreddine, Z. S., Phillips, N. A., Bédirian, V., Charbonneau, S., Whitehead, V., Collin, I., ... Chertkow, H. (2005). The Montreal Cognitive Assessment, MoCA: A brief screening tool for mild cognitive impairment. *Journal of the American Geriatrics Society, 53*(4), 695–699.

Panjwani, S., Narahari, A., Bains, A., & Lippmann, S. (2014). Frontotemporal dementia and its variants: What to look for. *Current Psychiatry, 13*(6), e1–e2.

Tindall, S. C. (1990). Level of consciousness. In H. K. Walker, W. D. Hall, & J. W. Hurst (Eds.), *Clinical methods: The history, physical, and laboratory examinations* (3rd ed.). Boston, MA: Butterworths.

# CHAPTER 2

# Defense Mechanisms

Derek William Gilbert ■ Rebecca L. Tamas

A 34-year-old male with a history of hypertension and anxiety presents to the emergency department (ED) accompanied by his wife. He complains of abdominal pain from an injury to the right upper quadrant of his abdomen secondary to a pellet gunshot. He is tachycardic but otherwise hemodynamically stable. The ED physician is suspicious that this may have been a self-inflicted gunshot wound. The man smells of alcohol and does not provide much information about how the injury happened. Routine laboratory tests are ordered, and a psychiatry consult is placed.

### What is the first step in evaluating this patient?

Given the aforementioned information it is important to obtain as much relevant information as possible, not only from the patient but from any collateral (in this case, his wife). Given the suspicion of alcohol involvement, getting a blood or breath alcohol level would contribute further objective evidence. You would also want to order an electrocardiogram (ECG). It is important to review routine laboratory tests commonly ordered in the emergency department (ED) because electrolyte imbalances could lead to confusion, seizures, or arrhythmias. A complete blood count (CBC), comprehensive metabolic panel (CMP), thyroid-stimulating hormone (TSH), and a urinalysis (UA) are ordered, and all are within normal limits. Also, there is no evidence of ECG changes that would require further cardiology workup. However, he does have a breath alcohol level of 0.12. Urine toxicology is positive for clonazepam, which appears on his medication reconciliation form from the pharmacy as a home medication.

Upon entering the room, the patient is sitting upright in bed and appears to be somewhat anxious. He reports that his wife and daughter left their home last night to stay with his in-laws. His wife has been increasingly argumentative about his alcohol use, and this has led to a strain on their relationship. When asked about why he is at the hospital, he replies, "I just came here because my wife wanted me to get help with anxiety." He denies recent alcohol use but when told about his alcohol level, the patient admits to consuming four or five beers. He becomes very guarded when asked about his alcohol use, frequently repeating: "My brother was the one with the problem. I just have a beer when I eat wings." Family history reveals his 36-year-old brother died from cirrhosis of the liver. When asked about the gunshot wound the patient reports that he was cleaning his pellet gun around 4 a.m. and accidently shot himself. He also acknowledges that he is prescribed clonazepam and may have taken more than the prescribed amount last night.

*If you suspect intentional self-injury and the use of unhealthy defense mechanisms, what elements of the history or what diagnostics would you order?*

A timeline beginning with the events leading up to his injury is important to establish, as well as the patient's previous means of coping with similar situations. It is crucial to understand the patient's past coping strategies to have a better understanding of his behavioral tendencies (not only in this acute situation, but also over the course of his life). What his behavioral tendencies are can be obtained by gathering a past history of response to stressful situations, a thorough mental status examination (MSE), and observing how the patient interacts with hospital personnel and his wife. It is also necessary to assess the patent's safety and determine whether he is having thoughts of self-harm while in the ED.

Furthermore, given his alcohol and benzodiazepine use, it is important to monitor for withdrawal signs and symptoms (e.g., tachycardia, diaphoresis, shakiness, tremor, formication, or seizures).

---

**CLINICAL PEARL**                                                            **STEP 1,2,3**

There is a plethora of theories regarding defense mechanisms. The most well-known theories come from the writings of Sigmund and Anna Freud. They described defense mechanisms as unconscious thoughts or feelings that are used to decrease anxiety or other unwanted emotions related to a potentially harmful stimuli. Although there is no consensus on the exact number of defense mechanisms, the Freuds ultimately laid the foundation for them. Sigmund Freud's structural theory of the mind included the id, ego, and superego (Table 2.1).

---

Anna Freud spent a significant amount of her career researching her father's work on defense mechanisms. She wrote about repression, regression, projection, reaction formation, and sublimation (all of these are commonly tested and will be described in detail later).

Categorizations of defense mechanisms that are frequently tested on examinations are listed later in the Beyond the Pearls section.

---

The patient and his wife are interviewed both separately and together after agreeing to do so. The patient is placed on the Clinical Institute Withdrawal Assessment for Alcohol protocol because of his alcohol and benzodiazepine use. The patient minimally divulges more information about his alcohol use but frequently points out that it was his brother who had a drinking problem. He remains focused on his anxiety and reports that he has been on clonazepam. He stopped taking it 2 months ago but filled a prescription this week. He asks how soon he can leave the hospital. When asked to quantify his alcohol use he says, "I got shot. Can we talk about that instead of everyone talking about alcohol?"

Throughout the interview his wife is tearful. She describes her husband as a fun-loving man and an incredible husband when he is not drinking alcohol. She is very concerned that his combination of a benzodiazepine and alcohol could have resulted in a fatal outcome. Her quantification of her husband's alcohol use is that he can drink enough "to fill the trash can with beer cans every night." He began to drink even more after the passing of his brother and has never acknowledged needing help to stop drinking. She also reports that he often accuses her of being jealous when he goes out drinking with his friends, and he will call her 20 to 30 times if she does not pick up her phone on the first attempt. Recently he yelled at their daughter because he was upset that his wife was complaining about his drinking, and this led his wife to take their daughter to her mother's house. His wife also mentions that when he visits his primary care doctor he is fixated on his liver enzymes ("My AST and ALT have always looked good, Doc") after he learned about them from his brother's situation. She also says he looks up the amount of alcohol that he has to drink to do damage to his liver and often refers to these statistics.

TABLE 2.1 ■ **Three Parts of the Psyche**

|          | Definition                                    | Example                                |
|----------|-----------------------------------------------|----------------------------------------|
| Id       | Primitive and instinctual unconscious thoughts | Eating, reproducing, surviving         |
| Ego      | Mediator between id and superego              | Balancing survival with societal norms |
| Superego | Moral conscience                              | Ideal self or form                     |

*Are there any additional considerations?*
Obtaining information from collateral sources is imperative in this case. Being able to understand the defense mechanisms that the patient has used in the present scenario, as well as in the past, is critical when formulating his psychological construct. Most of the defense mechanisms that the patient has used would be categorized as immature or neurotic. Obtaining a history from other family members would also be helpful because hearing only from the wife gives a limited view. The patient and his wife have been arguing, which could lead to the wife employing her own defense mechanisms.

*What defense mechanisms has this patient displayed?*
Step examinations focus on a few of those defense mechanisms described by the patient and his wife. Most notably:

**Denial:** the act of not accepting things too difficult to handle. In this particular case the patient consistently employs this defense. He does not acknowledge that his drinking is a problem or that it contributes to his injury, which could have been fatal.

**Displacement:** shifting emotions from an unwanted situation into a more tolerable one. In this case when the patient is upset with his wife he takes it out on their daughter.

**Intellectualization:** using facts, logic, and statistics to avoid feeling. This patient focuses on his liver enzymes and the amount of alcohol intake that would damage his liver, which exemplifies this defense.

**Rationalization:** the act of using explanations that are acceptable to one's self to justify an action or thought. The example in this case would be the patient's explanation of only drinking beer when eating wings, casually drinking, and, most notably, that his drinking is insignificant compared with that of his brother who died of cirrhosis. Because the patient doesn't have cirrhosis he rationalizes that he doesn't have a drinking problem.

**Projection:** the process of shifting one's own unacceptable thoughts or emotions to another person. The example in this case would be calling his wife several times while out with friends, then describing her as the jealous one (when in reality he is experiencing jealousy).

**BEYOND THE PEARLS:**

**Immature or Primitive Defenses**
**Denial:** (discussed earlier)
**Projection:** (discussed earlier)
**Acting out:** to avoid being conscious of the result of an action, there is a direct expression of an unconscious impulse or thought.
**Regression:** reverting back to earlier developmental stages when faced with stressful situations
**Somatization:** changing psychiatric complaints (e.g., depression, anxiety) into bodily symptoms (e.g., headaches, heartburn, back pain)
**Dissociation:** removing one's own identity to avoid emotional responses, which can manifest in fugue states (reversible amnesia of self)

**Neurotic Defenses**

**Displacement:** (discussed earlier)

**Intellectualization:** (discussed earlier)

**Rationalization:** (discussed earlier)

**Reaction formation:** managing unacceptable urges by essentially doing the opposite (e.g., showing exuberant excitement about seeing someone you deeply dislike). Some classify this as an immature defense mechanism.

**Repression:** removing a thought or feeling from conscious awareness that is likely to provoke an unwanted response (which occurs unconsciously; this is unlike suppression, which is done consciously).

**Mature Defenses**

**Altruism:** providing service or doing things for others at the sacrifice of self (e.g., a very rich person works at a homeless shelter to avoid feeling guilty)

**Humor:** adaptive way of expressing feelings without fear of undesirable effects, being able to accept consequences in a lighthearted manner. Humor helps alleviate stressful situations.

**Sublimation:** shifting a possibly negative emotion or thought into a positive action (e.g., working out to relieve tension)

**Suppression:** consciously putting a thought out of your mind, knowing you will have to deal with it eventually (e.g., finding out you failed a test when you are about to participate in a wedding).

## References

Ganti, L., Kaufman, M. S., & Blitzstein, S. M. (2016). *First aid for the psychiatric clerkship* (4th ed., pp. 180–182). New York: McGraw Hill Education.

Sadock, B. J., Sadock, V. A., & Ruiz, P. (2015). *Kaplan & Sadock's Synopsis of Psychiatry* (11th ed., pp. 159–162). Baltimore, MD: Lippincott Williams & Wilkins.

Shaw, J. M., Kolesar, G. S., Sellers, E. M., Kaplan, H. L., & Sandor, P. (1981). Development of optimal treatment tactics for alcohol withdrawal. I. Assessment and effectiveness of supportive care. *Journal of Clinical Psychopharmacology*, *1*(16), 382–389.

# CHAPTER 3

# Neuropsychological Testing

Tiffany Martinez ■ Daniel Martinez

A 63-year-old male is brought in by ambulance to the emergency room for new onset weakness and confusion. His last known well time was 1 hour before presentation. He was having dinner with his family when suddenly he developed weakness and confusion, and the family called 911. He has a past medical history of type 1 diabetes, hypertension, and a strong family history of cerebral infarctions. He has not had any recent head trauma, major bleeding, strokes, or blood thinners.

On physical examination his vital signs are within normal limits. He is awake and alert but confused and not answering questions appropriately. He is noted to have hemiparesis of the left lower face, left arm, and left leg. The remainder of the examination is normal.

The emergency room physician is concerned about a stroke, consults neurology, and orders a computed tomography (CT) head noncontrast stat. The CT head does not show any evidence of acute bleeding. The patient is evaluated by the neurologist. Because his last known well time was 1 hour ago he has no absolute contraindications for tissue plasminogen activator (tPA). Because his CT head did not show any evidence of bleeding he is given tPA and admitted to the stroke unit.

He does well during the hospitalization. A magnetic resonance imaging (MRI) and magnetic resonance angiogram (MRA) of the brain confirm a right middle cerebral artery stroke, which his clinical presentation originally suggested (Fig. 3.1). Once medically stable, he is then discharged to a rehabilitation center and started on daily aspirin.

### What are the risk factors for a stroke?

Although a stroke can happen to anyone at any age, it is more common as age increases. Medical risk factors for stroke include diabetes, hypertension, dyslipidemia, atrial fibrillation, and coronary artery disease. Behavioral risk factors include smoking and a sedentary lifestyle.

### Why was the patient sent to a rehabilitation center?

Even though the patient has survived the stroke, he may go to a rehabilitation center to help him regain functioning or adapt to lost functioning. A stroke can result in weakness or loss of muscular function, impaired speech production or comprehension, impaired cognitive abilities, impaired attention or judgment, changes to emotions or personality, and chronic pain. The specialists at the rehabilitation center will need to assess the patient's current level of functioning and use information from the patient's past, gathered from interviews with the patient and possibly the patient's family and friends, to identify areas where the patient's functioning has changed or been impaired likely because of the stroke. Physical and cognitive rehabilitation can then be used to help the patient regain functioning or adapt to lost functioning. Further assessment can then be used to mark the patient's functional change over time in the days, weeks, and months after the stroke.

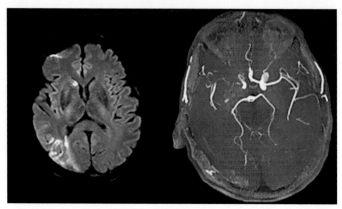

**Fig. 3.1** Example of a magnetic resonance image (MRI) and magnetic resonance angiogram (MRA) in a patient with a right middle cerebral artery (MCA) ischemic infarction. Note the severe stenosis at the right middle cerebral artery on the angiogram.

### What is neuropsychological testing?

Neuropsychological testing is an examination to identify current cognitive functioning as it relates to brain activity and to track changes in that functioning over time. Generally, changes in physical and emotional functioning also are considered and assessed. Neuropsychological testing involves several steps. A clinical interview is conducted with the patient and often with the patient's family. These interviews have several goals: One goal is to understand the patient's and family's goals for neuropsychological testing and what, if any, changes in functioning they have experienced, both of which can assist in selecting an appropriate battery of tests. In the case of an experienced change in functioning, another goal is establishing a baseline for before the event that presumably has caused change in functioning (e.g., stroke, onset of dementia, accident). Establishing rapport with the patient is also an important goal of the interview because it can help the patient during the testing process to feel safe and comfortable in completing tasks to the patient's best ability, thus increasing the likelihood of valid results. Neuropsychological testing can be done in one or more sessions, depending on the goals of assessment, and it can involve various types of tests. Some of the most common tests include: questionnaires that the patient fills out by selecting the most appropriate answer; verbal measures where the neuropsychologist presents various visual or auditory stimuli and the patient responds verbally; and physical/spatial measures where the patient manipulates objects with the hands or draws a response. Table 3.1 presents a list of common neuropsychological tests.

After the battery of tests has been completed, the neuropsychologist compares the patient's performance with standardized norms for the population, typically determined by age and sometimes by gender or race. The neuropsychologist then uses this information in conjunction with interviews and doctors' reports (when appropriate) to suggest where functioning seems to be different from the patient's population and where functioning seems to have changed from the patient's baseline. This information is compiled into a report that typically includes which tests were conducted, the patient's comparison with the population, and the neuropsychologist's professional assessment of what these tests mean for the patient and the patient's specific goal. The neuropsychologist then discusses the assessment with the patient and family, as appropriate, and next steps are discussed, including steps such as rehabilitation, therapy, or appropriate accommodations. Neuropsychological testing can be useful for a wide variety of patients; thus the next steps will be determined by the goals and the patient's individual situation. For example, a patient being assessed for dementia will have a different prognosis and treatment plan than a patient being assessed for possible attention-deficit hyperactivity disorder.

TABLE 3.1 ■ **List of Neuropsychological Tests**

| Measure | Summary |
| --- | --- |
| Beck Anxiety Inventory (BAI) | A 21-item, self-report measure of anxiety |
| Beck Depression Inventory-II (BDI-II) | A 21-item, self-report measure of depression |
| Finger Tapping Task | A task in which the patient taps a small mechanical device with the index finger as many times as possible in a predefined amount of time. Typically the task is completed several times on both hands, and a mean number of taps for each hand is calculated. |
| Halstead-Reitan Neuropsychological Battery | A neuropsychological battery that can be used to identify and locate brain dysfunction |
| Patient Health Questionnaire | This self-administered screening tool screens for eight mental disorder diagnoses, including major depressive disorder, which is assessed by the Patient Health Questionnaire-9 (PHQ-9) portion of the tool. This questionnaire is based on the *Diagnostic and Statistical Manual of Mental Disorders*, Fourth Edition (DSM-IV), thus the clinician should keep in mind that diagnostic criteria and categorization may change as the manual is updated in new editions. |
| Rorschach Inkblot Test | A projective test in which a series of nine inkblots are presented to the patient, who states what they see. Projective tests are used to determine a patient's unconscious drives, motivations, and feelings. The Rorschach has very specific scoring and interpretation guidelines, whereas other projective tasks may be interpreted more subjectively within broad conventions. |
| Trail Making Test | Trail making tests include several numbers and/or letters to connect in ascending order scattered on a page. The time to correctly complete the task is recorded for the purpose of comparing to normative values. The test administrator also will observe the patient completing the task and note any physical difficulties or unexpected behaviors. An example is favoring one side of the page, such that the patient does not see that the next point is on the other side of the page. |
| Wechsler Adult Intelligence Scale, Fourth Edition (WAIS-IV) | An intelligence test that includes scales of verbal comprehension, perceptual reasoning, working memory, and processing speed. Due to the inclusion of several individual tests and scales it is useful for neuropsychological testing beyond just intelligence testing. |
| Wechsler Memory Scale, Fourth Edition (WMS-IV) | A scale that assesses both auditory and visual memory. Due to the wide variety of tasks within the scale it can be useful in determining the specific nature of memory problems. |

Interviews conducted by neuropsychologists at the rehabilitation center with the patient and family members indicate that the patient is an English literature professor at a local university. He has been an active member of a faculty running club for 5 years. His family and friends describe him as a generally happy and energetic individual. Although the patient notes that learning new names at church can be difficult, his wife suggests that he is exaggerating and remembers new people just as well as anyone else does. He has no history of previous stroke, neurologic malfunction, or mental illness.

*What can the patient's vocation and hobbies tell us as we proceed to neuropsychological testing?*
Most neuropsychological tests have standardized norms to which the neuropsychologist will compare patient performance. However, the goal for this case is to understand how the stroke event itself has affected the patient's functioning. Information about whether the patient's performance is average, above average, or below average compared with the population on individual measures of the neuropsychological battery is useful but less relevant. It is important to know how the patient compares with himself before the stroke and whether he has lost functioning. Because premorbid neuropsychological testing is not available, it must be inferred from the interview what his functioning was before the ischemic incident.

> Proceeding to testing, it is noted from his history that the patient has above-average intelligence. As an English literature professor at a university his verbal perception, production, and reasoning is expected to be above average. The patient is an active member of a running club, suggesting that his physical abilities would be average to above average before the stroke.
> The patient is given a battery of neuropsychological and psychological tests and measures so that the neuropsychological team can infer any change in functioning. This battery includes testing of emotional, physical, and cognitive functioning.

*Why is testing of emotional functioning included for a patient who has suffered a stroke?*
One of the various problems that can occur after a stroke is depression. If a patient develops depression after a stroke it is important to encourage treatment of the depression, because this represents a change in emotional functioning. Furthermore, research suggests a correlation between depression and the prognosis for other functions, such as activities of daily living.

**CLINICAL PEARL**                                                                **STEP 2/3**

Meta-analyses suggest prevalence of poststroke depression is approximately one-third of patients. Thus when treating patients after a stroke, it is prudent to maintain a high index of suspicion for poststroke depression. Additionally, its presence can predict impairment in activities of daily living one or more years poststroke.

> The patient completes the Beck Depression Inventory-II (BDI-II) and his score screens for moderate depression. The patient also completes the Beck Anxiety Inventory (BAI), and his score indicates low to no anxiety symptoms. Although the clinical interview indicates no past history of depression and anxiety, the patient does discuss feeling a loss of interest in his hobbies since the stroke. He also discusses changes in sleep and appetite after the stroke.

**BASIC SCIENCE PEARL**                                                            **STEP 1**

The *Diagnostic and Statistical Manual of Mental Disorders, Fifth Edition*, states that five out of nine symptoms must be met for major depressive disorder to be diagnosed, one of which must be depressed mood or loss of interest in previously enjoyed activities. Those symptoms include: depressed mood; loss of interest or pleasure in previously enjoyed activities; increase or decrease in appetite; increase or decrease of sleep; physical restlessness or sluggishness; fatigue or loss of energy; feelings of guilt or worthlessness; difficulty concentrating, thinking, or making decisions; thoughts of death or suicide.

CLINICAL PEARL                                                              STEP 2/3

Although there are nine symptoms in the *Diagnostic and Statistical Manual of Mental Disorders, Fifth Edition*, for major depressive disorder and five must be present for a diagnosis, the presence of any symptoms as a change from previous functioning (even if less than five) should be considered clinically relevant and followed closely.

### How are depression and anxiety screened?

Screening tests can be either self-administered or clinician-administered. Both the BDI-II and BAI can be completed by the patient with paper and pen or administered verbally by the trained clinician. Another common screening test is the Patient Health Questionnaire (PHQ), which is a self-administered test that screens for eight specific diagnoses using criteria from the *Diagnostic and Statistical Manual of Mental Disorders*, Fourth Edition (DSM-IV). The Patient Health Questionnaire-9 (PHQ-9) is the specific tool within this larger test used to screen for major depressive disorder and contains nine items specific to the nine symptoms of depression. Of note, there were not significant changes in the diagnostic criteria for major depressive disorder from DSM-IV to DSM-5, making the PHQ-9 still a clinically useful screening tool. This test's brevity and direct inquiry into the severity of each of the nine symptoms of depression makes it an excellent screen. Additionally, because it is short and self-administered the patient can complete the screen before appointments or in the waiting room. The clinician can then delve deeper into a patient's specific answers to determine whether a diagnosis of major depressive disorder or another mood disorder is appropriate.

CLINICAL PEARL                                                              STEP 2/3

Screening measures like the Patient Health Questionnaire-9 can be administered regularly to monitor change in depressive symptoms and symptom severity. The questionnaire asks patients how often they have experienced each of the symptoms of depression, thus the clinician can quickly note if symptoms are occurring more or less often.

The patient completes a finger tapping task, a strength of grip task, and the trail making test. Additionally, the neuropsychologist has the patient walk down a hallway and notes any gait abnormalities. The patient, who is left-handed, has fewer finger taps on the left hand compared with the right hand in the same amount of time, and his grip strength is weaker on the left hand than on the right hand. The trail making test has two separate tasks: First, the patient connects numbered circles in order; second, the patient connects numbered and lettered circles in alternating order. The patient completes the trail making test with his left hand, and the neuropsychologist notes that the lines drawn by the patient are uneven. The neuropsychologist notes that the patient shows weakness in his left leg while walking down the hallway.

BASIC SCIENCE PEARL                                                          STEP 1

The Halstead-Reitan Neuropsychological Battery is a group of neuropsychological tests that includes such tests as the finger tapping test and trail making test that can help identify physical impairment related to brain dysfunction.

### Why did the patient complete these tasks?

Strokes can affect emotional, cognitive, and physical functioning. Particularly, strokes can result in muscle weakness or other impairments of muscular functioning. The fact that the patient, who is left-handed, performed more poorly on these tasks when using the left hand suggests that there is change in functioning due to the stroke. This is consistent with the initial reports and imaging showing right middle cerebral artery stroke.

### What is the next step for this patient, physically?
Both the initial physician reports and neuropsychological testing indicate a change in motor functioning in the limbs on the patient's left side. At the rehabilitation clinic the patient will work with other professionals, such as physical therapists, to further assess the nature of this motor deficit and to work toward regaining function. The neuropsychological team will reassess the patient using these same tests in the weeks and months that follow, to assess the patient's progression over time.

---

**CLINICAL PEARL**                                                      **STEP 2/3**

The well-known FLAME trial showed that patients who were prescribed fluoxetine after a stroke had greater recovery of motor function after 3 months compared with patients who received a placebo. Both groups also engaged in physiotherapy during the trial.

---

The patient also completes several measures of cognitive functioning, including the Wechsler Adult Intelligence Scale, Fourth Edition (WAIS-IV) and the Wechsler Memory Scale, Fourth Edition (WMS-IV). The patient's scores are well above average for verbal comprehension and are at or above average for tasks of perceptual reasoning, working memory, and processing speed. The patient's scores are average on memory tasks.

---

### Why did the neuropsychologist give the patient an intelligence test?
The WAIS-IV includes scales of verbal comprehension, perceptual reasoning, working memory, and processing speed. These scales can combine to suggest a full-scale intelligence quotient (FSIQ); they also can be considered individually to determine how those particular aspects of cognition may have changed in the patient. For example, if the patient had below-average verbal comprehension on the WAIS-IV, then the neuropsychologist would expect this to be a change from previous functioning because it is known that the patient is an English literature professor. The patient's average to above-average performance on cognitive tasks, including both the WAIS-IV and WMS-IV, is consistent with the right middle cerebral artery stroke, because a significant change in cognitive functioning would not be expected at this time.

---

The patient spends 2 weeks at the rehabilitation center engaging in physical therapy and cognitive behavioral psychotherapy, primarily focused on depressive symptoms. He also is prescribed fluoxetine. After 2 weeks of treatment he is given the same neuropsychological battery that he completed upon admission to the rehabilitation center. He shows improvement in motor functioning, though his left side remains weaker than the right. The patient's score on the BDI-II remains in the moderate depression range, with some improvement in symptoms.

---

**CLINICAL PEARL**                                                      **STEP 2/3**

Antidepressants such as fluoxetine may exert side effects, but not their therapeutic effects, immediately. It may take up to 4 to 8 weeks for antidepressants to reach their full therapeutic effect.

**BEYOND THE PEARLS:**

- Neuropsychologists work hard to keep test materials secure so that tests remain valid to as many potential patients as possible. However, the famous Rorschach test images are available in their entirety on the Internet, calling the test's validity into question. In the United States the Rorschach images are almost ubiquitous in media representations of neuropsychology.
- Neuropsychological testing can be helpful in locating dysfunctional areas of the brain, as research into brain function has helped in understanding functional patterns of brain regions.
- Just as doctors in training work under licensed physicians in hospital training programs during medical school, graduate students in clinical psychology and neuropsychology programs work with licensed practitioners throughout graduate school. Expect to work with these PhD or PsyD graduate students in rehabilitation centers or other sites that use neuropsychological testing. It is not uncommon for graduate students to administer neuropsychological batteries and to write the neuropsychological report while under the supervision of a licensed psychologist.

## References

American Psychiatric Association. (2013). *Diagnostic and statistical manual of mental disorders* (5th ed.). Washington, DC: American Psychiatric Association.

Ayerbe, L., Ayis, S., Wolfe, C., & Rudd, A. G. (2013). Natural history, predictors and outcomes of depression after stroke: Systematic review and meta-analysis. *British Journal of Psychiatry, 202*(1), 14–21.

Beck, A. T., Epstein, N., Brown, G., & Steer, R. A. (1988). An inventory for measuring clinical anxiety: Psychometric properties. *Journal of Consulting and Clinical Psychology, 56*(6), 893–897.

Beck, A.T., Steer, R.A., & Brown, G.K. (1996). *Manual for the Beck depression inventory-II*. San Antonio, TX: Psychological Corporation.

Centers for Disease Control and Prevention. (2018). Stroke. Retrieved from www.cdc.gov/stroke/index.htm.

Chollet, F., Tardy, J., Albucher, F. J., Thalamas, C., Berard, E., Lamy, C., ... Loubinoux, I. (2011). Fluoxetine for motor recovery after acute ischaemic stroke (FLAME): A randomised placebo-controlled trial. *Lancet Neurology, 10*(2), 123–130.

Exner, J. E. (2002). *The Rorschach: A comprehensive system* (4th ed.). Hoboken, NJ: Wiley.

Kroenke, K., Spitzer, R. L., & Williams, J. B. W. (2001). The PHQ-9: Validity of a brief depression severity measure. *Journal of General Internal Medicine, 16*(9), 606–613.

Loring, D. W. (Ed.). (1999). *INS dictionary of neuropsychology*. New York, NY: Oxford University Press.

Mitrushina, M., Boone, K. B., Razani, J., & D'Elia, L. F. (2005). *Handbook of normative data for neuropsychological assessment* (2nd ed.). New York, NY: Oxford University Press.

Ogden, J. A. (2005). *Fractured minds: A case-study approach to clinical neuropsychology* (2nd ed.). New York, NY: Oxford University Press.

Pohjasvaara, T., Vataja, R., Leppävuori, A., Kaste, M., & Erkinjuntti, T. (2001). Depression is an independent predictor of poor long-term functional outcome post-stroke. *European Journal of Neurology, 8*(4), 315–319.

Reitan, R. M., & Wolfson, D. (1993). *The Halstead-Reitan neuropsychological test battery: Theory and clinical interpretation* (2nd ed.). Tucson, AZ: Neuropsychology Press.

Robinson, R. G., & Jorge, R. E. (2016). Post-stroke depression: A review. *American Journal of Psychiatry, 173*(3), 221–231.

Sweeney, J. E., & Johnson, A. M. (2019). Halstead-Reitan characteristics of nonimpact and impact mTBI litigants and insurance claimants. *Applied Neuropsychology: Adult, 26*(1), 65–75.

Vogel, C. H. (1995). Assessment and approach to treatment in post-stroke depression. *Journal of the American Academy of Nurse Practitioners, 7*(10), 493–497.

Wechsler, D. (2008). *Wechsler adult intelligence scale (WAIS-IV)* (4th ed.). San Antonio, TX: Pearson.

Wechsler, D. (2009). *Wechsler memory scales (WMS-IV): Administration and scoring* (4th ed.). San Antonio, TX: Pearson.

Whyte, E. M., Mulsant, B. H., Vanderbilt, J., Dodge, H. H., & Ganguli, M. (2004). Depression after stroke: A prospective epidemiological study. *Journal of the American Geriatrics Society, 52*(5), 774–778.

# CHAPTER 4

# Depression

Kimberly Shain

A 16-year-old female presents to the emergency department with her parents after telling them earlier in the day that she didn't want to be alive anymore. The patient reports that for the past 6 months she has been "feeling down," and has been having thoughts of killing herself throughout the last week. She has a plan to kill herself that involves taking all of the medications in her family's medicine cabinet. The patient says that in the past 6 months she also has experienced a decrease in energy, saying that "it feels like I'm never able to sleep." Her parents tell you that she was previously on the track team at her school, and that she stopped going to practice 2 months ago because she "didn't see the point" any longer. Despite quitting the track team the patient reports a weight loss of 5 pounds in the past 6 months because of a decrease in her appetite. She denies fevers, chills, dizziness, lightheadedness, headache, vision changes, chest pain, palpitations, shortness of breath, cough, abdominal pain, nausea, vomiting, dysuria, auditory hallucinations, and visual hallucinations. She has no significant past medical, surgical, or psychiatric history.

***Given this patient's presentation, what initial diagnoses would be important to consider in a differential?***

Based on the vignette discussed previously, this patient is experiencing a major depressive episode. A major depressive episode is defined as an episode that meets diagnostic criteria for major depressive disorder (Table 4.1), is causing significant distress or impairment in functioning, and is not due to substance use or another medical condition. Several different conditions can initially present with a depressive episode, so it is important to obtain the relevant history to distinguish between these. The differential diagnosis for a patient presenting with a depressive disorder is vast and includes: major depressive disorder, schizoaffective disorder, bipolar disorder, persistent depressive disorder, substance/medication induced depressive disorder, and adjustment disorder with depressed mood.

Some important historical questions to ask patients presenting with a major depressive episode include questions about a history of substance use, a history of hypomanic or manic episodes, the duration of the current episode, the recent occurrence of a profound life-altering event, and a thorough medical history. It is important to distinguish between major depressive disorder and other diagnoses due to the sometimes vastly different treatment approaches for each (see Table 4.1). With roughly 350 million people around the globe affected by depressive disorders, these disorders are collectively one of the top three causes of morbidity worldwide. Lifetime prevalence for depression has been estimated anywhere from 10% to 25%, and approximately 2% to 9% of these patients will die by suicide. With such high prevalence, and potential for mortality, it is important to identify and appropriately treat depression.

TABLE 4.1 ■ Depressive Disorders

| Disorder | Presentation | Distinguishing Features |
|---|---|---|
| Major depressive disorder | A major depressive episode | |
| Persistent depressive disorder | Depressed mood in addition to two of the following: increased or decreased appetite, hypersomnia or insomnia, fatigue, low self-esteem, decreased concentration, feelings of hopelessness | Must be present for 2 years (1 year for adolescents) |
| Substance/medication-induced depressive disorder | Significant and persistent depressed mood or loss of interest | Mood symptoms occur in close temporal proximity to the initiation or withdrawal of a medication capable of producing the symptoms |
| Bipolar disorder | Can present with a hypomanic (bipolar II), manic (bipolar I), or major depressive episode | Manic symptoms |
| Schizoaffective Disorder | 2 or more of the following during a 1-month period: delusions, hallucinations, disorganized speech, grossly disorganized or catatonic behavior, negative symptoms, in addition to a major mood episode (manic or depressive) | Delusions or hallucinations must be present for 2 weeks without mood symptoms during the illness |
| Adjustment disorder with depressed mood | Low mood, tearfulness, or feelings of hopelessness that is out of proportion to the stressor | Develops within 3 months of the onset of the stressor |

*What medical conditions are associated with depressive symptoms?*

There are several medical conditions that have been shown to have a high incidence of depressive symptoms. The most common are Parkinson disease, Huntington disease, cardiovascular accidents (CVAs), traumatic brain injuries, and neuroendocrine disorders (Cushing disease and hypothyroidism).

Parkinson disease studies have shown prevalence as high as 22.5 %, 36.6 %, and 24.8 % of dysthymia, minor depression, and major depression respectively. In many instances, mood symptoms appear years before motor symptoms in Parkinson disease, and untreated depression can negatively affect the course of the disease. Although it may be hard to distinguish Parkinson disease from major depressive disorder when mood symptoms appear first, the development of rigidity, bradykinesia, tremor, and postural instability can assist in the differentiation.

Huntington disease is an autosomal dominant disease that is due to a trinucleotide CAG expansion on chromosome 4 in the gene that encodes the Huntingtin protein. This disorder is characterized by movement abnormalities such as bradykinesia, dystonia, rigidity, and chorea. Psychiatric manifestations are common as well for this disorder and can include irritability, anxiety, psychosis, and depressed mood; and it is not uncommon for these psychiatric symptoms to precede motor symptoms by more than a decade. This disease should be considered in patients with a family history of the disease and genetic testing should be offered.

A CVA is another common medical event associated with depression, with the prevalence of any depressive disorder after a CVA as high as 33.5% of patients. A thorough neurologic examination can help elicit new neurologic sequelae of a stroke, but neuroimaging, such as a head computed tomography (CT) and magnetic resonance imaging (MRI), commonly are used to diagnose the extent of neurologic injury.

Cushing disease and hypothyroidism have been associated with depressive symptoms as well. If Cushing disease is suspected, a 24-hour urine free cortisol test, followed by a high-dose dexamethasone suppression test, and an MRI of the sellar region can be performed. To evaluate hypothyroidism the following can be tested: thyroid-stimulating hormone (TSH), free triiodothyronine (T3), and thyroxine (T4).

It is important to identify and treat comorbid depression in individuals with these medical conditions, because untreated depression can worsen the clinical course of these diseases and result in a worse quality of life.

---

**CLINICAL PEARL**                                                              **STEP 1/2/3**

Major depressive disorder (MDD) is a clinical diagnosis based on nine symptoms outlined in the *Diagnostic and Statistical Manual of Mental Disorder,* Fifth Edition. In order to meet the criteria for MDD, the patient must have five out of nine of the following symptoms during a 2-week period. These symptoms must be different from previous functioning, exist for most of the day nearly every day, and one symptom must be either depressed mood or loss of interest or pleasure.
1. Depressed mood (can be irritable mood in children/adolescents)
2. **S**leep-insomnia or hypersomnia
3. Loss of **I**nterest or pleasure in all/almost all activities
4. Feelings of **G**uilt or worthlessness
5. Loss of **E**nergy (or fatigue)
6. Decreased ability to **C**oncentrate
7. Increase or decrease in **A**ppetite, or weight gain or loss
8. **P**sychomotor retardation or agitation
9. **S**uicidal ideation, suicide attempt, or recurrent thoughts of death
(***SIGECAPS*** is a common mnemonic used to remember eight out of nine of the diagnostic criteria.)

---

Upon further interview, the patient denies any history of substance use, any history of manic or hypomanic symptoms, or any identifiable recent life stressors. Her laboratory results reveal no abnormalities in thyroid-stimulating hormone levels, comprehensive metabolic panel, or complete blood count. Her urine drug screen is negative. Vital signs show her blood pressure is 102/70 mm Hg, respiration rate is 15/min, heart rate is 72/min, and temperature is 37.1°C (98.8°F).

---

*What are some other considerations in a case like this?*
Women are statistically more likely to attempt suicide, whereas males are more likely to die of a suicide attempt. In the past decade in the United States the male-to-female suicide death ratio was 3.7:1, making suicide the seventh leading cause of death for men and the 15th leading cause of death for women.

---

**CLINICAL PEARL**                                                                  **STEP 3**

In the month leading up to their death, 50% of those who completed suicide attempts saw a physician, and 24% saw a mental health care provider. This suggests that more comprehensive screening methods from both general practitioners and mental health professionals can help lower suicide rates.

Based on the patient's presenting symptom burden, and the lack of other criteria necessary for other diagnoses, she is diagnosed with major depressive disorder without psychotic features. Due to her suicidal ideation with a plan, she is admitted to the adolescent behavioral health unit for further evaluation and stabilization.

### *What are the treatment options for patients with major depressive disorder?*

- **Medications:** The first-line medications for major depressive disorder are typically selective serotonin reuptake inhibitors (SSRIs), due to their effectiveness and relatively lower side-effect profile. Other appropriate alternatives to SSRIs include serotonin norepinephrine reuptake inhibitors (SNRIs), tricyclic antidepressants (TCAs), and atypical antidepressants (bupropion, mirtazapine, trazodone). All of these have been shown to have comparable efficacy, and more importance is placed on follow-up and medication adjustment than initial medication choice.
- **Therapy:** Cognitive behavioral therapy (CBT) and interpersonal psychotherapy are both considered appropriate and effective treatments for major depressive disorder.
- **Combined medication and therapy:** The combination of pharmacotherapy and psychotherapy has been shown to be more efficacious than either treatment modality alone. In isolation, psychotherapy and pharmacotherapy appear to be similar in effect, although each offers distinct advantages. Pharmacotherapy is generally more widely available and affordable, but in terms of follow-up after cessation of treatment, the effects of psychotherapy tend to be longer lasting.
- **Electroconvulsive therapy (ECT):** Indications include refractory depression/mania/psychosis, psychotic depression, severe suicidality, and catatonia. ECT is most often delivered two to three times a week with a goal of 6 to 12 treatments in total. Although this treatment is very safe and effective, side effects can include anterograde amnesia, adverse reactions to anesthesia, arrhythmias, headache, and confusion.

### *What are the ethical considerations for involuntary hospitalization?*

One of the most important ethical considerations in a patient who presents with major depressive disorder arises when they express suicidality and present a danger to themselves. Although many patients seeking treatment may be agreeable to hospitalization, a percentage of this patient population will be resistant to this treatment option. When this happens, two of the guiding principles of medicine come into conflict: patient autonomy and nonmaleficence. In this clinical scenario, which is all too often an actual scenario that clinicians face, the patients in question may lack decision-making capacity. Capacity evaluation includes an evaluation of the patients' understanding of their illness, the consequences of refusing treatment, and the reliability in decision making. An important distinction to be made is that capacity must be evaluated in relation to a decision. Patients may have the capacity to make decisions in one domain and lack it in another, based on the understanding of each illness or situation. In the situation where a physician determines a patient lacks the capacity to refuse psychiatric hospitalization, the physician can balance nonmaleficence with autonomy by hospitalizing the patient (nonmaleficence) while committing to constant reevaluation of the patient's decision-making capacity (autonomy). Other steps that can be taken to minimize the potential trauma and humiliation of involuntary hospitalization include limiting coercive tactics, encouraging cooperative measures, and allowing patients to make decisions within the limitations of their illness.

**CLINICAL PEARL**                                                **STEP 2/3**

One rare but potentially fatal complication of selective serotonin reuptake inhibitor therapy and other serotonergic medications is serotonin syndrome. The most widely accepted criteria for diagnosing serotonin syndrome is the Hunter Serotonin Toxicity Criteria. To meet the criteria, the patient has to have been exposed to a serotonergic medication in the past 5 weeks, and one of the following conditions must be met:
1. Spontaneous clonus
2. Inducible clonus and agitation
3. Inducible clonus and diaphoresis
4. Ocular clonus and agitation
5. Ocular clonus and diaphoresis
6. Tremor and hyperreflexia
7. Muscle rigidity and temperature >38°C and ocular clonus
8. Muscle rigidity and temperature >38°C and inducible clonus

Treatment for serotonin syndrome is supportive and includes cessation of the offending medication, fluid resuscitation, and benzodiazepines for agitation. In more severe cases, sedation, paralysis, and intubation might be indicated.

---

The patient remained on the adolescent behavioral health unit for 4 days while she participated in group therapy, a family meeting, and daily individual meetings with the treatment team. She was started on 10 mg of fluoxetine daily. By the time of discharge, the patient denied suicidal ideation and felt she would be safe at home. The patient was provided with appointments to see both a psychiatrist and a therapist for follow-up after discharge. At her follow-up appointment she continued to deny suicidal ideation and reported an improvement in her depressive symptom

---

**BEYOND THE PEARLS:**

- Double depression is defined as a major depressive episode in a patient with comorbid persistent depressive disorder. This condition has a poorer prognosis than a major depressive episode alone.
- Research on the gut microbiota-brain axis is ongoing (specifically on the role of the hypothalamic-pituitary-adrenal (HPA) axis, nutrients available to the gut microbiome, and the resulting inflammation in the brain) and suggests there could be a connection to the development of diseases such as mood disorders.
- A 12-month prevalence of major depressive disorder is three times higher in the 18-year-old to 29-year-old age range than in individuals 60 years or older.
- Antidepressants all have a controversial black box warning about the possibility of increased suicidal thinking, particularly in youth and young adults. The risk of untreated depression far outweighs the risk of suicidal thoughts, but the warning still must be discussed with patients.
- Transcranial magnetic stimulation (TMS), vagus nerve stimulation (VNS), and ketamine are also being used to treat depression, particularly in people with treatment-resistant depression.

## References

American Psychiatric Association. (2013). *Diagnostic and statistical manual of mental disorders*, (5th ed., pp. 155–188). Washington, DC: Author.

Bartlett, D. (2017). Drug-induced serotonin syndrome. *Critical Care Nurse*, *37*(1), 49–54.

Buliman, A., Tataranu, L. G., Paun, D. L., Mirica, A., & Dumitrache, C. (2016). Cushing's disease: A multidisciplinary overview of the clinical features, diagnosis, and treatment. *Journal of Medicine and Life*, *9*(1), 12–18.

Cuijpers, P., van Straten, A., Warmerdam, L., & Andersson, G. (2009). Psychotherapy versus the combination of psychotherapy and pharmacotherapy in the treatment of depression: A meta-analysis. *Depress Anxiety*, *26*(3), 279–288.

Danzer, G., & Wilkus-Stone, A. (2015). The give and take of freedom: The role of involuntary hospitalization and treatment in recovery from mental illness. *Bull Menninger Clin.*, *79*(3), 255–280.

King, C., Horwitz, A., Czyz, E., & Lindsay, R. (2017). Suicide risk screening in healthcare settings: Identifying males and females at risk. *Journal of Clinical Psychology in Medical Settings*, *24*(1), 8–20.

Le, T., Bhushan, V., Chen, V., & King, M. (2016). *First aid for the USMLE step 2 CK* (9th ed., pp. 432–436). New York, NY: McGraw Hill.

Marsh, L. (2013). Depression and Parkinson's disease: Current knowledge. *Current Neurology and Neuroscience Reports*, *13*(12), 409.

Mitchell, A. J., Sheth, B., Gill, J., Yadegarfar, M., Stubbs, B., Yadegarfar, M., & Meader, N. (2017). Prevalence and predictors of post-stroke mood disorders: A meta-analysis and meta-regression of depression, anxiety and adjustment disorder. *General Hospital Psychiatry*. *47*, 48–60.

Petra, A., Panagiotidou, S., Hatziagelaki, E., Stewart, J., Conti, P., & Theoharides, T. (2015). Gut-microbiota-brain axis and its effect on neuropsychiatric disorders with suspected immune dysregulation. *Clinical Therapeutics*, *37*(5), 984–995.

Simon, G., & Perlis, R. (2010). Personalized medicine for depression: Can we match patients with treatments? *American Journal of Psychiatry*, *167*(12), 1445–1455.

Smithson, S., & Pignone, M. (2017). Screening adults for depression in primary care. *Medical Clinics of North America*, *101*(4), 807–821.

Zhang, X., Zhou, S., Hou, Y., & Liu, D. (2017). Effect of cognitive behavioral therapy versus interpersonal psychotherapy in patients with major depressive disorder: A meta-analysis of randomized controlled trials. *Chinese Medical Journal*, *130*(23), 2844.

# CHAPTER 5

# Bipolar

Amy Bischoff ■ Rif S. El-Mallakh

A 45-year-old female is brought to the emergency department by her husband. He says his wife has been up late at night for 8 days redecorating the interior of their house. She has been excitedly painting and refurnishing the living room and kitchen until around 5 a.m. each day, and she wakes up 3 hours later only to start again. Her husband says nothing like this has happened to his wife before. Upon examination, the patient is euphoric, and her speech is fast and difficult to interrupt.

*What are the first steps in evaluating the behavioral changes in this patient?*

This patient is exhibiting abnormally elevated mood, reduced need for sleep, and increased goal-directed activity for multiple days. This behavior is concerning for a manic episode, which is a psychiatric emergency because the patient can be a danger to herself or others due to severely impaired judgment. Your first job is to ensure safety. You may need to hospitalize the patient, or you may decide that there is sufficient support in her environment to attempt to manage her as an outpatient in a partial hospitalization program. Either way it is important to determine whether the cause of the manic episode is secondary to a medical issue, substance-induced, or a primary psychiatric diagnosis (bipolar I disorder). Possible medical causes include hyperthyroidism, temporal lobe seizures, neoplasms, and systemic infections such as human immunodeficiency virus (HIV). Substance/medication-induced causes may include antidepressants, sympathomimetics (e.g., cocaine, amphetamines, levodopa), corticosteroids, and bronchodilators. To exclude some of the more common organic causes of mania, the physician should order a urine drug/toxicology screen, serum levels of thyroxine, thyroid-stimulating hormone, vitamins $B_{12}$ and folate, an electroencephalograph (EEG), and brain imaging such as computed tomography (CT) of the head.

When asked if there is any family history of mood disorder, the patient replies that her deceased father had "extreme mood swings" for which he was hospitalized multiple times and started on many different medications.

---

**CLINICAL PEARL**        **STEP 1/2/3**

Of all the major psychiatric disorders, bipolar I has the strongest genetic link. A first-degree relative of someone with bipolar disorder is at a 10 times greater risk of developing the illness than the general population.

*How do you diagnose bipolar I disorder?*

Bipolar I disorder requires a history of at least one manic episode. Depressive episodes, hypomanic episodes, or euthymia (normal mood) may occur between manic episodes, but their presence is not necessary for the diagnosis of bipolar I.

A manic episode consists of a persistently elevated, expansive, or irritable mood accompanied by an unusual increase in activity or excess energy that lasts at least 1 week (or any duration if the person needs inpatient treatment). In addition, there need to be at least three of the following symptoms (or four of the following if the person's mood is only irritable):

1. Pressured speech or much more talkative
2. Flight of ideas or racing thoughts
3. Easily distracted
4. Inflated self-esteem
5. Very little sleep but well rested
6. Increase in activities and completing tasks, or psychomotor agitation/restlessness
7. Doing things that are very risky or may cause negative consequences

Bipolar II disorder requires a history of at least one major depressive episode and at least one hypomanic episode. Hypomania differs from mania in that symptoms last at least 4 days rather than a week, and the episode does not cause any major problems with social or occupational functioning. If the person has experienced psychosis during the episode, then the episode is considered manic. A patient cannot have both type I and type II bipolar illness; if the patient has ever experienced a full manic episode, bipolar I is the diagnosis.

---

**CLINICAL PEARL**                                                      **STEP 1/2/3**

Despite the shared name, bipolar I and II disorder have different diagnostic criteria and do not share genetic heritage. Nonetheless, treatment regimens are very similar. Whereas both disorders tend to be chronic and require long-term treatment, bipolar II frequently has a better functional prognosis. Unfortunately, the suicide risk is similar for both disorders.

---

*What are the acute and maintenance pharmacotherapeutic treatment options for bipolar disorder?*

For acute bipolar manic symptoms, certain mood stabilizers and/or atypical antipsychotics may be used. The most effective mood stabilizers for acute mania are lithium, valproic acid, and carbamazepine. Lithium is associated with a moderate reduction in symptoms in 40% to 80% of patients after 2 to 3 weeks of treatment for acute mania. However, lithium has a low therapeutic index and needs to be monitored closely to avoid toxicity. Furthermore, the active fraction of lithium is the intracellular fraction, and the delay in accumulation of intracellular lithium delays the time to response. Valproic acid and carbamazepine have a faster onset of action, and more than half of patients experience significant improvement in manic symptoms. Atypical antipsychotics are also effective as monotherapy or in combination with a mood stabilizer. Combination therapy tends to show a greater and faster response than monotherapy.

**Atypical antipsychotics approved for acute mania:**

Aripiprazole
Asenapine
Cariprazine
Olanzapine
Quetiapine
Risperidone
Ziprasidone

For bipolar depression, antidepressants are discouraged as monotherapy because of concern for activating mania and destabilizing the illness (i.e., inducing cycling).

**Efficacious treatments for acute bipolar I depression:**

Quetiapine monotherapy

Lurasidone monotherapy

Pramipexole (not U.S. Food and Drug Administration [FDA]–approved)

Combination olanzapine/fluoxetine therapy

Combination lurasidone/lithium therapy

Combination lurasidone/valproic acid therapy

Only quetiapine monotherapy is approved for bipolar II depression. In addition to approved agents, placebo-controlled randomized clinical trials have demonstrated efficacy of lamotrigine, pramipexole, modafinil, and armodafinil in bipolar depression with evidence of illness destabilization in short-term studies.

For many patients the medications that were effective in the acute phase become the first choice for maintenance treatment. At optimal doses, lithium reduces the rate of recurrence of mood episodes by 50%. Valproic acid and carbamazepine may be especially useful for patients with rapid cycling or mixed states. The atypical antipsychotics approved for maintenance treatment are aripiprazole, quetiapine, olanzapine, risperidone, and ziprasidone. Although some of these agents are approved as monotherapy, the best practice is to combine them with a mood stabilizer.

---

The patient is hospitalized to control her mania. A workup reveals normal complete blood count (CBC) and complete metabolic panel (CMP), and a negative urine drug/toxicology screen. Imaging of her brain is unremarkable. The diagnosis of bipolar I disorder is made. She is prescribed 1200 mg of lithium per day, and she stabilizes. She fully recovers within 2 weeks and is discharged from the hospital, returning to work soon after.

---

**CLINICAL PEARL**                                                                           **STEP 1/2/3**

Lithium remains the gold standard treatment for bipolar disorder. It is the only mood stabilizer that reduces suicide risk when used long term. Risk may be reduced by up to sevenfold.

---

*What are the nonpharmacotherapeutic options for treatment of bipolar disorder?*

Psychotherapy can improve outcomes by prolonging remission. After the acute manic or depressive episodes are controlled the patient can benefit from supportive psychotherapy, group therapy, or family therapy. For refractory or life-threatening acute mania or depression, electroconvulsive therapy (ECT) is very effective. For a pregnant woman having a manic episode, ECT is one of the best treatment options and can be used with reasonable safety in all trimesters.

---

A month has passed, and she follows up in an outpatient clinic. She complains of hand tremors interfering with daily function. She has adhered to her 1200 mg/day lithium regimen. Her lithium dose is reduced to 900 mg/day. Subsequently, her tremors become much more tolerable.

---

**CLINICAL PEARL**                                                                             **STEP 2/3**

The therapeutic range for lithium is 0.6 to 1.2 mEq/L. Lower levels are considered ineffective, whereas higher levels lead to more side effects and possible toxicity. Blood lithium levels should be monitored regularly.

The patient is adherent to her new regimen (900 mg/day) and remains stable for 14 months with few symptoms and a small residual tremor. However, she returns to the emergency department with manic symptoms. At this time, her lithium level is 0.7 mEq/L, and she has no notable tremor on examination. Her lithium is increased to 1200 mg/day, resulting in a lithium level of 1.0 mEq/L without tremor, and she stabilizes without requiring hospitalization. Six weeks later, her disabling tremor has returned.

### How can lithium side effects be used to guide prevention of recurrent manic episodes?

Patients who experience disabling side effects from lithium therapy are often prescribed a lower dose to mitigate those side effects. However, by reducing the dose enough to lessen these symptoms, physicians are unintentionally increasing the risk for relapse and recurrence of mania. In this patient's case, the 1200 mg/day lithium dose was reduced to 900 mg/day to combat her debilitating tremor. Yet the resulting lithium level (0.7 mEq/L) was ultimately not high enough to prevent recurrence of manic symptoms, even though the level fell within the recommended 0.6–1.2 mEq/L range. Interestingly, manic patients tolerate higher lithium levels with fewer side effects than euthymic patients. This example demonstrates that there is an increased need for lithium during active manic episodes. An explanation for the increased need for lithium during periods of active mania is that acutely manic patients tend to retain more lithium ions than euthymic patients. In a prospective cohort study, acutely manic subjects retained more lithium than euthymic subjects while achieving the same serum lithium level. This could be due to an increase in intracellular lithium ions during active mania, resulting in lower levels of serum lithium.

One way to determine when the lithium dose should be increased in order to prevent a full-blown manic episode is by looking for a lack of or reduction of side effects. When the patient in this case presented with manic symptoms, her residual tremor was absent. Her lack of tremor was likely caused by the increased lithium retention that accompanies acute mania. Therefore patients should be educated to look for reduction of adverse drug reactions and return of subsyndromal symptoms as indications to rapidly increase their lithium dose. Once euthymia is reestablished, it is reasonable to reduce the dose only if adverse reactions return. By using lithium side effects to guide changes in dosing, patients can prevent the development of a manic episode, and they may have more prolonged periods of remission.

---

**CLINICAL PEARL**                                                          **STEP 2/3**

The daily dose of lithium is not a useful marker of effectiveness to prevent a manic episode or the incidence of adverse drug reactions. Patient education, close surveillance during patient visits, and flexible dosage of lithium may help optimize prophylaxis.

---

The patient remains stable on lithium for the next 10 years, changing the dose as needed to prevent manic episodes and balance drug side effects. However, her most recent routine labs are notable for an estimated glomerular filtration rate (eGFR) in the 50s (previously stable in the 70s mL/min/1.73m2), creatinine 1.5 mg/dL (previously stable at 1.0–1.1 mg/dL), and BUN 20 (previously stable at 12–15 mg/dL). A magnetic resonance image (MRI) of her kidneys (Fig. 5.1) is available for review.

### How can the etiology of renal dysfunction be identified as lithium-induced versus lithium-independent?

Patients with mood disturbance have higher rates of renal disease, independent of lithium use. Therefore it is important to be able to distinguish whether a patient's nephropathy is lithium-related or lithium-independent. However, lithium use is associated with two types of renal disease. Lithium may reduce the kidney's ability to concentrate urine or its ability to filter blood. Lithium reduces the concentrating ability of the kidney through interference with vasopressin or by reversible renal tubular damage. Because these are reversible, they are problematic but not of great

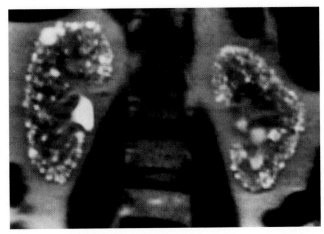

**Fig. 5.1**  T2-weighted magnetic resonance imaging (MRI) of the kidneys revealing numerous microcysts in the medullary and cortical regions (*Courtesy:* Farres, M., Ronco, P., et al. (2003). Chronic lithium nephropathy: MR imaging for diagnosis. *Radiology 229*(2), 570–574).

concern. However, reduction in creatinine clearance is much more worrisome. The most sensitive and specific screening tool for lithium-induced glomerular nephropathy is MRI evaluation for microcysts (see Fig. 5.1). Lithium-induced glomerular dysfunction usually occurs after 10 to 20 years of lithium use, and it is characterized by abundant renal microcysts that result in reduced GFR. These microcysts can be found anywhere in the kidney and show up as small hyperintense lesions on T2-weighted MRI. The mechanism for lithium-related microcyst formation is the phosphorylation and subsequent inhibition of the glycogen synthase kinase 3 beta (3βGSK-3b) enzyme. The phosphorylated version of this enzyme is associated with microcyst development in renal tubule epithelium. A mass effect is created as more and more microcysts develop, reducing GFR. Patients whose eGFR is greater than 40 mL/min/1.73 m2 have a higher chance of recovery of renal function after stopping lithium.

---

**CLINICAL PEARL**                                                              **STEP 2/3**

The main risk factor for the development of lithium-induced nephropathy is the duration of drug exposure. Chronic lithium exposure can stimulate microcyst formation, resulting in decreased estimated glomerular filtration rate.

---

Because of the confirmation of lithium-induced renal toxicity, the patient is slowly weaned off lithium. Over the next year and a half, she fails multiple different pharmacotherapy regimens (including valproic acid, carbamazepine, risperidone, and aripiprazole), ending up hospitalized five times for manic episodes. She has started smoking for the first time, two packs of cigarettes per day. She is desperate to find a medication that will work for her.

---

*How can pharmacogenomics be used to improve outcomes for patients with bipolar disorder?*
Certain genes can have significant effects on psychiatric treatment. Patients who fail multiple medication trials should undergo pharmacogenomic testing to identify drugs that may be metabolized too slowly (resulting in excessive side effects at typical doses) or too quickly (resulting in lack of efficacy at typical doses).

Because of her poor treatment response over the past year and a half, the patient decides to undergo pharmacogenomic testing to predict her response to olanzapine. A SULT4A1-1 haplotype is identified, as is a hyper-inducible allele at CYP1A2. Because of her smoking history, she is started on a 30 mg/day dose of olanzapine—twice the usual dose. On this single agent she has not been hospitalized and has shown significant improvement in outpatient follow-up.

There are few genes that predict response to a specific drug. The various sulfotransferase (SULT) gene products catalyze the biotransformation of many different neurotransmitters, hormones, drugs, and xenobiotics. Patients who have the SULT4A1-1 haplotype are more likely to have an effective response to olanzapine than those without the haplotype. Olanzapine is metabolized by the cytochrome enzyme CYP1A2. This gene product is induced by exposure to any burned hydrocarbon. However, a few individuals have a hyper-inducible variant. In these CYP1A2 hyper-inducers exposure to tobacco smoke will increase CYP1A2 enzyme activity. Patients with this variant may require significantly higher doses of olanzapine.

## BEYOND THE PEARLS:

- The lifetime prevalence of bipolar I disorder is approximately 1% to 2%, with women and men being equally affected. The onset is usually before age 30, with a mean age of 18 of the first mood episode. The lifetime prevalence of bipolar II is not clear, as some studies report higher whereas others report lower than bipolar I.
- Of patients with bipolar disorder, 25% to 50% attempt suicide at least once, and 5% to 15% die by suicide.
- An untreated manic episode usually lasts an average of 2 months, whereas an untreated depression may last 3 to 6 months. The course of bipolar disorder is typically chronic with relapses. The frequency of mood episodes increases as a function of the number of previous mood episodes.
- Bipolar I disorder may present with psychotic features. It is important to keep bipolar disorder on the differential in a patient with psychosis. Combination treatment with a mood stabilizer and an atypical antipsychotic is especially helpful for these patients.
- Patients who experience mania in the postpartum period have a high chance of relapse with future deliveries. These patients should be prophylactically treated with mood stabilizers in the peripartum period.
- Mood episodes appear to be toxic to the brain. Cognitive decline may occur as a long-term consequence of poorly controlled bipolar disorder. Onset of dementia may occur earlier than in the general population, unless patients are adequately controlled. Additionally, lithium may be neuroprotective in patients with bipolar disorder, resulting in a delay in the onset of dementia to match the general population.

## References

American Psychiatric Association. (2013). *Diagnostic and statistical manual of mental disorders* (5th ed.). Washington, DC: Author

Culpepper, L. (2014). The diagnosis and treatment of bipolar disorder: Decision-making in primary care. *The Primary Care Companion for CNS Disorders*, *16*(3), PCC.13r01609.

Greenspan, K., Goodwin, F., Bunney, W., et al. (1968). Lithium ion retention: Patterns during acute mania and normothymia. *Archives of General Psychiatry*, *19*, 664–673.

Khan, M., & El-Mallakh, R. S. (2015). Renal microcysts and lithium. *International Journal of Psychiatry in Medicine*, *50*(3), 290–298.

Larson, E., & Richelson, E. (1988). Organic causes of mania. *Mayo Clinic Proceedings*, *63*(9), 906–912.

Narahari, A., El-Mallakh, R. S., Kolikonda, M. K., Bains, A. S., & Lippmann, S. (2015). How coffee and cigarettes can effect the response to psychopharmacotherapy. *Current Psychiatry, 14*(10), 79–80.

Roberts, R. J., Lohano, K. K., & El-Mallakh, R. S. (2016). Antipsychotics as antidepressants. *Asia Pacific Psychiatry, 8*(3), 179–188.

Sutherland, C., Leighton, I. A., & Cohen, P. (1993). Inactivation of glycogen synthase kinase-3 beta by phosphorylation: New kinase connections in insulin and growth-factor signaling. *Biochemical Journal, 296,* 15–19.

Wilting, I., Heerdink, E.R., Mersch, , P.-P. A., Den Boer, J. A., Egberts, A. C. G., & Nolen, W. A. (2009). Association between lithium serum level, mood state and patient-reported adverse drug reactions during long lithium treatment: A naturalistic follow-up study. *Bipolar Disorders, 11*(4), 434–440.

# CHAPTER 6

# Generalized Anxiety Disorder

Tiya Johnson

A previously healthy 18-year-old female who is in her first year of college presents to your office with the complaint, "I'm having difficulty controlling my nerves." She describes worrying over "every little thing," which has become worse over the past 8 months. She feels this way on more days than not and generally feels "on edge," irritable, and unable to concentrate. Sometimes she experiences palpitations, tightness in her chest, and muscle tension. She has difficulty falling asleep on most nights because she cannot "turn off" her brain due to thinking about various things in her life. This causes her to not get enough sleep at night, and she feels tired all the time. She is concerned because the excessive worrying is affecting her ability to get her classwork done and keeps her from spending time with her friends. She tells you that she smokes marijuana a few nights each month to help with the anxiety and insomnia but adds that it sometimes makes her feel worse. She also drinks two to three alcoholic beverages on weekends with friends, but she has not been out in several weeks. She does not use any other substances and is not taking any over-the-counter or prescribed medications. She has never had anxiety this severe and is worried it will get worse.

### What would be the first thing you would want to know to help narrow the differential diagnosis?

This patient is experiencing symptoms of anxiety. Generally, having anxiety symptoms in response to some stressor is normal and, in some cases, necessary for survival. For example, becoming anxious when walking down a dark alley is normal because you become more aware of your surroundings. Anxiety becomes problematic or a "disorder" when the anxiety symptoms are severe enough to interfere with the ability to function normally in life.

Anxiety disorders typically include both emotional and physical symptoms. Also, many different substances and medical conditions can cause symptoms of anxiety. Because of this, it is important to make sure medical causes are ruled out first. Common nonpsychiatric causes of anxiety symptoms include but are not limited to: asthma, chronic obstructive pulmonary disease (COPD), congestive heart failure (CHF), ischemic heart disease, arrhythmias, hyperthyroidism, hypoglycemia, carcinoid tumors, pheochromocytoma, menopause, over-the-counter and prescribed medications, and substance intoxication and/or withdrawal.

### After obtaining a thorough history, what tests, if any, do you need to order to rule out medical causes of anxiety in this patient?

Although no laboratory test is required to diagnose a patient with an anxiety disorder, a medical workup should be done to ensure that the patient does not have any physical explanation for the symptoms. Diagnosing a person with an anxiety disorder is a diagnosis of exclusion, meaning that every other possible explanation must be ruled out before an anxiety disorder can be diagnosed.

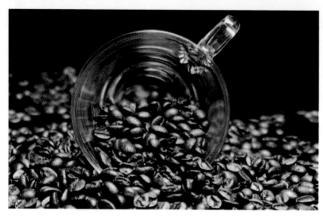

**Fig. 6.1**   Coffee beans.

The laboratory tests you decide to order will be guided by the reported symptoms and any abnormalities found during the physical examination. The following are the first laboratory tests you should consider ordering:

- **Thyroid function tests (thyroid-stimulating hormone [TSH], free thyroxine [free T4], and triiodothyronine [T3]):** Hyperthyroidism can cause symptoms of anxiety because of the overproduction of the thyroid hormones. There would be other symptoms described by the patient or found on physical examination, including heat intolerance, increased appetite with weight loss, tachycardia, palpitations, and tremors. The patient may also complain of hyperactivity, mood swings, insomnia, and difficulty concentrating. Laboratory results would reveal decreased TSH and elevated free T4 and possibly elevated T3.
- **Blood glucose testing:** Hypoglycemia (blood glucose level less than 50 mg/dL) can cause symptoms of anxiety along with tremors, palpitations, syncope, and fatigue.
- **Urine drug screen/blood alcohol level:** Intoxication with stimulants, such as amphetamine, methamphetamine, cocaine, and 3,4-methylenedioxymethamphetamine (MDMA), can cause anxiety symptoms. Marijuana use can worsen anxiety symptoms. Withdrawal from benzodiazepines and alcohol can also cause symptoms of anxiety. Testing for these substances is very important. Also be sure to ask about caffeine intake, because excessive caffeine use can cause significant anxiety symptoms as well (Fig. 6.1)

*What other laboratory tests do you want to order?*
Other laboratory tests are not likely to contribute any significant information when trying to rule out medical causes of anxiety. For example, ordering catecholamine (dopamine, epinephrine, norepinephrine) levels to rule out a pheochromocytoma should be reserved for patients with a family history of endocrine disorders/tumors or with severe episodic headaches and hypertension along with the anxiety symptoms. Again, let the history and physical examination guide which tests to order.

Anxiety disorders commonly co-occur with other psychiatric disorders. When evaluating a patient with anxiety symptoms, be sure to evaluate for symptoms of depression, suicidal ideation, specific fears (phobias), obsessions/compulsions, panic attacks, and substance abuse.

On examination, patient's temperature is 37 °C (98.6 °F), pulse is 110/min, blood pressure is 117/76 mm Hg, respiratory rate is 14/min, and oxygen saturation is 100% on room air. She is calm and cooperative throughout the interview; however, she rapidly taps her foot on the floor and shifts her position several times. She is oriented to person, place, time, and situation. Auscultation of the heart reveals tachycardia, but no other abnormalities. Laboratory work up includes complete blood count (CBC), comprehensive metabolic panel (CMP), and thyroid function tests. These are all within normal limits. Urine drug screen is negative.

***Based on the information from the physical and laboratory workup, how has the differential changed?***
Besides having some mild tachycardia, the patient's workup is negative for any medical causes of her anxiety. Her thyroid is not hyperactive, her blood glucose is normal, and despite telling you that she smokes marijuana a few times a month, her urine drug screen is negative. Also, she denies having any alcoholic beverage for several weeks. Therefore her anxiety appears to be due to a psychiatric illness or anxiety disorder.

***If you believe the patient has a psychiatric disorder, what information do you need to know that would help you correctly diagnosis the patient's condition?***
There are several different types of anxiety disorders that are possible in a person with anxiety symptoms. Because many anxiety disorders co-occur with one another, it may be difficult to choose just one diagnosis for your patient. As with most psychiatric diagnoses, obtaining a thorough history is imperative to proper diagnosis and treatment of each patient.

Because anxiety symptoms can be present in any of the anxiety disorders in Table 6.1, paying careful attention to the specific details of what symptoms the patient has and what triggers the symptoms is important. For example, with social anxiety disorder, one typically becomes anxious when faced with social situations, such as public speaking, meeting new people, or eating/drinking in front of others. This disorder is in contrast to panic disorder, which manifests as recurrent, unexpected episodes of intense anxiety with subsequent physical symptoms, such as palpitations, sweating, shaking, shortness of breath, chest pain, dizziness, or numbness/tingling.

### TABLE 6.1 ■ Common DSM-5 Anxiety Disorders Experienced in Adults

| | |
|---|---|
| Specific phobia | Intense fear or anxiety almost always experienced immediately when exposed to a specific object or situation |
| Social anxiety disorder | Intense fear or anxiety almost always about social situations where there may be exposure to embarrassment or humiliation by others |
| Panic disorder | Experiencing recurrent, unexpected panic attacks (a surge of intense fear with subsequent physical symptoms) |
| Agoraphobia | Intense fear or anxiety about being in situations where one might not escape easily or help might not be available if needed (public transportation, open spaces, enclosed places, standing in line, crowds, being outside of the home) |
| Generalized anxiety disorder (GAD) | Excessive anxiety and worry about different events or activities occurring more days than not for at least 6 months |
| Substance/medication-induced anxiety disorder | Panic attacks or anxiety proven (via history, physical, and/or laboratory tests) to develop during or shortly after intoxication or withdrawal of a substance/medication. Also, the substance/medication must actually be able to cause the anxiety symptoms |
| Anxiety disorder due to another medical condition | Evidence from history, physical, and/or laboratory tests proves panic attacks or anxiety are caused by the medical condition |

*Considering the different anxiety disorders typically experienced in adults, what is the most likely diagnosis in this patient?*
This patient has experienced symptoms of excessive worry about common stressors on most days for at least 6 months. She also has fatigue, difficulty concentrating, irritability, and insomnia. These symptoms are affecting her ability to function at school and socially (she is not spending time with her friends). She does not have any abnormalities on physical examination except for some mild tachycardia and psychomotor restlessness. Even though she uses marijuana and alcohol occasionally, her urine drug screen is negative. All other laboratory results are within normal limits. Based on careful consideration of all anxiety disorders in the *Diagnostic and Statistical Manual of Mental Disorders*, Fifth Edition (DSM-5), her symptoms appear most likely caused by generalized anxiety disorder.

---

Because of the specific symptoms experienced by the patient and the duration of those symptoms, she is diagnosed with generalized anxiety disorder (GAD). She is treated in the outpatient setting with both medication and psychotherapy.

---

Two quick screening tools for generalized anxiety disorder are the Generalized Anxiety Disorder 2-item and the Generalized Anxiety Disorder 7-item. They contain questions relating to the symptoms of GAD. The responses are in regard to symptoms occurring within the past 2 weeks. The patient responds to the questions by circling a number from 0 to 3, ranging from "not at all" to "nearly every day." The responses are then totaled, and a predetermined cutoff score determines the severity of the anxiety symptoms.

*What are the treatment options in a patient with generalized anxiety disorder?*
Treatment for generalized anxiety disorder is basically the same for most anxiety disorders (excluding specific phobias). Treatment for anxiety disorders includes two major categories: medication and psychotherapy.

- **Medications:** The first class of medications used to treat GAD (and other anxiety disorders) is antidepressants. The specific class of antidepressants that are generally tried first are selective serotonin reuptake inhibitors (SSRIs). However, of the four antidepressants with a federal drug administration (FDA) approval to treat GAD, only two of them are SSRIs (paroxetine and escitalopram). The other two FDA-approved medications for GAD are venlafaxine and duloxetine, both of which are serotonin norepinephrine reuptake inhibitors (SNRIs). Another medication particularly helpful in the treatment of GAD is buspirone (which binds to serotonin and dopamine receptors). Beta blockers, particularly low dose propranolol, and the antihistamine hydroxyzine are also useful anxiolytic medications.
- **Psychotherapy:** The most effective psychotherapy modality used to treat GAD is cognitive behavioral therapy (CBT). Research has shown that CBT has a major effect on worrying and anxiety symptoms in general. Also, CBT has been shown to have longer lasting effects for those with GAD even after treatment has ended, preventing the relapse of symptoms in this chronic disease. Other forms of therapy used to treat GAD are applied relaxation, mindfulness, and psychodynamic psychotherapy.

---

The patient decides, along with her primary care doctor, to take escitalopram and find a therapist to do weekly CBT sessions. At the 4-week followup appointment with her doctor she reports that her worrying has decreased and that her sleep has improved significantly. She feels that the combination of the medication and the therapy are helping; however, she feels that she could benefit more from the medication. The escitalopram dose is then increased, and she continues with her weekly CBT sessions. She will continue to have close followup appointments to evaluate the effectiveness of the treatment until her symptoms resolve.

**BEYOND THE PEARLS:**

- Uncontrollable worrying about everyday concerns is one major characteristic of GAD. Other anxiety disorders usually have a specific trigger or specific issue that causes the worry.
- GAD is a chronic medical condition in which symptoms wax and wane. Therefore a patient may be doing well with treatment then symptoms may worsen. Patients should remain in active treatment until symptoms are completely resolved and daily functioning has improved to prediagnosis levels. This causes problems for some patients because it can take a long time to accomplish.
- Many health care providers do not adequately recognize the symptoms of GAD. This leads to a delay in treatment, which can worsen the prognosis of this chronic disease. One of the reasons for this delay in recognition is the fact that GAD is usually co-occurring with other psychiatric diagnoses, which may overshadow the symptoms of GAD.
- As with all anxiety disorders, benzodiazepines should be avoided. If they are used, they should be prescribed only for brief periods of time and never long term.
- As a general rule, patients with anxiety disorders may require higher doses of antidepressants to obtain remission of symptoms compared with those patients with major depressive disorder.
- The Hamilton Anxiety Rating Scale (HAM-A) is used in research to determine the effectiveness of treatment for anxiety symptoms. This scale also can be used in the office to track improvement in anxiety symptoms over time.
- Most patients with anxiety symptoms will present to their primary care doctor for treatment of physical symptoms. Referral to a psychiatrist should occur when there is poor response to treatment, an unusual presentation of symptoms, or a severe psychiatric comorbid illness (such as suicidal ideation or intent, a personality disorder, or a substance use disorder).

## References

American Psychiatric Association. (2013). *Diagnostic and statistical manual of mental disorders* (5th ed.). Washington, DC: Author.

Crits-Christoph, P., Newman, M., Rickels, K., Gallop, R., Gibbons, M., Hamilton, J., Ring-Kurtz, S., & Pastva, A. (2011). Combined medication and cognitive therapy for generalized anxiety disorder. *Journal of Anxiety Disorders, 25*(8), 1087–1094.

Cuijpers, P., Sijbrandij, M., Koole, S., Huibers, M., Berking, M., & Andersson, G. (2014). Psychological treatment of generalized anxiety disorder: A meta-analysis. *Clinical Psychology Review, 34*(2), 130–140.

Garfinkle, E., & Behar, E. (2012). Advances in psychotherapy for generalized anxiety disorder. *Current Psychiatry Reports, 14*(3), 203–210.

Hayes, J. (2011). Generalized anxiety disorder. *InnovAiT, 4*(12), 685–690.

Kumar, V., Abbas, A., Fausto, N., et al. (2010). *Robbins and Cotran pathologic basis of disease* (8th ed.). Philadelphia, PA: Saunders/Elsevier.

Locke, A., Kirst, N., & Shultz, C. (2015). Diagnosis and management of generalized anxiety disorder and panic disorder in adults. *American Family Physician, 91*(9), 617–624.

Patel, G, & Fancher, T. (2013). In the clinic: Generalized anxiety disorder. *Annals of Internal Medicine, 159*(11).

Sadock, B., & Sadock, V. (2015). *Kaplan and Sadock's synopsis of psychiatry: Behavioral sciences/clinical psychiatry* (10th ed.). Waltham, MA: Wolters Kluwer Health.

Satterfield, J. M., & Feldman, M. D. (2014). Anxiety. In M. D. Feldman, J. F. Christensen, & J. M. Satterfield (Eds.), *Behavioral medicine: A guide for clinical practice,* (4th ed.). New York, NY: McGraw-Hill.

Solomon, C., Stein, M., & Sareen, J. (2015). Generalized anxiety disorder. *New England Journal of Medicine, 373*(21), 2059–2068.

Van der Heiden, C., Methorst, G., Muris, P., & Van der Molen, H. (2011). Generalized anxiety disorder: Clinical presentation, diagnostic features, and guidelines for clinical practice. *Journal of Clinical Psychology, 67*(1), 58–73.

# CHAPTER 7

# Panic Disorder

Emily Sykes ■ Lawson Wulsin

A 28-year-old female presents to an outpatient psychiatry clinic with a 1-month history of anxiety attacks. She has a past history of major depressive disorder (MDD) and is taking a low dose serotonin norepinephrine reuptake inhibitor (SNRI). During the panic attacks she experiences severe anxiety with the following symptoms: lightheadedness, accelerated heart rate, chest pain, shortness of breath, and nausea. The symptoms last between 2 and 20 minutes. She cannot identify any triggers for the panic attacks. She has been worrying about when the next panic attack will occur, and the symptoms are affecting her ability to function. She was previously effectively treated with venlafaxine and until now had experienced infrequent panic attacks.

*What history is essential to obtain when you suspect panic attacks?*

To understand the history required for this assessment, we must first define panic attacks. A panic attack is a period of intense anxiety that begins suddenly and can last from several minutes to an hour. It can begin from an anxious or calm state, and the intensity quickly escalates within minutes to a cluster of at least four symptoms of sympathetic arousal. The most significant feature is extreme anxiety or fear, and patients usually cannot identify the cause or trigger. Panic attack symptoms can dissipate rapidly or gradually over 30 to 60 minutes. Panic attacks can occur in a variety of psychiatric and other medical conditions, not just panic disorder. Panic disorder is characterized by two main features. The first is recurrent, unexpected panic attacks. The second feature is 1 month or more of either worry about future attacks (or their consequences) or a significant maladaptive behavior change due to the attacks.

History should be elicited about the following:

- Onset of symptoms
- Panic attack features, duration, frequency, and severity
- Triggers for the panic attacks or if they occur unexpectedly
- Persistent worry about additional attacks or their consequences
- Avoidance behaviors or other behavioral changes as a result of the panic attacks
- How the symptoms are affecting the patient's daily life, including work and relationships
- Recent stressors
- Beliefs about the reason for the symptoms
- Previous periods of having panic attacks, the duration of these periods, and treatment
- Medication and substance use
- Coping skills used

Additionally, it is important to screen for medical illnesses that could be causing the panic attacks and to explore other psychiatric conditions that could be the cause (or that may be comorbid with panic disorder).

**Panic Attack Symptoms**
1. Palpitations, pounding or racing heart
2. Sweating
3. Trembling or shaking
4. Shortness of breath or feeling like you are being smothered
5. Choking sensation
6. Chest pain or discomfort
7. Nausea or abdominal distress
8. Dizziness, unsteady gait, lightheadedness or faint feeling
9. Chills or heat sensations
10. Paresthesia (numbness or tingling sensations)
11. Derealization (feeling like the surroundings are not real) or depersonalization (feeling detached from self)
12. Fear of losing control
13. Fear of dying

---

| BASIC SCIENCE/CLINICAL PEARL | STEP 1/2/3 |
|---|---|

Panic attacks can occur in a variety of psychiatric illnesses (in addition to panic disorder): posttraumatic stress disorder, social anxiety disorder, specific phobias, and substance use disorders. The distinguishing feature of panic disorder is that the panic attacks are recurrent, unexpected, and do not occur solely in the context of a trigger relating to another mental illness. For example, the diagnosis of a patient with arachnophobia who has panic attacks every time she sees a spider would be "specific phobia (animal type) with panic attacks."

---

*What questions should you ask to exclude other possible diagnoses?*

The differential diagnosis for panic disorder is broad and includes cardiovascular, pulmonary, neurologic, endocrine-related conditions, substance intoxication, and substance withdrawal. It is important to screen for cardiac symptoms as well as both personal and family cardiac history. Other considerations are in Table 7.1.

It is also helpful to ask about substance use. If you suspect that the patient is not being forthcoming, obtain a urine toxicology screen. More specifically, consider the use of cocaine, amphetamines, or hallucinogens. You should also consider substance withdrawal, particularly from alcohol, opioids, or sedative-hypnotics. Withdrawal from these substances can increase adrenergic

---

TABLE 7.1 ■ Medical Differential Diagnosis of Panic Disorder with Additional Symptoms

| Diagnosis | Additional Symptoms |
|---|---|
| Arrhythmia | Racing or irregular heartbeat, chest pain, shortness of breath, lightheadedness, syncope |
| Asthma | Respiratory symptoms triggered by cold air or exercise |
| Ménière's disease or vestibular migraine | Vertigo, tinnitus, lightheadedness, nausea, hearing loss, unsteadiness |
| Seizure disorder | Aura, alterations in consciousness, bowel or bladder dysfunction |
| Hyperthyroidism | Diaphoresis, palpitations, tachycardia, tremor, weight loss, heat intolerance |
| Pheochromocytoma | Episodes of headache, diaphoresis, hypertension |
| Hypoparathyroidism | Muscle cramps, paresthesia |
| Reactive hypoglycemia | Panic attack symptoms after a high carbohydrate meal, relieved by intake of sugar |

activity and lower the threshold for panic attacks. It is important to ask about current and past substance use (not only as a potential etiology for the panic attacks but also in treatment considerations, because benzodiazepines have a very high abuse potential).

In addition to panic disorder, you should also consider other psychiatric conditions in the differential. Panic attacks can occur in many different psychiatric illnesses. It is essential to elicit a full psychiatric review of systems to identify the primary psychiatric condition causing the panic attacks and to identify possible comorbid conditions. This includes screening for depression, mania/hypomania, psychosis, generalized anxiety, obsessive-compulsive symptoms, social anxiety, specific phobias, posttraumatic stress disorder symptoms, cognitive impairment, eating disorders, and attention-deficit hyperactivity disorder (ADHD) symptoms.

Common psychiatric conditions comorbid with panic disorder include major depressive disorder, generalized anxiety disorder, social anxiety disorder, ADHD, and posttraumatic stress disorder. Additionally, agoraphobia often coexists with panic disorder but is classified as a separate condition.

---

**BASIC SCIENCE/CLINICAL PEARL**                                                      **STEP 1/2/3**

Agoraphobia is significant fear or anxiety about situations in which escape might be difficult or help might not be available in the event of developing paniclike or incapacitating symptoms (such as fear of falling in the elderly). The symptoms are severe, lead to avoidance behaviors, require assistance from loved ones, or cause significant distress and fear. Possible situations include using public transportation, being in wide open spaces, or standing in line. Agoraphobia can be present with or without panic disorder, in addition to other psychiatric conditions.

---

**CLINICAL PEARL**                                                                        **STEP 3**

For the Step 3 Computer-Based Case Simulations, think about a diagnosis of panic disorder if a patient has recurrent trips to the emergency department with acute anxiety, chest pain, and shortness of breath. The examination should include a focused physical examination, electrocardiogram (ECG), complete blood count, chemistry panel, arterial blood gas, thyroid function tests, and urine toxicology. Also consider cardiac enzymes based on cardiac risk factor stratification and ECG findings; chest x-ray depending on symptoms and vitals; and pulmonary embolism workup based on symptoms, history, and examination findings. A negative medical workup is supportive of a panic attack, with the exception of possible tachycardia, tachypnea, or hypertension. There could also be respiratory alkalosis or nonspecific ST and T wave abnormalities due to hyperventilation.

---

The patient reports numerous stressors at home, including conflicts with her husband, having a 7-month-old son, and recently taking in a friend who is homeless. She was restarted on venlafaxine 75 mg daily 5 months ago for depressive symptoms that reemerged after giving birth to her son. The venlafaxine had been stopped during her pregnancy to reduce the risk of teratogenicity. Psychiatric review of systems is positive for depression and generalized anxiety. She does not have any medical history or symptoms that would suggest a medical cause for her panic attacks. She denies any history of alcohol use or substance use and toxicology screen was negative for illicit substances.

---

*What is the natural course and prognosis of panic disorder?*
The onset of panic disorder is usually in late adolescence or early adulthood; however, this can vary. For the most part, panic disorder is a chronic and relapsing condition. Few patients will achieve complete lifetime remission of their symptoms. However, many patients will have ongoing mild symptoms that do not significantly affect their lives. Factors predicting remission include good functioning before symptom onset, low initial frequency and severity of panic attacks, brief

duration of symptoms, resolution of stressors, and being female. Factors predicting a chronic course include comorbid major depressive disorder, agoraphobia, and personality disorders.

### What are the treatments for panic disorder?

Traditional treatment options for panic disorder include cognitive behavioral therapy (CBT), antidepressants, and anxiolytic medications. CBT is an evidence-based therapy for many psychiatric conditions. It focuses on identifying and changing maladaptive thoughts, feelings, and behaviors. The typical treatment course is 12 weeks, with sessions usually occurring once per week. For panic disorder, some elements of CBT are relaxation training, mindfulness training, cognitive restructuring (identifying anxiety-provoking thoughts and replacing them with calm ones) and exposure therapy (systematic exposure to anxiety-producing situations to decrease fear associated with these situations and to reduce avoidance behaviors). For panic disorder, the combination of an antidepressant and CBT has been found to be superior to either antidepressant treatment or CBT alone. However, based on patient preference, treatment availability, and symptom severity, one may start with a trial of an antidepressant or CBT. For patients with comorbid psychiatric conditions, suicidality, or severe symptom burden, combination therapy is recommended. Some patients with severe symptom burden may not be able to initially participate in CBT and may need to wait until they have some medication response before starting therapy (Fig. 7.1).

Several classes of antidepressants are effective in treating panic disorder. The selective serotonin reuptake inhibitors (SSRIs) that are U.S. Food and Drug Administration (FDA) for panic disorder are fluoxetine, paroxetine, and sertraline. The other SSRIs are also effective for treating panic disorder, although not FDA-approved. Common side effects of SSRIs include headaches, gastrointestinal distress, activation (e.g., insomnia, restlessness), and sexual dysfunction.

Another FDA-approved medication for panic disorder is venlafaxine, a serotonin-norepinephrine reuptake inhibitor (SNRI). In addition to having the possible SSRI side effects noted previously, SNRIs can also cause increased blood pressure.

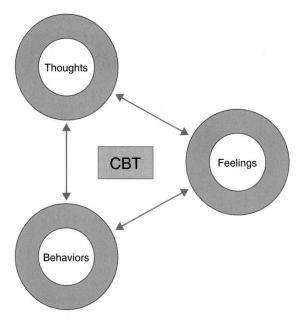

**Fig. 7.1** Cognitive behavioral therapy.

Mirtazapine, which has multiple mechanisms of action, has a small amount of evidence (in case reports and trials without a control group) for monotherapy or adjunctive treatment of panic disorder.

The tricyclic antidepressants (TCAs) imipramine and clomipramine have been found to be effective; however, they are used less often because of their side effect profile. TCAs block reuptake of norepinephrine and serotonin and also have activity at numerous different receptors (histaminergic, cholinergic, alpha-1 adrenergic, etc.), which accounts for their significant side effect profile. Although these medications are effective, TCAs have been largely replaced by SSRIs and SNRIs because of the TCAs' side effect profile and lethality in overdose.

Additionally, the irreversible monoamine oxidase inhibitors (MAOIs) phenelzine and tranylcypromine also are effective for treating panic disorder but are not commonly used because of dietary restrictions and potential side effects. These medications inhibit the activity of the enzyme monoamine oxidase (which metabolizes serotonin, norepinephrine, epinephrine, dopamine, tyramine, and other monoamines).

Patients with panic disorder may be sensitive to possible activating effects of antidepressants (e.g., insomnia, restlessness). For this reason, therapy should be initiated at low doses and titrated slowly. Once effective, the antidepressant should be continued for at least 8 to 12 months. If the medication is discontinued, it should be titrated off slowly because these patients may be more sensitive to discontinuation effects.

For patients with severely disabling symptoms, benzodiazepines may be used cautiously. FDA-approved benzodiazepines for the treatment of panic disorder include clonazepam and alprazolam. Longer acting benzodiazepines, such as clonazepam, are easier to taper off. Long-term use of a benzodiazepine is not recommended, and the medication should be titrated off as soon as possible.

Off-label alternatives to benzodiazepines include propranolol, prazosin, buspirone, gabapentin, hydroxyzine, low dose perphenazine, and low dose quetiapine. Propranolol has a quick onset of action, is well tolerated, and can be used up to three times per day. Low doses of this beta blocker greatly relieve the physiologic symptoms of anxiety (Fig. 7.2).

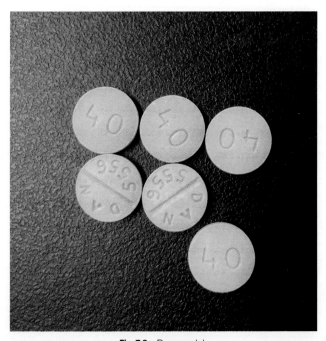

**Fig. 7.2** Propranolol.

| BASIC SCIENCE/CLINICAL PEARL | STEP 1/2/3 |
| --- | --- |

SSRIs act by blocking activity at the serotonin reuptake pump, which raises the availability of serotonin in circuits that regulate mood. This creates an immediate increase in somatodendritic serotonin levels; however, the full therapeutic effects of SSRIs (and other antidepressants) may take several weeks at the optimal dose. The delayed response is thought to be due to desensitization of somatodendritic serotonin autoreceptors to serotonin levels, thereby disinhibiting and "turning on" the serotonin neuron, leading to greater axonal serotonin release.

| BASIC SCIENCE/CLINICAL PEARL | STEP 1/2/3 |
| --- | --- |

If food or drink that is high in tyramine is ingested while monoamine metabolism is blocked by a monoamine oxidase inhibitor (MAOI), dangerous levels of tyramine can build up. This can lead to massive release of norepinephrine and epinephrine, which can precipitate a lethal hypertensive crisis. Food and drink high in tyramine content include dried, aged, smoked, fermented, spoiled, or improperly stored meat; aged cheeses; tap and unpasteurized beer; sauerkraut; and soy products. Additionally, sympathomimetic agents and serotonergic medications must be avoided with MAOIs because of the possibility of causing a hypertensive reaction or fatal serotonin syndrome.

---

For the patient's panic disorder comorbid with depression, her venlafaxine was increased to 150 mg daily, and she saw a psychologist for CBT and supportive therapy. In therapy, she worked on coping strategies for her anxiety, which included deep breathing, meditation, and communication strategies with her husband and houseguest. She responded well to combination pharmacologic treatment with CBT and had a significant reduction in her panic attack frequency and severity.

---

| BEYOND THE PEARLS: |
| --- |

- The pathogenesis for panic disorder is not yet known. The proposed neurobiological model suggests hyperexcitable areas in the fear circuit, namely the hypothalamus and amygdala.
- Panic disorder significantly affects a patient's quality of life and ability to function. Studies have demonstrated effects on social and occupational functioning comparable to that resulting from major depressive disorder.
- Panic disorder can increase the risk for both suicidal ideation and suicide attempts, even after controlling for comorbid psychiatric conditions.
- The Panic Disorder Severity Scale (PDSS) is a clinician-administered tool that is both valid and reliable for determining severity of illness and monitoring response to treatment. It assesses panic attack frequency, panic attack intensity, anticipatory anxiety related to panic attacks, avoidance of situations, avoidance of activities that may cause physical sensations similar to panic attacks, work impairment, and relationship impairment.

### References

American Psychiatric Association. (2013). *Diagnostic and statistical manual of mental disorders* (5th ed.). Washington, DC: Author.

Bakker, A., van Balkom, A. J., & Spinhoven, P. (2002). SSRIs vs. TCAs in the treatment of panic disorder: A meta-analysis. *Acta Psychiatrica Scandinavica, 106*(3), 163–167.

Batelaan, N. M., de Graaf, R., Penninx, B. W., van Balkom, A. J., Vollebergh, W. A., & Beekman, A. T. (2010). The 2-year prognosis of panic episodes in the general population. *Psychological Medicine, 40*(1), 147–157.

Furukawa, T. A., Watanabe, N., & Churchill, R. (2007). Combined psychotherapy plus antidepressants for panic disorder with or without agoraphobia. *Cochrane Database of Systematic Reviews, (1),* CD004364.

Goodwin, R. D., & Roy-Byrne, P. (2006). Panic and suicidal ideation and suicide attempts: Results from the National Comorbidity Survey. *Depression and Anxiety, 23*(3), 124–132.

Gorman, J. M., Kent, J. M., Sullivan, G. M., et al. (2000). Neuroanatomical hypothesis of panic disorder, revised. *American Journal of Psychiatry, 157*(4), 493–505.

Kessler, R. C., Chiu, W. T., Demler, O., & Coplan, J. D. (2005). Prevalence, severity, and comorbidity of twelve-month DSM-IV disorders in the National Comorbidity Survey Replication (NCS-R). *Archives of General Psychiatry, 62*(6), 617–627.

Roy-Byrne, P. P., & Cowley, D. S. (1994-1995). Course and outcome in panic disorder: A review of recent follow-up studies. *Anxiety, 1*(4), 151–160.

Sadock BJ, Sadock VA, Ruiz P. (2015). Panic disorder. In B. J. Sadock, V. A. Sadock, & P. Ruiz. *Kaplan & Sadock's synopsis of psychiatry: Behavioral sciences/clinical psychiatry* (11th ed.). Philadelphia, PA: Wolters Kluwer.

Sherbourne, C. D., Sullivan, G., Craske, M. G., Roy-Byrne, P., Golinelli, D., Rose, R. D., ... Stein, M. B. (2010). Functioning and disability levels in primary care out-patients with one or more anxiety disorder. *Psychological Medicine, 40*(12), 2059–2068.

Shear, M. K., Brown, T. A., Barlow, D. H., Money, R., Sholomskas, D. E., Woods, S. W., ... Papp, L. A. (1997). Multicenter collaborative panic disorder severity scale. *American Journal of Psychiatry, 154*, 1571–1575.

Stahl, S. M. (2013). *Stahl's essential psychopharmacology: Neuroscientific basis and practical applications* (4th ed.). Cambridge, UK: Cambridge University Press.

# CHAPTER 8

# Posttraumatic Stress Disorder vs Acute Stress Disorder

Sean Butterbaugh ■ Rebecca L. Tamas

A psychiatry consult has been requested on a 42-year-old white male who is recovering from a fractured left femur, pulmonary contusion, and mild concussion. His hospital course has been complicated by a deep vein thrombosis (DVT) in his right leg, and he is currently treated with heparin. The patient complains of poor sleep, recurrent nightmares, auditory hallucinations (hears son's voice), depressed mood, irritability, and feeling "on edge" with a heightened startle response.

*What is the first thing you would want to know about a patient presenting with sleep disturbance, nightmares, and an increased startle response?*

A patient presenting with these symptoms should be asked about a history of trauma, which could lead to a diagnosis of acute stress disorder (ASD) or posttraumatic stress disorder (PTSD). In addition, this patient should be evaluated for depression, psychotic disorders, and neurologic damage because these diagnoses also could present with sleep disturbances, increased startle responses, auditory hallucinations, and depressed mood.

*In suspecting PTSD, what is an important part of the history to determine?*

Asking about the timing of a trauma is important in differentiating between ASD and PTSD. ASD is diagnosed when symptoms occur between 3 days and 1 month after the exposure to trauma. PTSD is diagnosed when the exposure to trauma was more than 1 month before the onset of symptoms and the patient continues to experience symptoms.

*Diagnosing Trauma-Induced Stress Disorders*

The person is exposed to a traumatic actual or threatened death, serious injury, or a sexual assault. The trauma can be personally experienced or secondarily experienced (e.g., trauma happens to a close loved one, person witnesses it happening to another, or person is repeatedly exposed to traumatic stories or events). After the trauma there is a combination of symptoms that manifest. These symptoms tend to fall into one of the four categories shown in Table 8.1. A cluster of the symptoms discussed previously last for at least 3 to 30 days after the trauma exposure in ASD and persist for more than a month in PTSD. These symptoms interfere with the person's quality of life and are not due to other causes (e.g., alcohol use, traumatic brain injury).

TABLE 8.1 ■ Types of Symptoms in ASD and PTSD

| Intrusion Symptoms | Negative Symptoms | Avoidance Symptoms | Arousal Symptoms |
| --- | --- | --- | --- |
| Intrusive distressing memories | Inability to experience positive emotions | Avoiding thoughts associated with the trauma | Irritability and anger |
| Nightmares or bad dreams | Inability to remember things about the trauma | Avoiding feelings associated with the trauma | Self-destructive behavior |
| Flashbacks | Negative beliefs or expectations about self | Avoiding situations that are reminders of the trauma | Increased startle response (feeling on edge) |
| Psychological distress when exposed to reminders of trauma | Negative beliefs about life in general | Avoiding people associated with the trauma | Hypervigilance (extra aware, careful, and on guard) |
| Physiologic reactivity when exposed to reminders of trauma | Distorted thoughts leading to self-blame or blaming others | | Poor concentration |
| | No desire to do things | | Poor sleep |
| | Detachment from others | | |

*ASD,* Acute stress disorder; *PTSD,* posttraumatic stress disorder.

---

When asking the patient whether he has experienced any traumas, he informs you that his injuries were caused by a single-car motor vehicle accident that occurred 10 days ago. His 8-year-old son passed away from injuries sustained in the accident. The patient has never experienced any other traumatic event in his life. Although he does not remember the accident, he feels extreme guilt and anger over the death of his son.

---

*In consideration of this recent trauma and the symptoms this man is experiencing, what is the most likely diagnosis?*
This patient meets the criteria for ASD.

---

**CLINICAL PEARL**                                                              **STEP 1/2/3**

Alexithymia, the inability to identify or verbalize emotional states, is common in survivors of severe trauma.

---

*What therapy should be recommended to this patient?*
There is some evidence that early intervention with trauma-focused cognitive behavioral therapy (CBT) can prevent the development of PTSD. This therapy begins with psychoeducation of response to trauma and in anxiety management. Throughout the sessions, the patient is asked to reimagine the traumatic event, using particular skills and techniques. There is no strong evidence supporting the use of pharmacologic agents to prevent PTSD.

---

**CLINICAL PEARL**                                                              **STEP 1/2/3**

Increased activity and responsiveness of the autonomic nervous system occurs in some individuals with PTSD, specifically in the hippocampus and amygdala.

After being diagnosed with ASD and being educated on the risk of developing PTSD, the patient agrees to begin trauma-focused CBT after his discharge in the coming days.

### What are the first-line medical treatments for patients with PTSD?

First-line pharmacologic treatment for patients with PTSD are selective serotonin reuptake inhibitors (SSRIs), particularly paroxetine and sertraline. Both are U.S. Food and Drug Administration (FDA)–approved for acute treatment of PTSD, but only sertraline is approved for long-term treatment. PTSD symptoms generally show a slow response to SSRI therapy, and 6 to 12 weeks of treatment is recommended to determine full effectiveness of the medication.

Other antidepressant medications have shown some benefit as well. The serotonin norepinephrine reuptake inhibitors (SNRIs), particularly venlafaxine, have been shown to improve symptoms of PTSD (although hyperarousal did not show significant improvement).

Off-label use of atypical antipsychotics (such as quetiapine) also have been used, particularly if the patient is also experiencing psychotic symptoms (in this case, he had auditory hallucinations). These are usually used in combination with the SSRI or SNRI.

Tricyclic antidepressants (such as amitriptyline) also can be used to help with sleep, anxiety, depressive symptoms, and pain. These antidepressants should be used with caution in geriatric populations because of the anticholinergic effects that can lead to delirium.

Antiadrenergic agents (such as prazosin and propranolol) have been helpful in reducing hyperarousal symptoms and nightmares. These agents can be taken either as needed or as regularly scheduled medications.

Other antidepressants, such as mirtazapine and trazodone, can help with insomnia and sometimes provide additional anxiolytic and antidepressant effects.

Of note, benzodiazepines are contraindicated in the treatment of PTSD. Benzodiazepines have been shown to lead to a worsening of symptoms, cause worse psychotherapy outcomes, lead to more aggression and depression, and increase substance abuse.

---

**CLINICAL PEARL**                                                                **STEP 2/3**

Approximately 25% of PTSD cases are delayed-onset with symptoms presenting 6 months or longer after trauma exposure.

---

Following discharge, the patient underwent six sessions of trauma-focused CBT and no longer experiences the severe symptoms of auditory hallucinations, flashbacks, sleep disturbances, or startle response. He continues to see a therapist to cope with the passing of his son.

---

**BEYOND THE PEARLS:**

- There are many scales to diagnose and quantify the severity of PTSD, but a commonly used scale is the Clinician-Administered PTSD Scale for DSM-5 (CAPS-5).
- Patients presenting with a trauma history and possible PTSD also should be screened closely for substance use disorders because these are common among this population.
- 3,4-Methylenedioxymethamphetamine (MDMA) has shown some efficacy in phase 2 trials for treating PTSD, and phase 3 trials have begun for MDMA-assisted psychotherapy treatment.

## References

Alexander, W. (2012). Pharmacotherapy for post-traumatic stress disorder in combat veterans. *Pharmacy and Therapeutics, 37*(1), 32–38.

American Psychiatric Association. (2013) *Diagnostic and statistical manual of mental disorders,* (5th ed.) Washington, DC: Author.

Brady, K., Pearlstein, T., Asnis, G. M., Baker, D., Rothbaum, B., Sikes, C. R., & Farfal, G. M. (2000). Efficacy and safety of sertraline treatment of posttraumatic stress disorder: A randomized controlled trial. *Journal of the American Medical Association, 283*(14), 1837–1844.

Dass-Brailsford, P., & Myrick, A. C. (2010). Psychological trauma and substance abuse: The need for an integrated approach. *Trauma, Violence, & Abuse, 11*(4), 202–213.

Guina, J., Rossetter, S. R., DeRhodes, B. J., Nahhas, R. W., & Welton, R. S. (2015). Benzodiazepines for PTSD: A systematic review and meta-analysis. *Journal of Psychiatric Practice 21*(4), 281–303.

Marshall, R. D., Beebe, K. L., Oldham, M., & Zaninelli, R. (2001). Efficacy and safety of paroxetine treatment for chronic PTSD: A fixed-dose, placebo-controlled study. *American Journal of Psychiatry, 158*(12), 1982–1988.

Mithoefer, M. C., Mithoefer, A. T., Feduccia, A. A., Jerome, L., Wagner, M., Wymer, J., ... Doblin, R. (2018). 3,4-Methylenedioxymethamphetamine (MDMA)-assisted psychotherapy for post-traumatic stress disorder in military veterans, firefighters, and police officers: A randomised, double-blind, dose-response, phase 2 clinical trial. *Lancet Psychiatry, 5*(6), 486–497.

Weathers, F. W., Bovin, M. J., Lee, D. J., Sloan, D. M., Schnurr, P. P., Kaloupek, D. G., ... Marx, B. P. (2018). The Clinician-Administered PTSD Scale for DSM-5 (CAPS-5): Development and initial psychometric evaluation in military veterans. *Psychological Assessment, 30*(3), 383–395.

# CHAPTER 9

# Obsessive-Compulsive Disorder

Lauren H. Marasa

A 25-year-old female presents to the outpatient psychiatry office for emetophobia (a fear of vomiting). She reports her symptoms have been going on for "as long as I can remember." She describes that even thinking about vomiting will make her feel nauseated. She avoids food for days at a time to have an empty stomach to circumvent throwing up. She constantly washes her hands in an effort to avoid germs that could potentially lead to emesis from a gastrointestinal illness. She reports that these symptoms control her life.

***What would be the differential diagnosis based on the information you have?***
In this case the patient has a specific phobia, which she tells you in her chief complaint. However, more history is warranted for a complete diagnosis. For example, the patient mentions she will go days without eating (to have an empty stomach) to avoid any potential for emesis to occur. This would warrant further questioning into any history of an eating disorder. Furthermore, the patient has a known specific phobia. Specific phobias are frequently comorbid with other anxiety disorders, so this should be explored. Additionally, you would want to delve further into the patient's thoughts and behaviors revolving around her excessive handwashing to determine whether she also has obsessive-compulsive disorder (OCD). Lastly, OCD is quite impairing and affecting her quality of life, so you would want to assess for comorbid major depressive disorder.
**Differential Diagnosis:**
Obsessive-compulsive disorder
Generalized anxiety disorder
Specific phobia
Major depressive disorder
Eating disorders such as anorexia nervosa
Body dysmorphic disorder
Obsessive-compulsive personality disorder
Psychotic disorders
Tic disorder
Anxiety due to another medical condition
Substance-induced anxiety disorder

***If you suspect an underlying anxiety disorder, eating disorder, mood disorder, or obsessive-compulsive disorder, what initial history element is critical to obtain?***
The first priority is to assess the patient's safety. In particular, you should assess for suicidal thoughts. Anxiety and related disorders put patients at greater risk of self-harm than age-related controls without an underlying mental illness.

Individuals with a specific phobia are up to 60% more likely to attempt suicide than those without a specific phobia. Suicidal thoughts are reported to occur in up to half of individuals with OCD at some point in their lifetime. Up to one-fourth of patients with OCD report a suicide attempt, with comorbid major depression increasing that risk. Furthermore, individuals diagnosed with anorexia nervosa have an elevated rate of suicide. The mortality rate for anorexia is the highest, among any form of mental illness, due to the medical complications that accompany the suicide attempt.

---

Upon further evaluation of the patient, she endorses washing her hands constantly throughout the day (whenever she touches anything) to avoid any germs that may cause her to get sick. She will wash her hands three to four times an hour because she constantly worries about exposure to any pathogen. She points to her hands to show how red, dry, and cracked they are due to using the strongest antibacterial soap she can buy. She states that she will constantly clean her house due to her germophobic tendencies. The patient continues to state her parents are "clean freaks," but she feels her tendency to clean is even more excessive. She also sanitizes her cell phone throughout the day and places it in a UV light to decontaminate her phone at night. The patient states she "can't feign normalcy" and feels her thoughts are irrational, but she feels helpless in trying to control her compulsions. The patient feels her symptoms are affecting her relationship with her husband. She will not eat at restaurants if she cannot witness how the chefs prepare meat or how sanitary the kitchen is, which has limited her social interaction with friends. Furthermore, her husband wants to start a family; however, hearing many pregnant women experience some "morning sickness," she does not desire to ever get pregnant. When they have discussed the possibility of adopting a child, she points out that children bring home germs that parents catch, which causes further disagreements with her husband leading to feelings of guilt.

---

### What are additional considerations?
It can be helpful to delve further into why this fear has developed and to ask about childhood development. In addition, it is equally important to ask about a family history of mental illness, including OCD and other anxiety disorder symptoms.

| CLINICAL PEARL | STEP 1/2/3 |
| --- | --- |

The defense mechanisms of isolation and undoing are frequently described in obsessive-compulsive disorder (OCD). The isolation defense involves unconsciously disowning thoughts that are unwanted or intrusive—in other words, creating a separation between the unpleasant thought and other thoughts. The undoing defense relates to compulsions. Behaviors are performed to cancel out or undo the unwanted desire or behavior.

### What is the heritability of OCD?
The rate of OCD among first-degree relatives of adults with OCD is approximately two times that of age-matched controls without the disorder. However, if OCD is diagnosed in childhood or adolescence, the rate is 10-fold in their first-degree relatives. Genetic factors influence familial transmission with twin studies showing concordance rates of 57% in monozygotic twins and 22% in dizygotic twins.

Biologically, neuroimaging studies reveal increased perfusion and metabolism in the orbitofrontal cortex, anterior cingulate gyrus, caudate, and thalamus. There may be impaired inhibition in these areas of the brain, mediating strong emotional and autonomic responses.

This patient was given a diagnosis of obsessive-compulsive disorder. Upon further questioning, she remembers that when she was 7 years old, her sister got sick. This led to worrying that she, herself, would vomit, so she locked herself in her room and watched *Peter Pan* for days, thinking that it would somehow keep her from getting sick. Because she did not vomit, this led to magical thinking about controlling vomiting with rituals. She had two episodes of emesis in her entire life. One episode was from stomach acid causing her to gag, and since then she has avoided any foods, restaurants, and textures that remind her of that occasion. She feels the act of vomiting itself is not terrible; it is the lead-up to vomiting (the smell, the taste, the queasiness) that brings about intense anxiety and panic. This leads to washing her hands and watching *Peter Pan* for protection. Furthermore, she avoids alcohol because she associates those who consume alcohol as more likely to vomit after excessive use. She went a year eating only crackers to avoid feeling sick. Currently she denies symptoms of an eating disorder but remains very regimented in her diet. She eats a large variety of food but is consistent in what foods she does eat and when. If she eats too late at night, she associates the feeling of fullness with nausea. She denies any family history of anxiety or OCD, but her younger sister has a history of anorexia nervosa.

### How is OCD diagnosed?
A person reports having obsessions, compulsions, or both. The obsessions are recurrent and persistent thoughts, urges, impulses, or images. At some point these feel intrusive and unwanted by the person. Often the person will try to ignore the thoughts or actions. Sometimes he or she will try to counter the thoughts or behaviors with some other thought or behavior. Compulsions are repetitive behaviors or mental acts that a person feels compelled to do in response to an obsessive thought. These compulsive behaviors are performed to reduce anxiety and feelings of distress, are not always connected in a realistic way, and can sometimes be excessive. The symptoms of the disorder cause impairment in the person's life and are not due to any other cause or disorder. The diagnosis is further specified by how much insight the person has about the disorder.

### What are the percentage of symptoms seen in OCD?
Individuals with OCD have different obsessions and different compulsive behaviors. The graphs below (Figs. 9.1 and 9.2) show the most common obsessive and compulsive types in percentages.

### What are the treatment options?
OCD is best treated by a combination of psychotherapy and medication. For mild to moderate symptoms, one may choose to start with cognitive behavioral therapy (CBT) or a selective serotonin reuptake inhibitor (SSRI). Of the SSRIs, fluvoxamine is used almost exclusively for patients with OCD, although fluvoxamine generally is not chosen as a first-line therapy. In more severe or treatment resistant cases, you can treat with both CBT and an SSRI or tricyclic antidepressant (TCA). Of the TCAs, clomipramine has the greatest efficacy in the treatment of OCD. From a therapeutic perspective, CBT aims at identifying and correcting irrational beliefs.

---

**CLINICAL PEARL**                                                                 **STEP 2/3**

The use of exposure and response prevention, or ERP, involves exposing the patient to stimuli that triggers the obsession or compulsion until the anxiety subsides. It is one of the most effective therapeutic approaches for treating OCD.

---

SSRIs are shown to be moderately effective in decreasing symptom severity by 25% to 35% in approximately half of patients with OCD. Response is typically slow with medication, taking up to 16 weeks to achieve maximum benefit, and higher doses of medication are generally needed. If

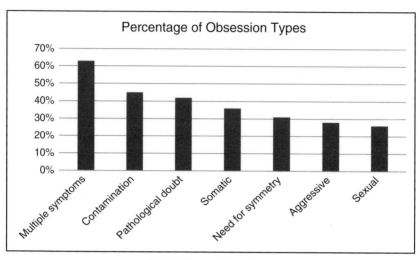

**Fig. 9.1**   Types of obsessions.

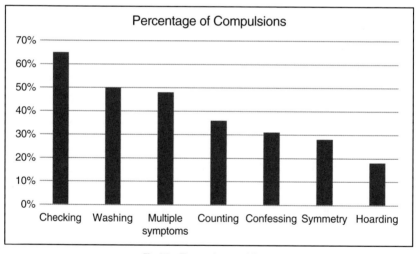

**Fig. 9.2**   Types of compulsions.

using clomipramine, you should be aware that this medication can be more lethal in overdose than SSRIs. You should caution the patient about the potential cardiac effects, seizure risks, weight gain, and anticholinergic side effects. Relapse rates are common with medication discontinuation; therefore the majority of patients need lifelong treatment. In severe, refractory cases, you may consider inpatient treatment involving intensive exposure therapy or electroconvulsive therapy (ECT). Although ECT is not as effective as psychosurgery, it is much less invasive. Lastly, you could consider referral to a neurosurgeon for deep brain stimulation (DBS) or an anterior cingulotomy; both have been shown to improve symptoms (by disrupting hyperactive neural networks) in up to half of patients.

She is maintained on fluoxetine for 3 months. On follow-up, she reports significant improvement in her symptoms. She has gone from washing her hands approximately 40 times a day down to 10 times a day. Her husband and friends have noticed an improvement. She now goes out to dinner without having a panic attack or obsessing over the fear of contamination. She reports that she has not used her phone sanitizer in over a month. In addition, she has not had a panic attack recently and reports feeling much calmer with a better quality of life.

### BEYOND THE PEARLS:

- The 12-month prevalence of OCD in the United States has been reported between 1.2% and 2.5% with approximately half of the cases reported as severe. Adult females are affected at a slightly higher rate than adult males. Males are more commonly affected in childhood. In the United States, the mean age of OCD onset is about 20 years, and one-fourth of cases start by age 14.
- Individuals with OCD commonly have comorbid psychopathology. Anxiety disorders are reported in up to three quarters of patients with OCD and mood disorders are reported in more than 60% of those with OCD. Furthermore, a comorbid tic disorder has been reported in many people with OCD. Some patients may turn to substance use, especially alcohol and sedatives, in an attempt to mediate symptoms. Others may become avoidant and isolative as a result of their symptoms.
- Given the potentially debilitating impairment from OCD, many patients remain symptomatic even when combining CBT with SSRIs or clomipramine. Therefore novel approaches are continuously being researched. Studies have shown efficacy using second-generation antipsychotics as augmenting agents, and others are investigating medications that target glutamate. A 2012 trial did not support the use of ketamine in the treatment of OCD, but a randomized trial in 2013 reported that half of patients responded to treatment with a single dose of ketamine. A study in 2016 supports the use of d-cycloserine, a partial agonist of the N-methyl-D-aspartate (NMDA) receptor, in combination with CBT to treat OCD.

### References

American Psychiatric Association. (2013). *Diagnostic and statistical manual of mental disorders* (5th ed.). Washington, DC: Author.

Burgy, M. (2005). Psychopathology of obsessive-compulsive disorder: A phenomenological approach. *Psychopathology, 38*, 291–300.

Comprehensive review of psychiatry (Initial Certification Edition). Westmont, IL: American Physician Institute, 2011.

De Silva, P., & Rachman, S. (2006). *Obsessive-compulsive disorder: The facts.* New York, NY: Oxford University Press.

Fineberg, N. A., Reghunandanan, S., Simpson, H. B., Phillips, K. A., Richter, M. A., Matthews, K., ... Accreditation Task Force of the Canadian Institute for Obsessive Compulsive Disorders. (2015). Obsessive-compulsive disorder (OCD): Practical strategies for pharmacological and somatic treatment in adults. *Psychiatry Research, 227*(1), 114–125.

Grant, J. E., Fineberg, N., van Ameringen, M., Cath, D., Visser, H., Carmi, L., ... van Balkom, A. J. (2016). New treatment models for compulsive disorders. *European Neuropsychopharmacology, 26*(5), 877–884.

Rodriguez, C. I., Kegeles, L. S., Levinson, A., Feng, T., Marcus, S. M., Vermes, D., ... Simpson, H. B. (2013). Randomized controlled crossover trial of ketamine in obsessive-compulsive disorder: Proof-of-concept. *Neuropsychopharmacology, 38*(12), 2475–2483.

Rodriguez T. Emerging treatments for obsessive-compulsive disorder. *Psychiatry Advisor.* Retrieved from https://www.psychiatryadvisor.com/home/topics/anxiety/emerging-treatments-for-obsessive-compulsive-disorder/

Sadock, B. J., & Sadock, V. A. (2007). *Kaplan and Sadock's synopsis of psychiatry* (10th ed.). Philadelphia, PA: Lippincott Williams & Wilkins.

Veale, D., Miles, S., Smallcombe, N., Ghezai, H., Goldacre, B., & Hodsoll, J. (2014). Atypical antipsychotic augmentation in SSRI treatment refractory obsessive-compulsive disorder: A systematic review and meta-analysis. *BMC Psychiatry, 14*, 317.

# CHAPTER 10

# Illness Anxiety Disorder/Somatic Symptom Disorder

Rebecca L. Tamas ■ Charlene McAndrews

A 35-year-old female with no known health problems presents to the emergency department and reports that over the past 5 months, she has been experiencing more and more dizziness. She went to an urgent care center 3 months ago complaining of dizziness and was discharged with no medication. She spends an hour or two daily searching the Internet for all of the serious illnesses that can lead to dizziness. A head computed tomography (CT) scan and electrocardiogram (ECG) are ordered; both return as normal. Despite these findings, she is certain there is something terribly wrong with her. She asks anxiously, "Are you sure it's not a cardiac sarcoma?" The patient shows no signs of intoxication and has no neurologic deficits. She appears visibly anxious and is noted to be diaphoretic and tremulous.

### What additional testing would you want to get?

Vital signs would help rule out a cardiopulmonary etiology. Other than a toxicology screen and pregnancy test, laboratory testing generally is not helpful for the purpose of diagnosing the problem. Radiographic testing usually will yield no helpful findings when working up dizziness in the absence of neurologic abnormalities (see Table 10.1).

She returns to the emergency room (ER) with a complaint of persistent, intermittent dizziness. Blood pressure, heart rate, and oxygen saturation are all in the normal range. The ER physician prescribes lorazepam, recommends she see a psychiatrist, and sends her home. She continues to be convinced that she has undiagnosed cardiac disease. She arrives at a psychiatry office for an initial assessment. A thorough psychiatric history is performed, and the following symptoms are described: poor sleep, middle-of-the-night awakenings with shortness of air, irritability, fatigue, low motivation, decreased concentration, and sad mood. She denies having flashbacks, nightmares, suicidal thoughts, paranoia, or hallucinations. Her primary concern is the intermittent dizziness. She explains that she is very concerned that there is something seriously wrong with her, and she is frustrated that the ER doctors could not figure out what's wrong with her heart.

### TABLE 10.1 ■ Types of Dizziness

| Type | Description | Percentage |
|---|---|---|
| Vertigo | False sense of motion, spinning sensation | 45%–54% |
| Disequilibrium | Off balance or wobbly | Up to 16% |
| Presyncope | Feeling one might lose consciousness or black out | Up to 14% |
| Lightheadedness | Vague description, feeling disconnected | Approximately 10% |

| CLINICAL PEARL | STEP 1/2/3 |
|---|---|

Lorazepam is available as an oral, intravenous, or intramuscular medication. It can cause anterograde amnesia and is therefore used as an anesthetic agent. It should not be used long term because of the development of tolerance, the possibility of withdrawal, and the effect on memory formation.

She has worried about having a serious health problem for many years and has worried about having a variety of serious illnesses. When she was put on birth control pills in her early 20s, she constantly worried about getting blood clots. This led to multiple visits to her primary care doctor. With her current dizziness, she is certain there is something wrong with her heart. Over the years, headaches have caused her to believe she has a brain tumor.

### What are somatoform disorders?

People with somatoform disorders are very anxious and preoccupied with physical symptoms. The main areas of concern are usually related to pain, gastrointestinal issues, and neurologic problems. The prior diagnoses of hypochondriasis, pain disorder, undifferentiated somatoform disorder, and somatization disorder were used for years to describe individuals who had excessive preoccupation with having a serious medical illness. There are now two new diagnoses that represent the prior somatoform disorders: somatic symptom disorder (SSD)and illness anxiety disorder (IAD).

### What is Illness Anxiety Disorder?

People with IAD have a preoccupation with having a serious disease or getting a serious disease. They have no identifiable medical problems other than perhaps mild physical symptoms. The worry is not specifically about a symptom but about what that symptom could mean. The anxiety is excessive and disabling. Reassurance with negative tests or normal medical findings does not help the anxiety go away. Even if the person has a medical illness (e.g., diabetes) the worrying is out of proportion to what would be expected. These individuals are quite sensitive to hearing about other people's physical problems and hearing news about epidemics and outbreaks. They seek out medical help or avoid medical settings all together, or fluctuate between the two. The perceived illness is not always the same; the person may think he or she has brain cancer 1 month, lupus the following month, and multiple sclerosis after that. The prevalence between males and females is similar.

### How is somatic symptom disorder different from illness anxiety disorder?

Somatic symptom disorder differs in that the person worries about particular symptoms rather than worrying about having an illness (Table 10.2).

TABLE 10.2 ■ Differences between IAD and SSD

| Illness Anxiety Disorder (IAD) | Somatic Symptom Disorder (SSD) |
|---|---|
| Excessive worry about having a terrible disease | One or more physical symptoms that are distressing (e.g., pain, fatigue, weakness) |
| High anxiety | High anxiety |
| >6 months duration | >6 months duration |
| Males = females prevalence | Females > males prevalence |
| Focus is on a specific illness | Focus is on symptoms |

The patient's family history reveals that her father was diagnosed with chronic myeloid leukemia when the patient was in the 10th grade. The father had multiple chemotherapy treatments that failed to put him in remission, and he declined a bone marrow transplant. After a long struggle, he finally achieved remission from a clinical trial when the patient was in college. She also reports having a distant relative who died prematurely of a myocardial infection at the age of 29. Despite never knowing the relative personally, she often thinks about the death.

**CLINICAL PEARL**                                                        **STEP 1/2/3**

It is very important to avoid excess testing and exploratory procedures. You may want to appease the person with negative test findings, but it should be remembered that the findings will not alleviate the anxiety. These tests increase health-related costs and can reinforce that there is something actually physically wrong (otherwise, why would a doctor order the tests?). Remember that the suffering is real, and the person is not acting or pretending. Such patients are often incredibly frustrated that the health care provider is not finding the illness they are convinced they have.

The patient is started on a selective serotonin reuptake inhibitor (SSRI) and titrated up to a therapeutic dose. At a 3-month follow-up appointment she reports that her symptoms have resolved, and she is no longer worrying about any health problems.

### What kind of prognosis does illness anxiety disorder have?

Approximately one-third of patients with IAD improve significantly. Good prognostic factors include a higher socioeconomic status, response to treatment of anxiety or depressive symptoms, and having no comorbid medical conditions and no comorbid personality disorder. Unfortunately, people with IAD are more likely to have a personality disorder than the general population.

### What would the differential diagnosis list include?

In addition to SSD there are other disorders that can appear similar to IAD: conversion disorder, body dysmorphic disorder, obsessive-compulsive disorder, generalized anxiety disorder, delusional disorder (somatic type), and factitious disorder. And there is a possibility the person may be malingering.

**CLINICAL PEARL**                                                        **STEP 2/3**

Individuals with conversion disorder (also known as *functional neurologic symptom disorder*) can sometimes show a lack of concern, known as *la belle indifférence*. For instance, despite explaining that they have suddenly gone blind, they seem calm and unaffected by the new condition. There is no strong evidence to use *la belle indifférence* to discriminate between conversion symptoms and organic disease. Conversion disorder is usually a loss of motor or sensory function without a medical cause.

**Body dysmorphic disorder (BDD)** involves a ruminative focus on a perceived flaw in appearance. This differs from IAD because the person has no concern about an underlying illness. Of note, BDD used to be considered a somatoform disorder but has more recently been moved to the Obsessive-Compulsive and Related Disorders section in the newest addition of the *Diagnostic and Statistical Manual of Mental Disorders*, Fifth Edition (DSM-5).

**Obsessive compulsive disorder** differs from IAD in that the intrusive thoughts and worries are not just focused on illness, and sometimes there are behavioral compulsions that accompany the obsessions.

**Generalized anxiety disorder** individuals have persistent anxiety that may include illness but also involves many other areas of their lives. These individuals tend to have excessive worry about a variety of things (e.g., doing something wrong, getting fired, forgetting something important).

**Delusional disorder, somatic type,** is also known as *delusional parasitosis* or *Ekbom's syndrome*. This disorder involves the belief that the person is infested with parasites or bugs without any evidence of infestation. People with this disorder usually seek care from primary care physicians or dermatologists.

**Factitious disorder** involves being deceptive about symptoms to receive internal gain or reward. The individual is cared for and nurtured, which is internally rewarding. Factitious disorder by proxy is diagnosed when the harm is perpetrated on someone else for the benefit of the perpetrator. In these cases, the caregiver gets praise and love for being there for the injured or sick patient.

---

**CLINICAL PEARL**                                                                     **STEP 2/3**

Factious disorder imposed on oneself is also known as *Munchausen syndrome*. When this involves one person harming another for internal gain, it is known as *Munchausen syndrome by proxy*.

---

**Malingering** is the intentional act of faking symptoms for the purpose of getting something external (e.g., getting disability, not having to go to school, etc.). Malingering is *not* a disorder because it is a willful act. One should be careful making this diagnosis too hastily. Proper evaluation for other causes should be done before jumping to a conclusion that someone is feigning symptoms.

*How would you treat this patient?*

Selective serotonin reuptake inhibitors (SSRIs), selective norepinephrine reuptake inhibitors (SNRIs), and tricyclic antidepressants (TCAs) can be helpful in ameliorating symptoms of anxiety and depression that accompany IAD. In addition, the beta blocker propranolol can help with anxiety symptoms experienced by these individuals. Mirtazapine might also be helpful for some people, particularly for those who have nausea or insomnia. Generally speaking, antipsychotics (dopamine antagonists) should be reserved for very severe cases that have not shown improvement with other medications. In addition to medication, cognitive behavioral therapy (CBT) and mindfulness-based therapy have been shown to be helpful. And usually a combined approach of medication with therapy will have better outcomes than just medication alone.

---

**BEYOND THE PEARLS:**

- Some studies have found that many people with IAD have comorbid personality disorders (common ones are: histrionic, paranoid, obsessive-compulsive, and avoidant personality disorders).
- People with a history of childhood abuse are more likely to have IAD (although not all patients with IAD have a history of abuse).
- SSD usually begins before age 30.
- A caring and patient primary care provider is very important. Realistic expectations should be established, and only appropriate referrals and testing should be performed. Education, reassurance, and a strong therapeutic alliance will lead to better outcomes.
- When referring to a mental health provider, do so in a manner that is compassionate rather than judgmental or dismissive. Imagine what you would feel like if you were convinced you had a serious medical illness and no one could figure out what was wrong with you.

## References

American Psychiatric Association. (2013). *Diagnostic and statistical manual of mental disorders* (5th ed.). Washington, DC: Author

Blitt, C. D. (1983). Clinical pharmacology of lorazepam. *Contemporary Anesthesia Practice, 7*, 135–145.

Kahn. D., & Xiong, G. (2018). Illness anxiety disorder (formerly hypochondriasis). In: D Bienenfeld (Ed.). *Medscape*. Retrieved from emedicine.medscape.com/article/290955

McManus, F., Surawy, C., Muse, K., Vazquez-Montes, M., & Williams, J. M. (2012). A randomized clinical trial of mindfulness-based cognitive therapy versus unrestricted services for health anxiety (hypochondriasis). *Journal of Consulting and Clinical Psychology, 80*(5), 817–828.

Newby, J. M., Hobbs, M. J., Mahoney, A. E. J., et al. (2017). DSM-5 illness anxiety disorder and somatic symptom disorder: Comorbidity, correlates, and overlap with DSM-IV hypochondriasis. *Journal of Psychosomatic Research, 101*, 31–37.

Olatunji, B. O., Kauffman, B. Y., Meltzer, S., Davis, M. L., Smits, J. A., & Powers, M. B. (2014). Cognitive-behavioral therapy for hypochondriasis/health anxiety: a meta-analysis of treatment outcome and moderators. *Behaviour Research and Therapy, 58*, 65–74.

Post, R. E., & Dickerson, L. M. (2010). Dizziness: A diagnostic approach. *American Family Physician, 82*(4), 361–368.

Stone, J., Smyth, R., Carson, A., Warlow, C., & Sharpe, M. (2006). La belle indifference in conversion symptoms and hysteria: systematic review. *British Journal of Psychiatry, 188*, 204–209.

# CHAPTER 11

# Delirium

Aarti Chawla Mittal ▓ Walter Klein

---

A 79-year-old male was admitted 1 day ago to the medical intensive care unit (ICU) for septic shock from a urinary tract infection. His past medical history includes hypertension, diabetes mellitus type 2, major neurocognitive disorder due to vascular dementia, generalized anxiety disorder, benign prostatic hyperplasia, and osteoarthritis of the knees. His hospital course includes placement of a central venous catheter into the right internal jugular vein and an arterial catheter in the right radial artery. The nurse reports that the patient seemed restless all night. Normally he is a kind, soft-spoken man, but this morning he seems agitated, is using foul language, and states that his brother (who passed away 4 years ago) visited him last night.

---

*What is your diagnosis for his change in mental status?*

Although it is easy to mix up the words *delirium* and *dementia* (major neurocognitive disorder), they are vastly different diseases. The acute period in which this patient had this mental status change is consistent with delirium. The American Psychiatric Association's *Diagnostic and Statistical Manual of Mental Disorders*, Fifth Edition (DSM-5) identifies five key features that characterize delirium:

1. A disturbance in attention and awareness.
2. The disturbance develops over a short period of time (hours to days), represents a change from baseline, and tends to fluctuate during the course of the day.
3. An additional disturbance in cognition (memory deficit, disorientation, language, visuospatial ability, or perception).
4. The disturbances are not better explained by another preexisting, evolving, or established neurocognitive disorder and do not occur in the context of a severely reduced level of arousal, such as coma.
5. There is evidence from the history, physical examination, or laboratory findings that the disturbance is caused by a medical condition, substance intoxication or withdrawal, or medication side effect.

---

**BASIC SCIENCE PEARL**                                                                      **STEP 1**

Delirium is an acute fluctuation in attention and awareness occurring with a disturbance of cognition. The neurotransmitter hypothesis postulates that reduced cholinergic function and excess release of dopamine, norepinephrine, and glutamate underlies the core behaviors of delirium. Decreased or increased serotonin and gamma-aminobutyric acid (GABA) activity may underlie different hypoactive and hyperactive subtypes.

---

**CLINICAL PEARL**                                                  **STEP 2/3**

A key clinical factor to distinguish delirium from major neurocognitive disorder (dementia) is time course: delirium is acute or subacute, whereas the latter condition is insidious and chronic.

---

Delirium can be subdivided into three types based on a patient's state of arousal: hypoactive (withdrawn, quiet), hyperactive (agitated, combative), and mixed (alternation between hypoactive and hyperactive delirium). The most common types are hypoactive delirium, and mixed type, which accounts for approximately 80% of cases.

Table 11.1 helps to differentiate delirium from dementia (major neurocognitive disorder).

### What is your differential diagnosis for the cause of delirium?

Many factors can contribute to the development of delirium. A handy mnemonic to remember for these causes is **ICU DELIRIUMS** (www.icudelirium.org).

**I**atrogenic exposures: consider any diagnostic procedure or therapeutic intervention that may have resulted in an adverse reaction that was not a natural consequence of the patient's illness

**C**ognitive Impairment: preexisting dementia (major neurocognitive disorder) or mild neurocognitive impairment (MCI) or depression

**U**se of restraints and catheters

**D**rugs: evaluate use of sedatives (i.e., benzodiazepines or opiates) and medications with anticholinergic activity, and consider abrupt cessation of smoking or alcohol and withdrawal from chronically used sedatives

**E**lderly: patients older than 65-years have the greatest risk

**L**aboratory abnormalities: especially hyponatremia, azotemia, hyperbilirubinemia, hypocalcemia, and metabolic acidosis

**I**nfection: sepsis and septic shock

**R**espiratory: consider respiratory failure, chronic obstructive pulmonary disease, acute respiratory distress syndrome, and pulmonary embolism

**I**ntracranial perfusion: consider presence of hypotension or hypertension, hemorrhagic or ischemic stroke, or tumor

---

**TABLE 11.1 ■ Differentiating Delirium from Dementia (Major Neurocognitive Disorder)**

|  | Delirium | Dementia (Major NCD) |
|---|---|---|
| Consciousness | Decreased or hyperalert "Clouded" | Alert |
| Course | Fluctuating | Steady slow decline |
| Onset | Acute or subacute | Chronic |
| Attention | Impaired | Usually normal |
| Psychomotor | Agitated or lethargic | Usually normal |
| Hallucinations | Perceptual disturbances May have hallucinations | Usually not present |
| Sleep–wake cycle | Abnormal | Usually normal |
| Speech | Slow, incoherent | Aphasic, anomic Difficulty finding words |

*NCD*, Neurocognitive disorder.
Adapted from: Saint Louis University Geriatrics Evaluation Mnemonics Screening Tools (SLU GEMS). Developed or compiled by: Faculty from Saint Louis University, Division of Geriatrics Medicine, and US Department of Veterans Affairs, Geriatric Research Education and Clinical Center (GRECC), St. Louis, Missouri.

Urinary/fecal retention

Myocardial: myocardial infarction, acute heart failure, arrhythmia

Sleep and sensory deprivation: consider alterations in sleep cycle or sleep disturbances, and consider the nonavailability of glasses (poor vision) or hearing aids (poor hearing)

Although the list of causes is long, the development of delirium is often multifactorial and will have causes from more than one category. In our patient, for example, he has a history of preexisting major neurocognitive disorder due to vascular dementia, is elderly, is in septic shock, and has had sleep disturbances that are all contributing to his delirium.

---

On physical examination, the patient has no focal neurologic deficits.

---

### Are there any other tests you would like to order to further your workup?

It would be prudent to ensure that there are no other metabolic abnormalities present. With a complete metabolic panel, the sodium, potassium, creatinine, and liver enzymes can be checked. Confirming normal thyroid function with a thyroid-stimulating hormone and free T4 would be warranted. An electrocardiogram would rule out any arrhythmia. A chest radiograph, repeat urinalysis, and blood culture may be considered to evaluate for a new infection. Luckily our patient does not have any focal neurologic deficits on examination, but if present, a computed tomography of the head would be warranted to evaluate for a stroke.

---

The patient's adult children come to visit him in the ICU. They ask you about the long-term effects of delirium.

---

### What are some of the negative short- and long-term consequences from developing delirium in the ICU?

In ICU patients, delirium is an important independent predictor of negative clinic outcomes, including increased mortality, hospital length of stay (LOS), cost of care, and long-term cognitive impairment.

---

His family asks you what medications the patient is currently receiving. They tell you that he normally takes diphenhydramine for sleep, hydroxyzine for anxiety, and opioids as needed for knee pain. They ask you whether these medications should be restarted while in the ICU.

---

### What steps should be taken to treat this patient's delirium in the acute setting?

Delirium treatment and prevention strategies can be categorized as pharmacologic, nonpharmacologic, and combined pharmacologic/nonpharmacologic.

### What are the pharmacologic strategies for treating delirium?

Although rigorous evidence is lacking, the use of antipsychotic medications (i.e., atypical antipsychotics and haloperidol) are endorsed by various international guidelines, and most critical care specialists use these medications in the treatment of delirium on an as-needed basis. Benzodiazepine use may be a risk factor for the development of delirium in adult ICU patients and, with few exceptions (i.e., acute alcohol withdrawal, status epilepticus), its use should be avoided. In mechanically ventilated patients at risk for developing delirium, dexmedetomidine infusions for sedation may be associated with a lower prevalence of delirium compared with benzodiazepine infusions. Additionally, use of anticholinergic and opioid medications should be limited due to their deliriogenic effects. As for this patient, it is best to not restart diphenhydramine, hydroxyzine, and opioids, as they may worsen his delirium.

---

**BASIC SCIENCE PEARL**                                                    **STEP 1**

Acetylcholine is biosynthesized from choline and acetyl-CoA, catalyzed by the enzyme choline acetyltransferase, and stored in vesicles at the ends of cholinergic neurons. The nucleus
basalis of Meynert is the major source of cholinergic innervation to the neocortex.

---

**CLINICAL PEARL**                                                        **STEP 2/3**

Oral haloperidol is preferred for targeting the symptoms of delirium; however, intravenous
(IV) haloperidol is often given due to convenient assess in delirious patients. It is important to
continuously monitor cardiac function with each IV dose, and goal is for QTc to be no greater
than 450 milliseconds. If greater than 500 milliseconds, then haloperidol should be discontinued.

---

### What about nonpharmacologic therapy?

An important nonpharmacologic intervention is to promote the patient's sleep. This is achieved
by optimizing the patient's environment, using strategies to control light and noise, clustering
patient care activities and decreasing stimuli at night. Early mobilization is the best-studied nonpharmacologic intervention for reducing the incidence and duration of delirium. Early and aggressive mobilization of ICU patients has been shown to be safe and, in addition to reducing rates
of delirium, has been shown to reduce cost of care and hospital LOS. Finally, if the patient uses a
corrective lens or hearing aid to assist with vision or hearing impairment, these devices should be
brought from home to facilitate interaction with hospital staff.

### What type of "protocols" should be put in place to control the patient's pain and agitation while simultaneously reducing the occurrence of delirium in the ICU?

As noted previously, iatrogenic (exposure to sedative and opioid medications) or environmental
(prolonged physical restraints or immobilization) may contribute to delirium in ICU patients. It
is therefore important to:

1. Frequently monitor pain, depth of sedation, and delirium using valid and reliable assessment tools. (A detailed discussion of the monitoring tools is beyond the scope of this
   text.)
2. Limit sedation and opioid infusions when possible (while still adequately controlling the
   patient's pain).
3. Limit restraints and mobilize patients when possible.

Patients should receive adequate and preemptive treatment for pain. For patients on mechanical ventilation and unable to provide a numeric pain score, validated scoring systems such
as the Critical-Care Pain Observation Tool (CPOT) and the Behavioral Pain Scale (BPS) can
be used.

Patients should receive sedation only if required (i.e., an "analgesia first" protocol). If patients
do require sedation, the sedatives should be minimized to allow patient responsiveness and awareness, which is are demonstrated by their ability to respond purposely to commands (i.e., a combination of any three of the following actions upon request: open eyes, maintain eye contact, squeeze
hand, stick out tongue, wiggle toes). Sedation should be monitored with a validated tool such as
the Richmond Agitation Sedation Scale (RASS) and also should be interrupted on a daily basis;
this daily interruption of sedation is termed a *spontaneous awakening trial* (SAT). If the patient is
mechanically ventilated, this should be done in combination with a spontaneous breathing trial
(SBT) to facilitate liberation from mechanical ventilation.

Delirium monitoring is achieved by routine assessment of the Confusion Assessment Method for the ICU (CAM-ICU) or the Intensive Care Delirium Screening Checklist (ICDSC). If delirium is detected, it is treated and prevented by the mechanisms previously discussed (including both pharmacologic and nonpharmacologic methods).

Finally, the patient's family should actively participate during ICU rounds. The patient's family is integral to the patient's recovery by providing the emotional support and cognitive stimulation necessary for the patient to recover from the critical illness. Family engagement is fostered and encouraged by a multidisciplinary approach to patient care. The team includes not only the physician, nurse, and respiratory therapist, but the rehabilitation specialists, pharmacists, social workers, and chaplains.

These interventions are combined in what is termed the *ABCDEF protocol* (Fig. 11.1), which has been shown to improve outcomes (including reducing the rate of delirium, ventilator days, and ICU LOS) in adult ICU patients.

### Assess, prevent & manage pain

- CPOT or BPS to assess pain, insure adequate pain control
- Use of regional anesthesia and nonopioid adjuncts
- Analgesia-based sedation techniques with fentanyl

### Both SAT & SBT

- Daily linked SAT and SBT
- Multidisciplinary coordination of care
- Faster liberation from MV

### Choice of sedation

- Targeted light sedation when sedation necessary
- Avoidance of benzodiazepines
- Dexmedetomidine if high delirium risk, cardiac surgery, MV weaning

### Delirium monitoring & management

- Routine CAM-ICU or ICDSC assessments
- Nonpharmacologic intervention, including sleep hygiene
- Dexmedetomidine or antipsychotic if hyperactive symptoms

### Early mobility & exercise

- Physical and occupational therapy assessment
- Coordinate activity with SAT or periods of no sedation
- Progress through range of motion, sitting, standing, walking, ADLs

### Family engagement & emprowerment

- Reorientation, provision of emotional and verbal support
- Cognitive stimulation, participation in mobilization
- Participation in multidisciplinary rounds

**Fig. 11.1  Intensive care unit delirium: A review of diagnosis, prevention, and treatment.** *ADLs,* Activities of daily living; *BPS,* Behavioral Pain Scale; *BPSCAM-ICU,* Confusion Assessment Method for the ICU; *CPOT,* Critical-Care Pain Observation Tool; *ICDSC,* Intensive Care Delirium Screening Checklist; *MV,* mechanical ventilation; *SAT,* spontaneous awakening trial; *SBT,* spontaneous breathing trial. The ABCDEF protocol for ICU delirium reduction. Hayhurst, C.J., Pandharipande, P.P., Hughes, C.G. (2016). Intensive care unit delirium: A review of diagnosis, prevention, and treatment. *Anesthesiology 125*(6), 1229–1241.

As a result of medically stabilizing the patient, treating his underlying urinary tract infection, targeting the symptoms of delirium with low-dose haloperidol, avoiding deliriogenic medications, and using nonpharmacologic therapies, his delirium slowly improves over the course of 3 days.

## BEYOND THE PEARLS:

- Delirium affects 70% to 80% of intensive care unit patients and is associated with a 10-fold increase in rates of cognitive impairment at discharge and a 3-fold increase in mortality rates.
- Always keep delirium on your differential when being consulted for evaluation of depression or psychosis, as hypoactive and hyperactive delirium, respectively, may clinically look like psychiatric illness.
- Generalized slowing on routine clinical electroencephalographic (EEG) strongly correlates with delirium and should trigger elevated concern for the prognosis of patients with altered mental status.
- The Anticholinergic Risk Scale (ARS) is a validated clinical tool that can measure anticholinergic burden and risk for developing delirium. In a study by Zimmerman et al (2014), increased anticholinergic burden measured by the ARS was associated with a 40% greater likelihood for delirium in palliative care inpatients.
- In some cases, catatonia can co-occur with delirium. This complicates the treatment approach, as benzodiazepines are the first line treatment for catatonia, while they are avoided in delirium. For this treatment dilemma, memantine or amantadine can be used for targeting catatonia.
- The American Geriatric Society publishes the, "AGS Beers Criteria." It lists medications that are potentially inappropriate for older adults. Many of these medications have the potential to precipitate delirium.

## References

Barr, J., Fraser, G. L., Puntillo, K., Ely, E. W., Gelinas, C., Dasta, J. F., ...American College of Critical Care Medicine. (2013). Clinical practice guidelines for the management of pain, agitation, and delirium in adult patients in the intensive care unit. *Critical Care Medicine, 41,* 263–306.

Ely, E. W. (2017). The ABCDEF bundle: Science and philosophy of how ICU liberation serves patients and families. *Critical Care Medicine, 45,* 321–330.

Hayhurst, C. J., Pandharipande, P. P., & Hughes, C. G. (2016). Intensive care unit delirium: A review of diagnosis, prevention, and treatment. *Anesthesiology, 125,* 1229–1241.

Pandharipande, P. P., Pun, B. T., Herr, D. L., Maze, M., Girard, T. D., Miller, R. R., ... Ely, E. W. (2007). Effect of sedation with dexmedetomidine vs lorazepam on acute brain dysfunction in mechanically ventilated patients: The MENDS randomized controlled trial. *Journal of the American Medical Association, 298,* 2644–2653.

Pandharipande, P. P., Girard, T. D., Jackson, J. C., Morandi, A., Thompson, J. L., Pun, B. T., ... BRAIN-ICU Study Investigators. (2013). Long-term cognitive impairment after critical illness. *New England Journal of Medicine, 369,* 1306–1316.

Zimmerman, K. M., Salow, M., Skarf, L. M., Kostas, T., Paquin, A., Simone, M. J., & Rudolph, J. (2014). Increasing anticholinergic burden and delirium in palliative care inpatients. *Palliative Medicine, 28*(4), 335–341.

# CHAPTER 12

# Mild Neurocognitive Disorder

William H. Zhu

A 63-year-old male presents to his primary care physician complaining of forgetfulness for the past year. He reports he could not recall the name of a local street in a recent conversation and has forgotten his clothes in the washing machine several times. His cooking has gotten worse because he sometimes forgets steps or performs them in the wrong order. He continues to live independently and manage his groceries, finances, and medical care, but has begun carrying numerous index cards on which he writes reminders to himself. His medical history includes osteoarthritis and hypertension. He takes no medications and smokes a quarter of a pack of cigarettes daily. On physical examination, blood pressure is 137/86 mm Hg. The remainder of his vital signs and physical examination is normal.

### What are some potential causes of forgetfulness?

Forgetfulness is a common manifestation of cognitive impairment. There are many potential causes of cognitive impairment in older patients. Table 12.1 presents a list of reversible and irreversible etiologies related to neurologic, psychiatric, and medical diagnoses that can manifest as cognitive impairment. Reversible causes such as medication effect are most common and should not be overlooked because they may be addressed easily to provide significant symptomatic improvement. Irreversible causes are less common and are generally more difficult to treat.

| CLINICAL PEARL | STEP 2/3 |
|---|---|
| Reversible causes of cognitive impairment are common in older patients. They include the effects of medications and substances, impaired sleep due to another illness, depression, vitamin $B_{12}$ deficiency, hypothyroidism, and abnormal electrolyte levels. Basic screening tests for patients who present with cognitive impairment should include a vitamin $B_{12}$ level and a thyroid-stimulating hormone level. | |

The patient immigrated to the United States as an adult and has been living alone ever since his wife died 10 years ago. He telephones his sister regularly but has few social contacts who speak his native language. His sister tells him that he seems more forgetful. The patient questions this because he can still easily recall details from their childhood.

TABLE 12.1 ■ Causes of Cognitive Impairment in the Elderly

| | | |
|---|---|---|
| **Reversible** | | |
| | Medication/substance effect | Anticholinergics<br>Benzodiazepines<br>Alcohol |
| | Sleep problems | Obstructive sleep apnea<br>Benign prostatic hypertrophy<br>Aging-related sleep changes |
| | Depression | "Pseudodementia," also known as *dementia syndrome of depression* |
| | Vitamin B$_{12}$ deficiency | |
| | Hypothyroidism | |
| | Other medical conditions | Normal pressure hydrocephalus<br>Autoimmune processes<br>Metabolic derangements |
| **Irreversible** | | |
| | Traumatic brain injury | |
| | Vascular disease | Cerebral infarction<br>Hypertension<br>Atherosclerosis<br>Diabetes |
| | Neurodegenerative disease | Alzheimer disease<br>Lewy body disease<br>Frontotemporal lobar degeneration<br>Parkinson disease<br>Huntington disease |
| | Korsakoff syndrome | |
| | Human immunodeficiency virus infection | |
| | Prion disease | |

---

**BASIC SCIENCE PEARL**                                                                 **STEP 1**

Patients presenting with memory loss may report preserved recall of remote memories, such as memories from childhood. This is because the hippocampus, which encodes new memories, is often affected early in the progression of a neurocognitive disorder (e.g., Alzheimer disease). Because older memories have already been encoded, the formation of new memories may be affected before much older memories.

---

### *What are some risk factors for cognitive impairment?*

Recent studies have identified all of the following as risk factors for cognitive decline:

- Age
- Genetics (family history, specific mutations)
- Cardiovascular disease
- Obesity
- Lifestyle (smoking, physical inactivity, low education, social isolation)

Based on the information provided about the patient thus far, we know that he has multiple risk factors for cognitive impairment, including increased age, hypertension, smoking, and social isolation.

On neurologic and psychiatric examination, the patient's cranial nerves are intact, and gross motor and sensory testing reveals no deficits. He exhibits no tremors or rigidity. He walks with a steady gait. The patient's mental status examination is normal, and he is oriented to person, place, and time. He screens negatively for depression.

### How do these findings guide your diagnosis?

The patient's neurologic and mental status findings help us rule in and out various etiologies of cognitive impairment that may be related to the diagnosis of a neurocognitive disorder. For example, his neurologic examination is grossly normal, with no tremors, rigidity, or deficits. This makes diseases associated with abnormal neurologic findings less likely, including Huntington disease, Parkinson disease, Lewy body disease, normal pressure hydrocephalus, and cerebral infarction (stroke). The patient's mental status examination is also grossly normal, and he screens negative for depression. This makes it less likely that a psychiatric disorder such as depression is causing his cognitive impairment.

| CLINICAL SCIENCE PEARL | STEP 2/3 |
|---|---|

Cognitive impairment also can be a manifestation of underlying psychiatric illness. When this is seen in older adults it may mimic the presentation of major neurocognitive disorder (dementia). Therefore this presentation of a psychiatric illness is sometimes called *pseudodementia*, also known as *dementia syndrome of depression*.

### How is cognition assessed in the clinical setting?

There are many instruments that clinicians can use to assess a patient's cognitive functioning, such as in screening for neurocognitive disorders (Table 12.2). Brief assessment tools commonly used by physicians include the Mini-Mental State Examination (MMSE), the Montreal Cognitive Assessment (MoCA), and the Mini-Cog. Formal neuropsychiatric testing also is available but is more time intensive and is usually performed by neuropsychologists. Among the commonly used instruments for cognitive assessment, the MoCA is thought to be more sensitive in detecting subtle cognitive impairment than the MMSE. The Mini-Cog may be more easily employed with patients who have less formal education or less familiarity with the English language.

The clinician performs a Mini-Cog cognitive assessment with the patient. The patient is able to repeat the words *banana*, *sunrise*, and *chair* to the clinician and acknowledge the instruction to remember them. When asked to draw a clock showing a time of "10 past 11," the patient draws a clock with the correct placement and order of numerals, and hands pointing to the 11 and the 2. It takes the patient less than 1 minute to draw the clock. When asked to recall the three words he was asked to remember earlier, the patient says "banana" and "chair" but cannot recall the remaining item.

TABLE 12.2 ■ **Selected Cognitive Assessment Instruments**

| *Brief* | |
|---|---|
| Mini-Mental State Examination | More limited evaluation of executive function |
| Montreal Cognitive Assessment | More sensitive in detecting milder cognitive deficits |
| Mini-Cog | Easier to use with patients with less education/English |
| *Extended* | |
| Neuropsychologic testing | More extensive training and time required to perform |

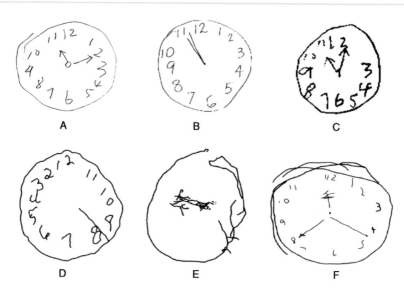

**Fig. 12.1** Clock drawing examples: (A) is normal, (B) through (F) are abnormal. (From Mini-Cog© Web site. https://mini-cog.com/mini-cog-instrument/scoring-the-mini-cog/ and http://mini-cog.com/wp-content/uploads/2018/05/Graphical-Mini-Cog-for-pocket-card-mar2018.pdf. Accessed July 27, 2019.

*How do you score and interpret the results of the patient's cognitive assessment?*

The patient scores 4 out of 5 total points on the Mini-Cog assessment. He correctly recalled two out of three words and drew a normal clock. One point is given for each word correctly recalled without cuing, and two points are given for drawing a normal clock.

Fig. 12.1 shows examples of clock drawing including a normal clock and various abnormal clocks. Any deviation from a normal clock is given zero points. A normal clock includes all numerals in the correct position and order, has hands pointing to the requested time, and is completed in less than 3 minutes.

A score of 3 or above on the Mini-Cog constitutes a negative screen. This makes a diagnosis of major neurocognitive disorder less likely but does not rule it out completely. It also does not rule out a less severe diagnosis of cognitive impairment such as mild neurocognitive disorder (see Fig. 12.1).

---

The patient is concerned that he missed one of the three items in the recall portion of the cognitive assessment. He fears that this may be a sign of a major neurocognitive disorder (dementia). He expresses worry because he had a friend who became severely disabled and passed away shortly after being diagnosed with dementia.

---

*Does the patient have major neurocognitive disorder (dementia)?*

To answer this question, it is important to first clarify the naming conventions for diagnoses of cognitive impairment. Different names have been used historically and in different fields to refer to clinically equivalent conditions. The *Diagnostic and Statistical Manual of Mental Disorders*, Fifth Edition (DSM-5), includes diagnoses of mild and major neurocognitive disorders. In some clinical settings and scientific literature, mild neurocognitive disorder may be referred to as *mild cognitive impairment*, and major neurocognitive disorder may be referred to as *dementia*.

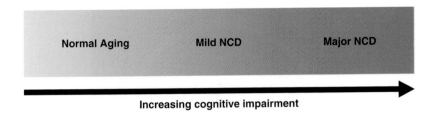

**NCD: neurocognitive disorder**

**Fig. 12.2**   Cognitive impairment exists on a spectrum.

Clinicians who assess cognitive impairment often are asked whether they think a patient has dementia. The diagnosis may carry a lot of meaning for patients and their families. The cognitive symptoms experienced by the patient may represent nonpathologic memory loss associated with normal aging, mild neurocognitive disorder, or major neurocognitive disorder (Fig. 12.2). To diagnose major neurocognitive disorder, a patient's presentation must meet several DSM-5 criteria. One key criterion is that symptoms must interfere with independent function in everyday activities. Because the patient is able to live and manage his affairs independently, he does not meet this criterion and therefore does not have major neurocognitive disorder. This also is supported by the patient's negative Mini-Cog screening for dementia. The patient should be counseled empathically regarding his concern and be reassured that he does not have dementia.

Laboratory tests are performed, including a complete blood cell count, a basic metabolic panel, a vitamin $B_{12}$ level, and a thyroid-stimulating hormone level. The results are all found to be within normal limits. A magnetic resonance imaging (MRI) scan of the patient's brain also is obtained (Fig. 12.3).

*How do you interpret the patient's laboratory tests?*
The patient's laboratory test results are all within normal limits. This makes it less likely for a reversible etiology of cognitive impairment to be causing the patient's symptoms (e.g., vitamin $B_{12}$ deficiency, hypothyroidism, metabolic derangements). Because the patient has a normal complete blood cell count, it is also less likely that an infectious etiology is causing his symptoms.

*How do you interpret the patient's imaging?*
The patient's MRI of the brain shows an axially oriented T2-weighted-fluid-attenuated inversion recovery sequence (*T2-FLAIR*). The cerebral contours within the skull show mild generalized cerebral atrophy. Additionally, there are seven small (<20 millimeters in diameter) white matter hyperintensities in different brain regions without a central focus. The overall pattern of these findings is consistent with mild changes in the brain associated with aging and vascular disease. The presence of white matter hyperintensities on this patient's MRI is not necessarily diagnostic, but their presence increases his risk for developing a major neurocognitive disorder due to vascular disease.

**BASIC SCIENCE PEARL**                                                         **STEP 1**

Different regions of the brain are correlated with different forms of memory. Working memory is linked to the prefrontal cortex. Declarative memory, comprising semantic memory (factual knowledge) and episodic memory (experienced events), relies mostly on the hippocampus, as well as the neocortex and amygdala. Nondeclarative memory, comprising procedural memory (physical skills) and associative memory (learned associations), is found in the cerebellum and basal ganglia.

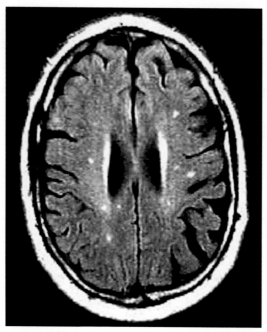

**Fig. 12.3**   Magnetic resonance imaging of the brain shows mild atrophy and multiple small white matter hyper-intensities. (From Inzitari, D., Pogessi, A., Carlucci, G., Barkhof, F., Chabriat, H., Erkinjuntti, T., ... Pantoni, L. (2009). Changes in white matter as determinant of global functional decline in older independent outpatients: three-year follow-up of LADIS (leukoaraiosis and disability) study cohort. *Br Med J 339*, b2477.)

### *What is the diagnosis?*

The patient's diagnosis can be elucidated by integrating the relevant history, examination findings, and test data presented thus far.

The patient is a 63-year-old man with a history of untreated hypertension and cigarette smoking who presents complaining of increased "forgetfulness" for the past year. He reports being forgetful at times, corroborated by a close contact, as well as having some executive and attentional impairment. He continues to live independently and to successfully manage his basic and instrumental activities of daily living, including medical care, groceries, and bills. Cognitive assessment shows a modest memory deficit. Basic laboratory tests, including a vitamin $B_{12}$ level and thyroid-stimulating hormone level, are normal. An MRI of his brain shows mild cerebral atrophy and white matter hyperintensities consistent with aging and vascular disease.

The patient's diagnosis is mild neurocognitive disorder due to vascular disease.

Mild neurocognitive disorder is a heterogeneous and clinical diagnosis that describes a syndrome in which patients exhibit "in-between" cognitive function. This diagnosis captures patients with cognitive impairment that is more severe than normal aging, with a noticeable decline from their prior baseline, but not yet severe enough to prevent independent function and meet criteria for major neurocognitive disorder (see Fig. 12.2). Table 12.3 presents a set of simplified diagnostic criteria for mild neuro cognitive disorder as adapted from DSM-5.

TABLE 12.3 ■ Simplified Diagnostic Criteria for Mild Neurocognitive Disorder (Adapted from DSM-5)

| | | |
|---|---|---|
| A) | Modest cognitive decline | As evaluated by the patient, a close contact, or a cognitive assessment |
| B) | Symptoms do not interfere with independence | The patient can manage all activities of daily living and more complex tasks, such as paying bills and managing medications |
| C) | Symptoms are not better explained by delirium | No acute fluctuations in mental status |
| D) | Symptoms are not better explained by another psychiatric diagnosis | For example, depression, bipolar disorder, schizophrenia |

DSM-5, *Diagnostic and Statistical Manual of Mental Disorders*, Fifth Edition

There are many etiologies that can lead to this clinical syndrome (see Table 12.1). This patient has multiple vascular risk factors, including untreated hypertension and cigarette smoking. His MRI shows potential signs of vascular disease affecting the brain. Therefore we can specify that his cognitive impairment diagnosis is likely due to vascular disease (Table 12.3).

---

**CLINICAL PEARL**                                                                 **STEP 2/3**

The diagnosis of mild neurocognitive disorder increases with age. Large studies estimate a prevalence of approximately 7% in individuals age 60 to 64. This rises rapidly to approximately 25% for individuals age 80 to 84. For those over age 70 the estimated incidence of mild neurocognitive disorder is 5% to 6% each year.

---

### *What treatment(s) do you recommend to the patient?*

Treatment for mild neurocognitive disorder is focused on preventing potential progression to major neurocognitive disorder and addressing any reversible factors contributing to the patient's cognitive impairment. There are no evidence-based specific treatments for mild neurocognitive disorder. Some studies have found aerobic exercise to have modest benefit on global cognitive ability. Cognitive interventions such as memory cues (like using index card reminders) can help improve functioning. Patients with mild neurocognitive disorder may even present a history of using similar compensatory strategies before receiving a formal diagnosis.

Medications such as anticholinesterase inhibitors are used in major neurocognitive disorder that is due to Alzheimer disease or dementia with Lewy bodies. However, these medications have not been consistently shown to provide symptomatic improvement in patients with mild neurocognitive disorder. Additionally, anticholinesterase inhibitors are not recommended because of the potential for medication-related side effects, and the risks seem to outweigh the benefits. With that said, the patient does have untreated vascular risk factors for further cognitive decline and progression to major neurocognitive disorder due to vascular dementia.

---

The patient's comorbid hypertension is treated, and he is educated on healthy lifestyle habits, including exercise and a balanced diet. He is also counseled on and prescribed smoking-cessation treatment. Six months later, re-administration of the Mini-Cog reveals a stable score. The patient continues to live independently and without impairment in his daily functioning.

**BEYOND THE PEARLS:**

- It is estimated that more than one-quarter of patients diagnosed with mild neurocognitive disorder may progress to major neurocognitive disorder within 5 years.
- Psychiatric symptoms are often associated with mild neurocognitive disorder and can include apathy, anxiety, and depressed mood.
- When mild neurocognitive disorders present with memory impairment, they are classified as "amnestic." There are also "nonamnestic" presentations with more predominant visuo-spatial, behavioral, or executive impairment symptoms.
- The most commonly identified causal etiology for diagnoses of neurocognitive disorders is Alzheimer disease. These patients may have inherited mutations in the genes *APOE4*, *PSEN1*, *PSEN2*, and *APP*.
- In addition to mild and major neurocognitive disorders, other diagnoses should be considered in patients with cognitive impairment. Delirium is an acquired form of cognitive impairment that usually presents with an acute and dramatic change in mental status. Nonacquired (congenital) forms of cognitive impairment usually present in childhood and include intellectual disability and specific learning disability.

## References

Petersen, R. C., Lopez, O., Armstrong, M. J., Getchius, T. S. D., Ganguli, M., Gloss, D., … Rae-Grant, A. (2018). Practice guideline update summary: Mild cognitive impairment: Report of the Guideline Development, Dissemination, and Implementation Subcommittee of the American Academy of Neurology. *Neurology, 90*(3), 126–135.

Smith, G. E., & Bondi, M. W. (2013). *Mild cognitive impairment and dementia: Definitions, diagnosis, and treatment.* New York, NY: Oxford University Press.

Steffens, D. C., Blazer, D. G., & Thakur, M. E. (2015). *The American Psychiatric Publishing textbook of geriatric psychiatry.* Arlington, VA: American Psychiatric Publishing.

Stokin, G. B., Krell-Roesch, J., Petersen, R. C., & Geda, Y. E. (2015). Mild neurocognitive disorder: An old wine in a new bottle. *Harvard Review of Psychiatry, 23*(5), 368–376.

# CHAPTER 13

# Major Neurocognitive Disorders: Alzheimer Disease, Vascular Dementia, and Frontotemporal Dementia

Kurtis S. Kaminishi

---

Mr. A is a 70-year-old male who presents to his outpatient primary care appointment with his daughter, who reports Mr. A's cognitive functioning has worsened over the past few months. Approximately 1 year ago Mr. A was seen by a geriatric psychiatrist, who diagnosed him with mild neurocognitive disorder, noting that he was functionally independent at the time. Mr. A is a retired accountant and lives a fairly comfortable but sedentary lifestyle. Recently his daughter noted that he required assistance with his finances. His past medical history is significant for hypertension, hyperlipidemia, peripheral vascular disease, and carotid artery stenosis, conditions for which he takes hydrochlorothiazide and atorvastatin. On physical examination, his blood pressure is 150/90 mm Hg, pulse rate is 90/min, respiration rate is 20/min, and oxygen saturation is 95% on room air. Generally his physical examination is unremarkable and within normal limits. Mr. A and his daughter are concerned about dementia or major neurocognitive disorder (NCD).

---

*What is the difference between mild NCD and major NCD?*

*Cognitive impairment* is a general term used to describe abnormalities in a patient's brain functioning. Cognition is typically measured by evaluating various "cognitive domains," such as memory, learning, executive functioning, orientation, language, social cognition, comprehension, calculation, judgment, visuospatial ability, and motor skills. Consciousness is not typically affected in NCDs compared with delirium.

Mild NCD, previously known as *mild cognitive impairment* (MCI), is characterized by modest impairment in one or more cognitive domains, preferably documented by neuropsychological testing or another quantified clinical assessment. Mild NCD *does not* present with problems with independence in everyday activities, but greater effort or compensatory strategies may be required. Additionally, cognitive deficits do not occur exclusively in the context of delirium and are not better explained by a major psychiatric disorder such as major depressive disorder or schizophrenia.

Major NCD, previously known as *dementia*, is characterized by impairment in one or more cognitive domains, preferably documented by neuropsychological testing or another quantified clinical assessment. Unlike mild NCD, major NCD *does* present with functional impairment and problems with independence and *does* require assistance with everyday activities; cognitive deficits do not occur exclusively in the context of delirium and are not better explained by a major psychiatric disorder such as major depressive disorder or schizophrenia (Table 13.1).

TABLE 13.1 ■ Comparison of Mild vs Major Neurocognitive Disorder

| Mild NCD | Major NCD |
|---|---|
| Modest cognitive impairment in at least one cognitive domain | Significant cognitive impairment in at least one cognitive domain |
| Retains functional independence with basic activities of daily living and instrumental activities of daily living | Requires assistance with basic activities of daily living and instrumental activities of daily living |
| Cognitive deficits do not occur exclusively in the context of delirium and are not better explained by an underlying psychiatric disorder (e.g., major depressive disorder, schizophrenia) | |

*NCD,* Neurocognitive disorder.

| CLINICAL PEARL | STEP 2/3 |
|---|---|

An acute change from baseline cognitive functionality is often key to confirming the diagnosis of delirium in patients with major or mild neurocognitive disorder (NCD); however, if acute worsening of cognition is accompanied by focal neurologic symptoms, cerebral vascular accidents or vascular dementia (VD) should also be considered in the differential diagnosis.

In both mild and major NCDs, it is also important to specify whether or not behavioral disturbances are present (psychotic symptoms, mood disturbances, agitation, apathy, wandering, or insomnia).

***What are activities of daily living (ADLs) and instrumental activities of daily living (IADLs)?***
Functionality is typically measured using the terms *basic ADLs* and *IADLs.* In mild NCD, patients retain functional independence without assistance, albeit they may engage in compensatory strategies or require more effort to complete tasks. Impairment in IADLs is detected at the transition from mild to major NCD, whereas impairment in basic ADLs is detected in the transition from mild to moderate or severe stage of major NCD. Examples of ADLs and IADLs are shown in Table 13.2.

***What are some causes of cognitive decline?***
The differential diagnosis for cognitive decline should include reversible and irreversible considerations. It is important to rule out modifiable risk factors and comorbid medical conditions before diagnosing a patient with major NCD. For instance, delirium, psychiatric disorders, and substance-related disorders may contribute to worsening cognitive functioning and may confound a diagnosis of major NCD. Table 13.3 outlines various differential diagnoses to consider when examining patients with worsening cognitive functioning.

TABLE 13.2 ■ Activities of Daily Living and Instrumental Activities of Daily Living

| ADLs | IADLs |
|---|---|
| Bathing | Food preparation |
| Eating | Finances |
| Ambulation/transferring | Shopping |
| Toileting | Telephone use |
| Hygiene | Medication management |
| Dressing | Driving/transportation |

*ADLs,* Activities of daily living; *IADLs,* instrumental activities of daily living.

TABLE 13.3 ■ **Differential Diagnoses of Cognitive Decline**

| Diagnostic Categories | Diagnoses |
|---|---|
| Neuropsychiatric and substance use disorders | Major depressive disorder/"pseudo dementia," also known as *dementia syndrome of depression* <br> Anxiety spectrum disorders <br> Schizophrenia <br> Insomnia (including sleep apnea disorders) <br> Bipolar Disorder <br> Posttraumatic stress disorder <br> Substance use disorders (prescription medications, alcohol, Wernicke-Korsakoff syndrome, chemotherapy agents, opiate analgesics, illicit drug use or withdrawal) |
| Neurocognitive disorders and encephalopathies | Delirium <br> Alzheimer disease <br> Lewy body disease <br> Parkinson disease <br> Huntington disease <br> Vascular dementia <br> Frontotemporal neurocognitive disorder (NCD) <br> Multiple sclerosis <br> Normal pressure hydrocephalus <br> Cerebral autosomal-dominant arteriopathy with subcortical infarcts and leukoencephalopathy <br> Seizure disorder |
| Infectious and inflammatory diseases | Herpes simplex <br> Urinary tract infections/other infections <br> Meningoencephalitis <br> Syphilis <br> Human immunodeficiency virus <br> Cerebral vasculitis <br> Temporal arteritis <br> Neurosarcoidosis |
| Immune diseases | Rheumatologic diseases <br> Systemic lupus erythematosus |
| Organic brain injuries | Traumatic brain injury <br> Chronic traumatic encephalopathy <br> Concussions <br> Cerebral vascular accidents |
| Tumors | Meningioma <br> Brain metastasis <br> Paraneoplastic syndrome <br> Cerebral tuberculoma |
| Metabolic disorders | Metabolic syndrome <br> Hyperthyroidism and hypothyroidism <br> Glucose metabolism disorders <br> Calcium metabolism disorders <br> Mitochondrial disease (e.g., mitochondrial encephalomyopathy with lactic acidosis and strokelike episodes) <br> Vitamin $B_{12}$, thiamine, and other nutritional deficiencies |

***Beyond meeting criteria for major NCD, what other information may be helpful to clarify the diagnosis?***
Diagnostic evaluation of major NCD requires a detailed history provided by the patient and a knowledgeable informant; a thorough physical examination including neurologic examination; and mental status examination preferably documenting standardized cognitive assessment screening scores, such as the Mini-Mental State Examination (MMSE), Montreal Cognitive

Assessment tool (MoCA), or formal neuropsychological testing batteries. Additional diagnostic investigations for major or mild NCD may include laboratory and radiologic studies along with genetic testing if a diagnosis is difficult to establish. A summary of potentially helpful diagnostic investigations is provided in Table 13.4.

---

Further history obtained from Mr. A's daughter reveals worsening agitation and apathy. She notes his cognitive symptoms appear to be slowly progressing but occasionally seem suddenly and markedly worse. Mr. A denies substance use and screens negative for depression using the Geriatric Depression Scale. He has a positive family history of a mother with Alzheimer disease. His physical and neurologic examinations are normal, except for elevated blood pressure on initial examination. Mental status examination reveals evidence of scanning speech, paraphasic errors, and difficulty with memory and recall, without fluctuations in consciousness or attention noted. All laboratory studies mentioned previously were obtained in addition to an electrocardiogram (ECG); all results are within normal limits and unremarkable.

---

### Once a diagnosis of major NCD is established, what are the characteristics of the four main etiologies of NCDs?

Although it is not necessary to establish a specific etiology when diagnosing major NCDs, it is important to be familiar with the most common types of NCDs to better counsel and educate patients and families about disease progression and prognosis, guide clinical management and treatment approaches, and develop future planning strategies. Characteristics of the main types of NCDs are outlined in Table 13.5.

---

Mr. A meets criteria for major NCD with behavioral disturbances because he displays functional impairment and requires assistance with his finances. His behavioral disturbances are agitation and apathy.

---

### What is the likely etiology underlying Mr. A's major NCD with behavioral disturbances?

Given the current history and unremarkable laboratory studies it is difficult to establish a clear working diagnosis or etiology underlying Mr. A's progressive cognitive decline beyond meeting criteria for major NCD. On one hand, his daughter notes a progressive slow decline in his cognitive functioning, which is suggestive of Alzheimer disease (AD), particularly given a positive family history of Mr. A's mother being diagnosed with AD. On the other hand, Mr. A's daughter also reports his cognition sometimes appears to be "suddenly worse," which is suggestive of a vascular dementia (VD) etiology or mixed AD/VD etiology, particularly given Mr. A's history of cardiovascular risk factors, including hypertension, hyperlipidemia, coronary artery disease, and peripheral vascular disease. Furthermore, the behavioral disturbances noted represent a change from his baseline. Frontotemporal dementia (FTD) should also be ruled out, because the management for FTD may differ compared with AD.

---

| BASIC SCIENCE PEARL | STEP 1 |
|---|---|

Alzheimer disease (AD) is the most common cause of mild and major NCD.

TABLE 13.4 ■ **Evaluation of Cognitive Impairment**

| Clinical history | Timing of initial symptoms |
|---|---|
| | Progression of disease |
| | Family history of NCDs |
| | Functional changes |
| | Behavioral changes |
| | Substance use |
| | Education history |
| | Premorbid baseline |
| Physical examination | Weight changes |
| | Blood pressure |
| | Dehydration |
| | Cardiovascular disease |
| | Cerebrovascular disease |
| | Metabolic illnesses |
| | Nutritional status |
| | Neurologic/gait symptoms |
| | Sensory impairments |
| Mental status examination | Screen for depression |
| | Cognitive functioning |
| | Suicide risk |
| | Psychosis |
| | Fluctuations in consciousness or attention, abnormal behaviors |
| | Abnormal speech |
| | Abnormal thought process |
| Laboratory studies | Complete blood panel |
| | Basic metabolic panel |
| | Thyroid-stimulating hormone |
| | Calcium |
| | Glucose |
| | Creatinine |
| | Vitamin $B_{12}$ and thiamine |
| | Homocysteine |
| | Liver function tests |
| | Urine toxicology |
| | Urinalysis |
| | Rapid plasma regain |
| | Human immunodeficiency virus |
| Electrocardiogram (optional) | Conduction abnormalities |
| | Arrhythmias |
| Radiologic studies (optional) | Magnetic resonance imaging |
| | Computed tomography (CT) |
| | Functional magnetic resonance imaging (MRI) |
| | Single positron emission computed tomography |
| | Positron emission tomography (PET) |
| | PET-Amyloid |
| | Pittsburgh compound B |
| Cerebral spinal fluid (optional) | Beta-amyloid levels |
| | Phosphorylated tau |
| Genetic testing (optional) | Apolipoprotein E epsilon4 allele (chromosome19) |
| | Amyloid precursor protein (chromosome 21) |
| | Presenilin1 (chromosome 14) |
| | Presenilin2 (chromosome 1) |
| | Microtubule-associated protein tau (MAPT) |
| | Progranulin |

*NCDs,* Neurocognitive disorders.

TABLE 13.5 ■ Etiologies and Characteristics of Neurocognitive Disorders

| NCD Type | Characteristics |
|---|---|
| Alzheimer disease | Progressive cognitive and functional decline<br>Early loss of insight (anosognosia)<br>Amnestic pattern typically observed<br>Cognitive domains commonly affected include memory, visuospatial, language, and executive functioning<br>Cortical and hippocampal atrophy on MRI<br>Older age of onset (often greater than 65 years old) |
| Lewy body disease | Parkinsonian neurologic changes<br>Cognitive impairment fluctuations<br>Visual hallucinations<br>Sleep disturbances<br>Autonomic changes<br>Antipsychotic sensitivity |
| Frontotemporal lobar degeneration | Focal atrophy in frontal/temporal lobes on MRI<br>Personality and behavior/language changes<br>Younger age of onset (often less than 65 years old)<br>Strong familial/genetic component |
| Vascular cognitive impairment | Stepwise progression often observed<br>Focal neurologic signs often observed<br>Often with comorbid hypertension, peripheral vascular disease, or atherosclerosis<br>Subcortical, ischemic changes often observed on MRI<br>Impairment in attention, processing speed, retrieval difficulties<br>Depression |

*NCD,* Neurocognitive disorder; *MRI,* magnetic resonance imaging.

---

**CLINICAL PEARL**                                                                              **STEP 2/3**

The onset of Alzheimer-type major NCD is typically over the age of 65, whereas the onset of frontotemporal major NCD is typically between ages 45 and 64.

---

**BASIC SCIENCE PEARL**                                                                          **STEP 1**

In AD, the spread of neurofibrillary tangle pathology in the brain correlates with synaptic and neuronal loss and cognitive decline. Accumulation of extracellular beta-amyloid plaques in the brain has also been implicated in the pathology of AD. Beta amyloid is derived from amyloid precursor protein.

---

**CLINICAL PEARL**                                                                              **STEP 2/3**

Frontotemporal dementia (FTD) should be considered when patients present with disinhibition or indifference/apathy in middle age; progressive unexplained aphasia; or neurocognitive impairment accompanied by vertical gaze palsy, falls, or motor neuron disease. FTD may be comorbid with amyotropic lateral sclerosis (ALS).

---

**CLINICAL PEARL**                                                                              **STEP 2/3**

FTD is the leading cause of NCDs in patients younger than 65 and presents with spontaneous and familial forms.

TABLE 13.6 ■ **Radiologic Findings in Neurocognitive Disorders**

| NCD Type | Radiologic Findings |
|---|---|
| Alzheimer disease | Generalized cortical atrophy<br>Hippocampal atrophy<br>Hippocampal hypometabolism |
| Frontotemporal lobar degeneration | Focal atrophy in frontal/temporal lobes<br>Hypoperfusion/hypometabolism in frontal/temporal lobes |
| Vascular dementia | Macro/microscopic cerebral infarcts<br>Subcortical ischemic changes<br>Periventricular white matter lesions |

*NCD,* Neurocognitive disorder.

*How might a brain magnetic resonance imaging (MRI) or head computed tomography (CT) help clarify the diagnosis or etiology underlying Mr. A's major NCD?*

Obtaining neuroimaging may help clarify the underlying etiology of a major NCD but is not required to meet criteria for major NCD. For instance, focal atrophy patterns differ between AD and FTD. Additionally, a brain MRI may help visualize cerebral infarcts, microvascular ischemic lesions, or other cerebrovascular abnormalities. Oftentimes, in addition to clarifying an NCD diagnosis, neuroimaging is helpful to rule out other causes of cognitive impairment, such as brain tumors, hemorrhages/hematomas, or inflammation. Radiologic patterns across various NCDs are outlined in Table 13.6.

---

**CLINICAL PEARL**                                                    **STEP 2/3**

Structural neuroimaging and lumbar puncture are not required to diagnose major NCD, although these procedures may be indicated in some cases to rule out other organic brain lesions that may confound a diagnosis of NCD, such as tumor, metastasis, encephalitis, etc.

---

Brain MRI reveals hippocampal atrophy with widespread cortical atrophy beyond that expected for normal aging. Additionally, multiple subcortical microvascular hyperintensities and patchy periventricular lesions are noted, which are suggestive of cerebrovascular disease. There is no evidence of disproportionate atrophy indicated in frontal or temporal lobes.

These neuroimaging findings are helpful in ruling out frontotemporal NCD and are most consistent with a diagnosis of mixed AD/VD etiology underlying his major NCD.

Given the consistent findings between Mr. A's structural imaging findings and his clinical history, there is no further indication for functional neuroimaging; functional neuroimaging may provide diagnostic clarification when structural neuroimaging does not reveal early atrophy patterns or significant findings.

---

**BASIC SCIENCE/CLINICAL PEARL**                                      **STEP 1/2/3**

Vascular dementia (VD) neuroimaging studies often show cerebral infarcts, white matter lesions, and microhemorrhages, which stem from arteriosclerotic changes, atherosclerosis, partial ischemia, and blood–brain barrier abnormalities. These changes are often multifactorial and due to the effects of aging, genetics, physiologic factors, metabolic factors, oxidative stress injury, and inflammatory factors.

---

**CLINICAL PEARL**                                                          **STEP 2/3**

In FTD, neuroimaging is most likely to be useful early in the disease course because the classic frontal lobe and temporal lobe focal atrophy pattern seen in the early stages of disease become more generalized at later stages of the disease, making the differentiation more difficult.

---

*What are nonpharmacologic management strategies for patients with major NCD?*
When a patient meets criteria for major NCD, it is important to provide the patient and caregivers with early education about the diagnosis or etiology of the patient's condition, prognosis, and treatment, and to schedule regular follow-up visits. It is important to evaluate whether it is safe for the patient to live at home, whether there are any new functional impairments, and whether the patient has additional needs for assistance. Clinicians should inform primary caregivers of the naturally progressive nature of neurodegenerative conditions; as cognitive and functional impairments progress, so too does the risk of behavioral disturbances in the patient and of caregiver responsibilities, thus increasing the risk of caregiver burnout. It is important to monitor caregivers for signs of depression, anxiety, or worsening medical conditions that may signal caregiver burnout, risking hospitalization or early institutionalization of their patient with major NCD. Future planning and education may help mitigate risk of caregiver burnout, reducing safety risks while improving patient and caregiver quality of life and health outcomes. Future planning strategies are outlined in Table 13.7.

---

**CLINICAL PEARL**                                                          **STEP 2/3**

AD typically follows a slowly progressive trajectory with median survival of 11.8 years after symptom onset and a cognitive decline of approximately 3 Mini-Mental State Examination (MMSE) points per year.

---

Mr. A and his daughter are provided information about major NCD due to AD/VD and are referred to a social worker for advanced care planning.

---

*What are pharmacologic treatment options available for major NCDs?*
It is important to be familiar with treatment options for patients with major NCD. In this case Mr. A has reported behavioral disturbances, which are commonly associated with major NCD and are the primary risk factor for caregiver burnout and early institutionalization. For AD,

---

TABLE 13.7 ■ Future Planning Strategies for Patients with Neurocognitive Disorders

| Advanced Care Planning | Examples |
|---|---|
| Legal | Advanced directives/code status |
| | Appointing a durable power of attorney (DPOA) |
| | Estate planning, living wills, trusts |
| Financial | Planning for costs of health care |
| | Home safety modifications |
| | In-home supportive services |
| | Adult day services/transportation |
| | Long-term care facility costs |
| Emergencies | Crisis planning |
| | Contact information of family, health care providers |
| | Local crisis line phone numbers |
| | Lists of diagnoses, medications, allergies |
| | List of triggers for agitation and helpful management strategies |

**TABLE 13.8 ■ Pharmacologic Considerations for Major Neurocognitive Disorders**

| Major NCD Type | Pharmacologic Considerations |
| --- | --- |
| Alzheimer disease | Cholinesterase inhibitors<br>Donepezil<br>Galantamine<br>Rivastigmine<br>Memantine |
| Frontotemporal lobar degeneration | Selective serotonin reuptake inhibitors<br>Trazodone<br>Antipsychotics<br>*Avoid cholinesterase inhibitors* |
| Vascular dementia | Antihypertensive medications<br>Antihyperglycemic medications<br>Antihyperlipidemic medications<br>Anticoagulation if atrial fibrillation is present |

*NCD,* Neurocognitive disorder.

cholinesterase inhibitors may modestly help mitigate symptoms of disease for mild-moderate severity; memantine is indicated for moderate-severe AD. However, it should be noted that currently there are no available treatments that modify the underlying pathophysiology of the disease. Regarding FTD, cholinesterase inhibitors are not recommended generally, as they may worsen agitation or disinhibition. Treatment strategies for VD typically target cardiovascular risk factors. Available treatment options for AD, FTD, and VD are outlined in the Table 13.8.

Mr. A demonstrates functional impairment with one IADL, consistent with a mild stage of major NCD. He was started and titrated on donepezil to 10 mg daily to slow progression of the disease. Additionally, he was instructed to follow-up with his primary care physician to optimize his elevated blood pressure of 150/90 mm Hg. At a follow-up visit, Mr. A and his daughter note that his agitation has diminished after meeting with the social worker, attending adult day health center activities, and starting donepezil. Both he and his daughter arranged for home safety modifications and addressed advanced care planning. Mr. A and his daughter note feeling more in control of his health, safety, and future living with major NCD.

**BEYOND THE PEARLS:**

- Magnetic resonance imaging (MRI) is more sensitive and accurate than a computed tomography (CT) scan for delineating cortical atrophy.
- Coronal MRI is the easiest way to detect temporal lobe atrophy or hippocampal atrophy.
- Positron emission tomography (PET) scans, such as fluorodeoxyglucose (FDG)-PET and amyloid PET, are not presently indicated in clinical practice but may be useful to help rule out causes of major or mild NCD.
- Memory and visuospatial functions are usually preserved in earlier stages of major FTD, in contrast to the clinical presentation in AD.
- There is significant overlap between AD and VD, which makes it challenging to establish accurate incidence and prevalence data for each form individually.
- When systemic medical conditions warrant starting delirium-provoking medications (e.g., opiate analgesics, anticholinergics, antihistaminergics, sedative hypnotics, corticosteroids, etc.), consider dosage tapering, switching, or discontinuing nonessential medications to reduce polypharmacy and risk of delirium.
- FTD is divided into two main subtypes: (1) behavioral variant and (2) primary progressive aphasias.

## References

American Psychiatric Association. (2013). *Diagnosis and statistical manual of mental disorders* (5th ed.). Washington, DC: Author.

Hachinski, V. C., Lassen, N. A., & Marshall, J. (1974). Multi-infarct dementia. A cause of mental deterioration in the elderly. *Lancet, 2*(7874), 207–210.

Hategan, A., Bourgeois, J. A., Hirsch, C. H., & Giroux, C. (2018). *Geriatric psychiatry—A case-based textbook* (pp. 369–466). Cham, Switzerland: Springer International Publishing.

Marshall, G. A., Amariglio, R. E., Sperling, R. A., & Rentz, D. M. (2012). Activities of daily living: Where do they fit in the diagnosis of Alzheimer's disease? *Neurodegenerative Disease Management, 2*(5), 483–491.

Mendez, M. F., Shapira, J. S., McMurtray, A., & Licht, E. (2007). Preliminary findings: Behavioral worsening on donepezil in patients with frontotemporal dementia. *American Journal of Geriatric Psychiatry, 15*(1), 84–87.

# CHAPTER 14

# Major Neurocognitive Disorder: Parkinson Disease vs Lewy Body Disease

Tammy Duong

A 59-year-old male presents to his primary care physician with complaint of bilateral hand tremor with insidious onset over the past year. He also has felt more unsteady on his feet. He tripped on the curb outside of his house three times in the last 6 months. His wife, who accompanies him, adds that he gets lost on his way to the local grocery store and has trouble reading the time on his wristwatch. He has a history of anxiety and hypertension, but both are well controlled. His medications include sertraline 100 mg daily and amlodipine 5 mg daily. His vital signs are blood pressure 127/83 mm Hg, pulse rate 78/min, respirations 16/min, and oxygen saturation 99% on room air. On neurologic examination, he has smooth vertical and horizontal bilateral eye saccades. On confrontation, he can see in all four quadrants. He has normal neck flexion and extension, and there is no evidence of apraxia. However, he has a stiff axial gait, increased muscle tone in his bilateral upper extremities, and a faint resting tremor worse in the right hand compared with his left hand. He is without evidence of myoclonus. His handwriting on his preclinic forms is also unusually small.

### What are causes of tremor?

There are various causes of tremor, summarized in Table 14.1. First, it is important to characterize the type of tremor. Generally, tremors can be categorized as action versus rest tremors. Action tremors occur when the patient engages in movement. Common action tremors include physiologic, essential, intention, and primary writing tremors. Physiologic tremors are triggered by increased sympathetic activity (i.e., anxiety, nicotine, caffeine, fatigue, and hypoglycemia). Many normal individuals can have physiologic tremors. **Essential tremors** are the most common type of action tremors. Up to 70% of patients with tremor have a family history of essential tremor. It usually affects the hands and arms but can also involve the head, trunk, or voice. The tremor worsens with goal-directed movements such as pointing or drinking a glass of water. **Intention tremors** also are common. They worsen over the course of the movement, whereas other action tremors remain constant, and further worsen as the hand approaches its target. Many action tremors worsen during hand-writing; however, if a tremor occurs exclusively during hand-writing then it is a primary writing tremor.

**Rest tremors** are apparent when the patient's extremity is resting against gravity and can abate during movement. These tremors tend to worsen in times of stress. Parkinson disease (PD) is a primary cause of rest tremors and is sometimes referred to as a *pill rolling tremor*. These tremors usually start as unilateral and progress to the other side as the disease progresses, or the tremor may start bilaterally but be worse on one side compared with the other.

Tremor is one feature of parkinsonian symptoms (Table 14.1).

**TABLE 14.1 ■ Differential Diagnosis of Tremor**

***Resting tremor***
- Idiopathic Parkinson disease

***Action tremor***
- Physiologic tremor
- Essential tremor
- Intention tremor

*What are parkinsonian symptoms?*

Parkinsonian symptoms or parkinsonism is a clinical syndrome that includes: (1) resting tremor, (2) muscle rigidity, and (3) bradykinesia. Slow movements can lead to other symptoms such as masked facies and reduced trunk and limb movements. Hand-writing can also become smaller than usual, which is called *micrographia*. Similarly a patient's voice can become quieter, which is called *hypophonia*. Other features include a shuffling gait, stooped posture, and postural instability, which can lead to falls.

This patient's symptoms of right-sided resting tremor, muscle rigidity, and micrographia can be classified as parkinsonism.

---

Two months ago the patient was prescribed olanzapine 2.5 mg at bedtime, because he told his wife he was seeing a brown cat with green eyes sitting on the couch. His wife grew concerned because they do not own a cat. He is unbothered by seeing the cat and thinks it is "cute." The medication was quickly stopped because his muscles felt more rigid and he was more confused shortly after starting it.

---

*How do you differentiate between medication-induced parkinsonism and neurodegenerative causes of parkinsonism?*

Antidopaminergic medications such as antipsychotics or metoclopramide can also induce parkinsonism. To distinguish between this etiology and neurodegenerative causes, in clinical practice antidopaminergic medications are stopped and symptoms are monitored for improvement. This is the most cost-effective and least invasive to the patient. In some cases it can take months for symptoms to resolve after the agent is stopped. In addition, there are certain situations in which it is not feasible to taper off the antidopaminergic agent.

In those cases, presynaptic dopamine transporter (DaT) imaging can be used as a diagnostic tool to differentiate neurodegenerative and nonneurodegenerative causes of parkinsonism. In neurodegenerative disease, there is a loss of dopaminergic projection from the substantia nigra to the striatum. This results in loss of DaT, which can be used as a surrogate for dopamine levels. In DaT imaging, radio-isotope is used to bind to presynaptic DaTs and is detected by either single-photon emission compute tomography (SPECT) or positron emission tomography (PET). This can be useful in early disease before other distinguishing clinical features emerge (Fig. 14.1).

| BASIC SCIENCE PEARL | STEP 1 |
|---|---|

Motor symptoms in Parkinson disease are implicated by a loss of dopaminergic neurons in the substantia nigra, which is in the basal ganglia of the midbrain. These structures are responsible for movement initiation.

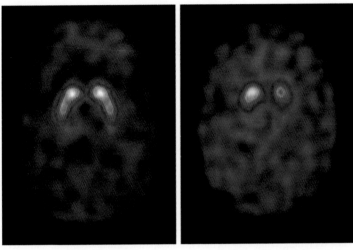

*DaTscan Normal*                    *DaTscan Abnormal*

**Fig. 14.1**  A normal DaT scan on the left and a positive DaT scan for neurodegenerative parkinsonism on the right.

---

| **CLINICAL PEARL** | **STEP 2/3** |
| --- | --- |

Dopamine transporter (DaT) imaging is the most useful when there is question of differentiating parkinsonian symptoms from nondegenerative (medications, essential tremor) and from degenerative causes (Parkinson disease). It may be difficult to delineate these etiologies in early disease before other symptoms appear.

---

The patient's muscle rigidity improves within a few weeks after stopping olanzapine. At this time, a DaT scan is deferred because he is not taking an antipsychotic.

| **CLINICAL PEARL** | **STEP 1/2/3** |
| --- | --- |

Extrapyramidal side effects (dystonia, muscle rigidity, akathisia, and tardive dyskinesia) from antipsychotics can sometimes continue for weeks and up to months after stopping the medication.

---

The patient's wife mentions that she has taken over the responsibilities of driving and buying groceries because the patient has been getting lost on his way to the neighborhood supermarket. A bedside cognitive screening test is administered. The patient scores 25/30 on the Montreal Cognitive Assessment (MoCA) test. Points are deducted from his score for his cube drawing, clock drawing, and delayed recall (Fig. 14.2). He is referred for a full battery of neuropsychological testing to assess cognitive and daily functioning. The report confirms below-average performance on tests of executive functioning and visuospatial abilities. His memory is slightly below average for his age.

---

*What are cognitive screening tests?*
Cognitive screening tests are standardized bedside tools that can help clinicians look for cursory cognitive deficits in patients. There are a variety of screening tests available, including the

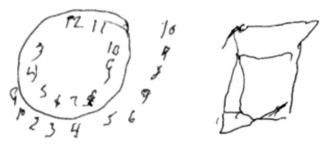

**Fig. 14.2**   Patient's clock drawing (left) and cube copy (right) on Montreal Cognitive Assessment Test.

MoCA, Mini-Mental Status Examination (MMSE), Saint Louis University Mental Status Examination (SLUMS), and the Mini-Cog. It can take just a few minutes or up to 15 minutes to administer a test in clinic or at the bedside. These tools have standardized instructions so that those unfamiliar with the tests can easily administer them. Each of these challenge various cognitive domains, including language, memory, visuospatial skills, attention, and executive functioning (planning, doing tasks in sequence, set shifting, inhibition). The MoCA, MMSE, and SLUMS are scored out of 30 points; however, the scores on these examinations are not equivalent to each other. This is because each one tests the cognitive domains differently. For example, the MMSE tests more heavily on language and relatively little executive functioning or visual spatial skills. In contrast, the MoCA is more sensitive to executive function deficits. Patients with high educational backgrounds may score higher than their counterparts with lower total education. In addition, these tests were validated in native English speakers, but the MoCA is available in a variety of languages. It is important to remember that these tests are for screening purposes, and for more in-depth information about cognitive deficits, patients should be referred to neuropsychological testing.

---

A basic metabolic panel reveals no electrolyte or renal abnormalities. Comprehensive blood counts show normal white blood cell counts and no evidence of anemia. Thyroid function tests and vitamin $B_{12}$ levels are normal. Rapid plasma reagin and human immunodeficiency virus antibody tests are negative.

---

### What is your differential diagnosis?

There are two different but equally valid ways to approach this case—either by creating a differential for cognitive impairment and then for parkinsonism, or vice versa. For this case, first consider the differential diagnosis for cognitive impairment.

It is important to establish whether this patient has a mild neurocognitive disorder (NCD, formerly known as *mild cognitive impairment* or *MCI*) or a major NCD (formerly known as *dementia*). In both mild and major NCD there must be a clinical history of worsening cognition and deficits in one or more cognitive domains (memory, language, visual spatial abilities, executive functioning, attention, learning, comprehension, calculation, orientation, or motor functioning) confirmed by neuropsychological testing. The difference between mild and major NCD is determined by a loss of functioning within a person's daily living; that is, for mild NCD there typically is no loss in daily functioning, whereas patients with major NCD begin to experience a gradual loss of their ability to function independently. Activities of daily living are divided into two categories: instrumental activities of daily living (IADLs) and basic activities of daily living (ADLs). IADLs consist of activities that are required for typical adult functioning,

TABLE 14.2 ■ **Differential Diagnosis of Parkinsonism**

Idiopathic Parkinson disease
Dementia with Lewy bodies
Medication-induced parkinsonism
• Antipsychotics
• Metoclopramide
• Prochlorperazine
• Reserpine
Parkinson-plus syndromes
• Multiple system atrophy
• Progressive supranuclear palsy
• Corticobasal degeneration

including paying bills, grocery shopping, cooking, cleaning, driving, and doing laundry. ADLs are basic necessities, including feeding, grooming, bathing, toileting, and transferring from one position to another.

This patient has a clinical history of worsening cognition in terms of becoming lost and having difficulty reading his wristwatch. These are both within visual spatial cognitive domain. Deficits in this domain are confirmed on formal neuropsychological testing along with other deficits in executive functioning and mild memory impairments. As he is yielding some of his IADLs to his wife (driving and finances), this patient also demonstrates a loss of functioning. As such, he qualifies for a diagnosis of major NCD.

Next, consider the various etiologies of major NCD. There are many contributors to cognitive decline, including nonneurodegenerative causes (psychiatric, infectious, tumors, vitamin deficiencies, metabolic and endocrine abnormalities) and neurodegenerative causes (Alzheimer disease, vascular disease sequelae, frontotemporal dementia, dementia with Lewy bodies [DLB], and PD dementia). This patient's laboratory results are normal, which points away from a nonneurodegenerative etiology.

Then, consider that this patient's other signs and symptoms are consistent with parkinsonism including tremor, postural instability, unsteady gait, increased muscle tone, and micrographia. The most common etiology is idiopathic PD; however, there are multiple other causes. These can be divided into neurodegenerative causes (PD, Parkinson plus syndromes, and DLB) and nonneurodegenerative causes (i.e., antidopaminergic medications). Medication-induced parkinsonism is less likely in this patient because he has not been taking antipsychotics for several months.

Alzheimer disease, vascular dementia, and frontotemporal dementia do not present with parkinsonism and may be ruled out of the differential diagnosis.

Parkinson plus syndromes are disease states that have parkinsonism as a main feature but have differing pathologies and other distinctive symptoms. They are less common than PD or DLB. Summary of Parkinson plus syndromes are listed in Table 14.2.

This patient does not have evidence of autonomic instability, impaired vertical or horizontal saccades, or hemineglect. Without these distinctive features, the diagnosis of a Parkinson plus syndrome is less likely. This narrows the differential diagnosis to PD or DLB.

### What is the diagnostic criteria for DLB?

DLB symptoms are categorized into core and suggestive diagnostic features. The core features include: (1) fluctuating cognition with variations in attention and alertness, (2) well-formed visual hallucinations, and (3) cognitive impairment that occurs before parkinsonian symptoms or 1 year from its onset. The suggestive features are: (1) rapid eye movement sleep behavior disorder (RBD)

**TABLE 14.3** ■ **Signs and Symptoms of Dementia with Lewy Body**

| Core clinical features | |
|---|---|
| | Fluctuating cognition |
| | Recurrent, well-formed visual hallucinations |
| | Parkinsonism |
| **Supportive clinical features** | |
| | REM sleep behavior disorder |
| | Severe sensitivity to antipsychotic agents |
| | Postural instability |
| | Hyposmia or anosmia |

*REM,* Rapid eye movement.

and (2) neuroleptic sensitivity. For a diagnosis of DLB, a patient must have at least two core features or one core feature plus one or more suggestive features (Table 14.3).

This patient exhibits two core features of DLB (visual hallucinations and cognitive decline at the same time of parkinsonism) and the suggestive feature of neuroleptic sensitivity.

---

The diagnosis is major NCD due to DLB.

---

DLB is the third most common cause of major NCD after Alzheimer disease and vascular dementia. Worldwide, approximately 1% to 2% of individuals over age 65 have the diagnosis of DLB.

The terminology for DLB may seem confusing initially. The term *dementia with Lewy bodies* denotes the clinical syndrome, whereas *Lewy body disease* denotes the underlying neuropathological findings. Hence, Lewy body *disease* causes DLB (Fig. 14.3).

**BASIC SCIENCE PEARL**                                                                          **STEP 1**

Lewy bodies are eosinophilic inclusion bodies inside of neurons. They are composed of α-synuclein proteins and are a pathologic feature in both dementia with Lewy bodies and Parkinson disease. As such, they are categorized as "α-synucleinopathies."

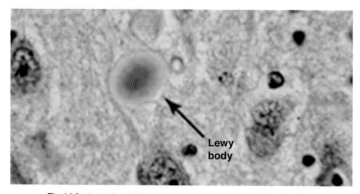

**Fig. 14.3**   Lewy body in patient with dementia with Lewy bodies.

It is common for patients with DLB to complain of fluctuating cognition. Patients describe the sensation as feeling more confused, mental fogginess, "out of it," or "in a daze" on certain days compared with other days. When visual hallucinations occur they tend to be detailed and of people or animals. Some patients are not distressed by these hallucinations (e.g., seeing animals in the house) because they are relatively benign, but other patients may find them very upsetting. Patients sometimes describe seeing family members coming out of ceilings or walls, which causes distress.

| BASIC SCIENCE PEARL | STEP 1 |
|---|---|

Fluctuations in dementia with Lewy bodies are thought to be due to a cholinergic imbalance and thalamic damage.

The cognitive impairment in patients with DLB occurs before or at the same time as the parkinsonian symptoms, which is a distinguishing feature from PD. The typically affected cognitive domains are executive functioning and memory. The visuospatial deficits can be pronounced. Patients can become easily lost or get "turned around." Reading the face of a clock can become confusing and very frustrating for patients. A simple bedside task to evaluate visual spatial skills is to ask the patient to copy a picture of intersecting pentagons or draw a clock. DLB patients tend to perform very poorly on this measure.

RBD is a phenomenon that occurs in DLB patients. Normally during rapid eye movement (REM) sleep, the brain sends inhibitory signals to skeletal muscle to produce paralysis or atonia. However, this is disrupted in RBD so the body loses its atonia during REM sleep. The result is that the individual is physically active during REM sleep and may act out dreams. Such patients may end up injuring themselves or their partners during sleep. Because these patients may not realize they are engaging in this behavior, information about it often is gathered via collateral reports from a spouse or partner. RBD can precede the other symptoms of DLB by years or decades. Other sleep disturbances such as insomnia or daytime sleepiness also can occur in patients with DLB.

Neuroleptic sensitivity can occur in patients with DLB as well. Very small doses of antipsychotic medications, which are usually subtherapeutic for most patients, cause marked side effects, usually extrapyramidal. This can cause additional muscle rigidity or dystonia that can lead to falls. However, only about half of all DLB patients experience neuroleptic sensitivity.

In DLB the autonomic nervous system can be affected. Lightheadedness, dizziness, hot flashes, and fluctuations in blood pressure can occur. In addition, urinary incontinence or retention can be problematic for some patients. Table 14.3 summarizes the signs and symptoms of DLB.

### How is DLB similar and different from PD?

Both, DLB and PD have many overlapping features. Pathologically, they are both referred to as *α-synucleinopathies* as Lewy bodies deposit in various parts of the central nervous system to cause symptoms. It is thought that relatively more peripheral structures such as the olfactory nerve and the enteric system are vulnerable to these neurodegenerative changes, which is why these patients may experience anosmia and constipation decades before the onset of motor symptoms.

| BASIC SCIENCE PEARL | STEP 1 |
|---|---|

Aside from Lewy bodies, β-amyloid and tau depositions may be seen in patients with DLB. Their presence is thought to be a variant of Alzheimer disease.

As DLB and PD share a similar pathology they may share similar symptomatology as well. Symptoms are usually divided into motor symptoms (parkinsonism) and nonmotor symptoms. For PD patients, tremor or another parkinsonian symptom may be the first presenting symptom.

However, for DLB patients, motor symptoms may be a later sign of the disease or may not occur at all. Up to 25% of DLB patients never develop parkinsonian symptoms. Tremor tends to be less prominent in DLB, and patients have poor balance compared with their PD counterparts.

Because DLB and PD patients both may experience significant cognitive dysfunction, the timing of these symptoms is important to delineate between these two diseases. As previously mentioned, one of the core features of DLB is the "1-year rule" (cognitive impairment precedes motor symptoms or begins within a year of parkinsonian symptom onset). Typically for PD, the average time to develop an NCD is 10 years but can be up to 20 years. Cognitive deterioration tends to progress more rapidly in DLB compared with PD. The areas of deficits are similar, though DLB patients tend to have more attentional difficulties.

Visual hallucinations occur spontaneously in any stage of DLB. Hallucinations may also occur in PD; however, in PD patients, psychotic symptoms such as visual hallucinations, auditory hallucinations, delusions, and paranoia occur either as late-stage symptoms or as a marker of more severe disease. These symptoms also can be a consequence of or exacerbated by dopaminergic agents (ropinirole, pramipexole or levodopa) used to control motor symptoms. Although these treatments enhance dopamine in the nigrostriatal pathway in order to initiate movement, dopamine excess in the mesolimbic pathway can lead to these problematic psychiatric symptoms. Striking a balance between these pathways is often a treatment challenge.

### *Aside from visual hallucinations, what are some comorbid psychiatric symptoms of DLB and PD?*

Psychiatric symptoms are very common in both DLB and PD. For some patients, these symptoms can be more distressing than the motor symptoms and can lead to significant functional impairment. Anxiety is one of the prominent symptoms occurring in up to 40% of patients with DLB or PD. These patients may qualify for a formal anxiety disorder diagnosis such as generalized anxiety disorder, panic disorder, social anxiety disorder, or an unspecified anxiety disorder, or patients may describe symptoms of anxiety but do not meet the full criteria for a diagnosis listed in the *Diagnostic and Statistical Manual of Mental Disorders*, Fifth edition (DSM-5). Depression is another common feature of DLB and PD. Many patients will experience depressive symptoms or an episode of major depressive disorder during their lifetimes. As previously mentioned, treatment with dopaminergic agents can precipitate psychotic symptoms or destabilize mood, which can lead to hypomania. Impulse control disorders such as gambling disorder, hypersexuality, and excessive shopping also can emerge.

---

The patient and his wife are surprised to hear the diagnosis. They want to know if there are any treatments to slow down or stop the cognitive decline.

---

### *What is the treatment of DLB?*

As with all major NCDs, there are no disease-modifying treatments. Treatment is focused on reducing symptoms, minimizing distress, future planning, and providing familial support in order to prevent care-giver burnout.

As DLB is thought to be a disease with a cholinergic deficiency, acetylcholinesterase inhibitors such as donepezil or rivastigmine can be helpful to address cognitive deficits and fluctuations. There are no differences between the acetylcholinesterase inhibitors, so if one medication in this class is not effective then it makes little sense to switch to another. The most common side effect is gastrointestinal distress and can also exacerbate heart block, so conduction abnormalities should be monitored.

If present, motor symptoms such as tremor, rigidity, and bradykinesia are treated similarly to patients with PD using dopaminergic agents.

In the case of RBD the goal of treatment is to minimize injury to the patient or spouse. As these patients act out their dreams, they are at risk of falling out of bed, or kicking or punching their partners during sleep. Low dose benzodiazepines such as lorazepam or clonazepam are first-line treatments. However, as DLB patients can be older and are at risk for falls, the use of these treatments may not be preferred. High-dose melatonin can be used as an alternative.

Visual hallucinations are treated only when distressing to the patient because use of antipsychotics can worsen motor symptoms. When psychotic symptoms are benign, caregiver education can be provided, advising the caregiver not to engage the patient in hallucinations or delusions, but also not to contradict the patient as to whether the hallucinations or delusions are real or not. However, if the symptoms are disruptive or upsetting, then psychosis should be adequately addressed. Psychotic symptoms can be debilitating to patients and are a leading cause of caregiver burnout. If symptoms are iatrogenic through dopaminergic agent use, then a dose reduction can be helpful. Additionally, acetylcholinesterase inhibitors can attenuate psychosis in this population. In 2016 a newer medication, pimavanserin, was approved by the Food and Drug Administration for psychosis related to PD. However, its effectiveness is still under debate. Clozapine and quetiapine, which are relatively dopaminergic sparing compared with other antipsychotics, are used off-label. These two agents tend not to worsen motor symptoms.

Depression and anxiety are treated with antidepressants such as selective serotonin reuptake inhibitors. There is little evidence to support or refute their use in this population, but their side-effect profile is relatively benign. Caution should still be taken as serotonergic agents can exacerbate extrapyramidal symptoms of PD or DLB. For cases of anxiety, buspirone, gabapentin, or low doses of benzodiazepines can be used as an alternative or augmenting strategy.

---

An echocardiogram is ordered that reveals normal sinus rhythm without signs of conduction abnormalities. Donepezil 5 mg daily is then started. During the next visit, the patient reports that his thoughts seem clearer and he feels less confused. Carbidopa/levodopa is started, which improves his muscle rigidity but does not worsen his visual hallucinations. He continues seeing the cat with green eyes but without distress or challenge from his wife. The patient and his wife join a support group for patients with DLB and their families. The patient begins seeing a physical therapist twice weekly and joins a dance class, both of which help with his balance.

---

**BEYOND THE PEARLS:**

- Parkinson disease (PD) usually presents with unilateral resting tremor or bilaterally with one side more dominant than the other. Drug-induced parkinsonism can present with a bilateral tremor.
- The Braak staging system is the most widely hypothesized model of staging symptoms of PD. Lewy bodies are thought to deposit in the central nervous system in a caudal-to-rostral fashion. They are found in the enteric and olfactory nerves initially and then progress to the brainstem, substantia nigra, and to cortical structures.
- Cognitive dysfunction is usually a late symptom of PD.
- "Off" depression or anxiety is described in patients with PD who experience these symptoms only in the context of when they feel their dopaminergic medication losing its effect before their next dose.
- All antipsychotics used for dementia-related psychosis carry a black-box warning for use in patients over 65 years old, for increased risk of all cause mortality but cardiovascular events and infections in particular.

## References

Ba, F., & Martin, W. R. (2015). Dopamine transporter imaging as a diagnostic tool for parkinsonism and related disorders in clinical practice. *Parkinsonism & Related Disorder, 21*(2), 87–94.

Bhatia, K. P., Bain, P., Bajaj, N., Elbel, R. J, Hallett, M., Louis, E. D., ... Tremor Task Force of the International Parkinson and Movement Disorder Society. (2018). Consensus statement on the classification of tremors from the task force on tremor of the International Parkinson and Movement Disorder Society. *Movement Disorders, 33*(1), 75–87.

DeLong, M. R., & Juncos, J. L. (2005). Parkinson's disease and other movement disorders. In D. L. Kasper, E. Braunwald, A. S. Fauci, S. L. Hauser, D. L. Longo, J. L. Jameson (Eds.), *Harrison's principles of internal medicine* (16th ed., pp. 2406–2417). New York, NY: McGraw-Hill.

Hassin-Baer, S., Sirota, P., Korczyn, A. D., Treves, T. A., Epstein, B., Shabtai, H., Martin, T., ... Giladi, N. (2001). Clinical characteristics of neuroleptic-induced parkinsonism. *Journal of Neural Transmission, 108*(11), 1299–12308.

Jellinger, K. A., & Korczyn, A. D. (2018). Are dementia with Lewy bodies and Parkinson's disease dementia the same disease? *BCM Medicine, 16*(34), 1–16.

Seritan, A. L., Ureste, P., Duong, T., & Ostrem, J. L. (2019). Psychopharmacology for patients with Parkinson's disease and deep brain stimulation: Lessons learned in an academic center. *Current Psychopharmacology, 8*(1), 41–54.

Weintraub, D., Siderowf, A. D., Troster, A. I., et al. (2011). Parkinson's disease and movement disorders. In C. E. Coffey, & J. L. Cummings (Eds.), *Textbook of geriatric neuropsychiatry* (3rd ed., pp. 569–570). Washington, DC: American Psychiatric Press.

# CHAPTER 15

# Alcohol Use

Elie G. Aoun ■ Lama Bazzi

A 53-year-old female comes into the clinic reporting problems with sleep for the past 5 months. She tells you that she has been using over-the-counter sleep aids but has not found them helpful. Even though they help her fall asleep, she wakes up multiple times every night. She also feels groggy for several hours in the morning.

*Given the information the patient provided, what should be included in your differential diagnosis?*
Insomnia or sleep deprivation is a very common medical complaint. Insomnia results from primary sleep disorders, or, more commonly, it may be a symptom of another condition. It manifests with a persistent difficulty in falling asleep or staying asleep and leads to daytime fatigue. Psychiatric manifestations of insomnia include depression, reduced motivation, reduced concentration, and musculoskeletal pains. In addition to ruling out primary sleep disorders, the differential diagnosis for insomnia should include general medical or neurologic conditions, psychiatric disorders including substance use disorders, poor sleep habits, and acute stress.

She later explains that in fact she has always had sleep issues. She used to drink a glass of wine in the evening and that was enough to put her to sleep. In recent years, one glass has not been sufficient, and even when she drinks three or four glasses of wine, that might not be enough.

*How does alcohol use affect sleep?*
Alcohol is a sedating substance and many patients claim it helps them fall asleep. However, alcohol also causes disruptions in sleep architecture, resulting in poor and fragmented sleep. Alcohol causes increased sleep latency and decreases in the rapid eye movement stage of sleep, sleep efficiency, total sleep time, and slow wave sleep. Heavy alcohol consumption also contributes to the development and/or worsening of obstructive sleep apnea by causing a reduction in muscle tone of the upper airways, increased episodes of desaturation, and decreased likelihood of arousal from an obstructive event.

As you inquire further about her alcohol use, you find out that on average, she drinks two glasses of wine on weekday evenings and three to four glasses of wine on weekend evening. She says that she never gets drunk and does not think that her drinking is problematic.

*How would you classify her drinking?*
The National Institute for Alcohol Abuse and Alcoholism (NIAAA) recommends that men under 65 years old drink no more than 4 drinks daily and 14 drinks weekly, and that women and men

over 65 years old drink no more than 3 drinks daily and 7 drinks weekly. Exceeding these limits is classified as "at-risk drinking." As such, the drinking patterns of the patient in this vignette may be classified as "at-risk drinking."

---

You remember that you attended a training on Screening, Brief Intervention, and Referral to Treatment (SBIRT) and decide to put it to good use. You administer an Alcohol Use Disorder Identification Test (AUDIT-C) screen and give her a score of 8.

---

### What are the components of SBIRT?

SBIRT is designed for patients without a known history of substance use disorders. The components are screening, brief intervention, and referral to treatment. Screening is usually performed by a health care professional using a standardized tool, such as the AUDIT (used to screen for maladaptive alcohol use) or Drug Abuse Screening Test (DAST, used to screen for illicit drug use). Screening can be done in an emergency room, urgent care center, doctor's office, or any other health care setting. If maladaptive substance use is identified, brief interventions (BI) are administered. Various models for BI have been proposed and typically use the principles of motivational interviewing (more on this later in this chapter). In BI a health care professional engages the patient in a short, meaningful conversation about the patient's risky substance use behaviors, listens actively to the patient's concerns, provides feedback, and gives the patient advice. Patients found to be at higher risk of complications from substance use or as in need of additional services are referred to treatment in clinics specializing in the management of addictions.

### What does the literature say about the effectiveness of SBIRT?

In primary care settings, SBIRT is a well-established, effective tool for patients with risky alcohol use but not for a moderate-to-severe alcohol use disorder (AUD). In patients who screened positive for risky alcohol use, brief interventions have been shown to reduce self-reported drinking. Brief interventions were shown to reduce risky drinking 1 year after administration compared with patients who received care as usual. Furthermore, BI decreased patients' health care utilization and led to significant cost savings. The efficacy of SBIRT for nonalcohol substance use disorders is not well established.

---

You perform BI and schedule her to return in 2 weeks for a follow-up.

---

### What laboratory tests would you want to check in patients with at-risk drinking?

In patients with at-risk drinking, the following blood tests should be obtained: complete blood count, basic metabolic panel, and liver function tests. A complete blood count with macrocytosis may indicate folate or vitamin $B_{12}$ deficiencies, whereas microcytosis may indicate bleeding from an ulcer, falls, etc. A basic metabolic panel may reveal electrolyte abnormalities, such as hypomagnesemia, hypokalemia, or hypophosphatemia, along with renal function. Liver enzymes, including aspartate aminotransferase (AST) and alanine aminotransferase (ALT), bilirubin, and albumin are needed to test for liver damage. Liver disease due to alcohol use usually results in an AST:ALT ratio of 2:1. A lipid panel and glycosylated hemoglobin (A1C) may also be clinically indicated.

---

Three days later, you receive a call from a nearby hospital. The patient was arrested for drunk driving, and during the encounter with law enforcement officers, she fell and hit her head. During transport, she had an episode of emesis, aspirated, and had to be intubated. The technicians found your card in her wallet.

---

*What are some of the acute risks of alcohol intoxication?*

Alcohol intoxication causes different signs and symptoms, depending on the level of intoxication. Patients can present with disinhibited behaviors, lack of coordination, memory impairment, impaired motor functioning, slurred speech or dysarthria, unsteady gait, respiratory depression, and eventually stupor and even coma or death. Incoordination and unsteady gait can lead to falls and head injuries. Disinhibition can lead to combative and violent behavior at times. Alcohol intoxication can cause intravascular volume loss, leading to peripheral vasodilation and resulting in tachycardia and hypotension. Nausea and vomiting can occur, exacerbating metabolic disturbances. Some metabolic disturbances that can result from alcohol intoxication are hypoglycemia, hypokalemia, hypomagnesemia, hypocalcemia, hypophosphatemia, and hyperlactatemia. Alcohol also causes dose-dependent vasodilation. Blood pressure and tissue perfusion is maintained until the intoxication-induced hypoventilation leads to hypoxemia.

---

Three days into her admission, the patient develops a generalized tonic-clonic seizure.

---

*What could be causing this seizure?*

Generalized tonic-clonic seizures can occur as part of alcohol withdrawal syndromes, usually between 12 and 48 hours after the discontinuation of heavy alcohol consumption. Alcohol withdrawal seizures typically indicate a more severe alcohol withdrawal syndrome and increase the likelihood of having future withdrawal seizures.

| CLINICAL PEARL | STEP 2/3 |
|---|---|

Other manifestations of severe alcohol withdrawal include delirium tremens; a rapid-onset delirium syndrome marked by agitation; cognitive impairments with poor concentration and disorientation, hallucinations, and autonomic disturbances such as fever, tachycardia, hypertension, and diaphoresis. These symptoms present between 72 and 96 hours after the patient's last drink. Untreated delirium tremens is often lethal and requires treatment in an intensive care unit.

Most individuals with AUD do not experience seizures or delirium tremens in withdrawal. Alcohol withdrawal typically presents with symptoms such as anxiety, restlessness, tremors, sweating, tachycardia, headaches, and urges to drink to relieve these symptoms.

*How do you manage alcohol withdrawal?*

The goal of treatment in alcohol withdrawal is to identify and correct metabolic abnormalities and alleviate symptoms. Benzodiazepines are key in preventing the progression of withdrawal and in reducing agitation and alleviating discomfort. Intravenous fluids and nutritional supplementation should be initiated whenever clinically indicated, and vital signs should be assessed frequently. Along with intravenous fluids, thiamine should be given to prevent the occurrence of Wernicke's encephalopathy (WE).

| BASIC SCIENCE/CLINICAL PEARL | STEP 1/2/3 |
|---|---|

Wernicke's encephalopathy (WE) occurs in individuals with chronic alcohol use disorder (AUD) due to the effects of thiamine deficiency on mammillary bodies. It presents with gait instability, oculomotor dysfunction, and confusion.

| CLINICAL PEARL | STEP 2/3 |
|---|---|

Parenteral repletion of thiamine (because gastrointestinal absorption may be impaired due to the effects of chronic alcohol use on the gastrointestinal mucosa) typically reverses the symptoms of Wernicke's encephalopathy (WE).

| CLINICAL PEARL | STEP 2/3 |
|---|---|

Thiamine has to be repleted before any ingestion of glucose-containing foods by the patient, because glucose metabolism can lead to a depletion of thiamine reserves, which could precipitate Korsakoff syndrome.

Patients presenting in moderate to severe alcohol withdrawal should be given benzodiazepines. Intravenous or intramuscular administration of benzodiazepines should be considered for patients at high risk of aspiration, including those with severe withdrawal symptoms. The patient's vital signs as well as other symptoms of withdrawal should be closely monitored. In clinical settings, the Clinical Institute Withdrawal Assessment for Alcohol Scale (CIWA), a formal assessment tool, is frequently used, and elevated CIWA scores result in benzodiazepine administration. Barbiturates also are effective in managing alcohol withdrawal; however, they have been used infrequently in recent years except in cases of severe alcohol withdrawal. Benzodiazepine-sparing protocols for alcohol withdrawal using gabapentin, other antiepileptic agents (such as carbamazepine or valproic acid), or adrenergic agents (such as clonidine or dexmedetomidine) have also been found to be effective in treating alcohol withdrawal, though they have not been approved by the Food and Drug Administration (FDA) for this indication.

---

After hospital discharge, the patient returns to your office and admits that she had minimized her alcohol drinking and that, in fact, she drinks more than twice as much as she had initially told you. She did not start drinking alcohol until her late 20s, but in her mid-40s her two best friends were killed in a car accident. She was the only survivor of the car crash, and she began drinking heavily afterward. The patient has tried to quit "cold turkey" on multiple occasions but each time would feel "sick" to the point where "only alcohol would make me feel better." She had made attempts to cut down but found that she would begin drinking more within a few days. The patient has never been in formal alcohol treatment. She thinks that her drinking makes her depression worse, because "it just makes me numb, but my life is still a mess when I sober up, so I feel even worse and drink again." Although she wakes up early, she feels anxious and shaky in the morning and then drinks alcohol to calm herself. She then has to wait at least 4 hours before she can start her day, and this affects her work. She has received several citations at work because of her behavior.

---

### Does this patient have a substance use disorder?

According to the American Psychiatric Association's *Diagnostic and Statistical Manual of Mental Disorders*, Fifth Edition (DSM-5), AUD is defined as a problematic pattern of alcohol use leading to clinically significant impairment or distress, as manifested by at least two behavioral symptoms within a 12-month period.

### What gender differences are there for AUD?

AUD is more common among men than among women. Women may be more sensitive to the effects of alcohol due to having lower levels of gastric alcohol dehydrogenase (resulting in larger amounts of alcohol being absorbed) and a lower total body water volume (resulting in alcohol being distributed in a smaller volume). Additionally, women may be more sensitive to stress-induced or cue-induced reinstatement (relapsing to alcohol use after being exposed to stressful situations or cues reminiscent of past alcohol use behaviors), whereas men may be more sensitive to drug-induced reinstatement (relapsing to habitual alcohol use after consuming a small amount of alcohol). Telescoping is the phenomenon whereby AUD severity progresses faster in women than in men. It is also associated with women more likely to seek treatment for AUD sooner than men.

### What are some of the most significant health consequences of severe AUD?
Severe AUD is linked to increased mortality. Excessive alcohol consumption is the third leading form of preventable death in the United States, resulting in the death of 1 in every 10 Americans. The risk of drowning is 3.5 times higher in people who drink. Almost 30% of all traffic fatalities are alcohol related. AUD increases the risk of suicidal ideation, suicide attempts, and completed suicides. The lifetime rate of suicide attempts in regular alcohol users is 7%, which is significantly higher than the 1% lifetime rate of suicide attempts in the general adult population.

AUD has adverse effects on virtually every organ system. The gastrointestinal tract is adversely affected by an increased risk for gastritis, stomach ulcers, and duodenal ulcers. Long-term, chronic alcohol consumption causes liver cirrhosis and pancreatitis in about 15% of users. Furthermore, alcohol increases the risk of many cancers, including those of the mouth, esophagus, throat, liver, and breast. Bone marrow suppression can occur, leading to infections and pneumonia. Hypertension is common in patients with AUD, and cardiomyopathy is more common in patients with AUD than in the general population. Alcohol causes an increase in low-density lipoprotein and triglycerides, increasing patients' risk of heart disease. As for the nervous system, alcohol increases the risk of peripheral neuropathy, leading to paresthesias, peripheral sensory abnormalities, and muscular abnormalities. Wernicke-Korsakoff syndrome is a rare but terrible alcohol-induced amnestic disorder in which the patient can no longer form new memories. Cognitive deficits with AUDs result from the direct effects of alcohol, from trauma related to falls, and from B-vitamin deficiencies, including thiamine. Cerebellar degeneration can occur as well.

### What are the physical findings you may find in persons with severe AUD?
Despite the many health repercussions of severe AUD, a patient's physical examination can be completely normal. We discussed Wernicke's encephalopathy and Korsakoff syndrome earlier. Other signs of AUD include broken veins around the nose. Some features of alcohol withdrawal include autonomic instability, agitation, tremor, and elements of delirium, including confusion and disorientation. Chronic and prolonged alcohol use can lead to testicular atrophy, Dupuytren's contractures, and gynecomastia. Advanced liver disease causes hepatic enlargement, splenic enlargement, spider angiomata, and palmar erythema. Hepatic encephalopathy would present with asterixis and confusion.

---

The patient tells you she wants help quitting alcohol and that she never wants to drink again.

---

### What are the components of treatment for AUD?
AUD treatment consists of psychosocial treatments and medication management. Although psychosocial treatments have been shown to be effective, more than 70% of patients treated for AUD without medication relapse into heavy alcohol use. A combination of structured, evidence-based psychosocial treatment and medication management is indicated in the treatment of severe AUD.

*What medications are effective in treating AUD?*

Three medications are approved by the FDA for the treatment of AUD: naltrexone (both as a daily oral formulation or as a long-acting injectable formulation), acamprosate, and disulfiram. Additionally, several other medications were found to be effective for the treatment of AUD (topiramate, gabapentin, baclofen, and odansetron) but have not been approved by the FDA for this indication.

Naltrexone is an antagonist at the mu-opioid receptor and an agonist at the kappa-opioid receptor. Because endogenous opioids modulate alcohol's reinforcing effects, blocking the mu-opioid receptors results in less pleasure from alcohol consumption. Furthermore, naltrexone functions by modulating the hypothalamic-pituitary-adrenal axis and decreases alcohol consumption. Naltrexone can be prescribed as a once-daily oral formulation or as a monthly injection and can be started in a patient who is still drinking. Naltrexone is metabolized through the liver, so patients who have elevated liver enzymes should be monitored carefully if prescribed naltrexone.

Acamprosate is an amino acid derivative that modulates glutamate neurotransmission. It is dosed three times daily, which can make adherence to treatment challenging. Acamprosate is excreted unchanged through the kidneys.

Disulfiram works by inhibiting alcohol dehydrogenase and preventing the metabolism of acetaldehyde. As acetaldehyde levels rise in the blood, patients begin to sweat; exhibit sympathetic nervous system activation; and can develop palpitations, headache, nausea, and vomiting. Flushing and shortness of breath are also common. The unpleasant effects discourage further drinking by acting as a deterrent.

| BASIC SCIENCE PEARL | STEP 1 |
|---|---|

Alcohol is metabolized via zero-order kinetics, which means that a constant amount of alcohol is cleared per unit time. Alcohol is metabolized into acetaldehyde by alcohol dehydrogenase (ADH) and further metabolized into acetate by aldehyde dehydrogenase (ALDH).

| BASIC SCIENCE/CLINICAL PEARL | STEP 1/2/3 |
|---|---|

Genetic polymorphism affecting the genes coding for ADH or ALDH can increase or decrease an individual's risk of developing AUD. For example, those with a hyperactive ADH or a hypoactive ALDH will see an accumulation of acetaldehyde and are less likely to drink alcohol or have AUD.

You discuss with the patient her drinking goals, and she tells you that at this point she would like to give up drinking completely, at least for a year or two. She is worried about "cheating" and asks if there are tests that you could do to make sure that she is not drinking.

*What are the biomarkers used to evaluate drinking in patients with AUD?*

There are indirect and direct biomarkers of alcohol use available for clinical practice. Indirect markers reflect alcohol-mediated organ damage indicating prolonged heavy alcohol use, including AST, ALT, and gamma-glutamyltransferase (GGT).

Direct biomarkers of alcohol use can be metabolites of ethanol or compounds modified by the presence of ethanol. These include ethyl-glucuronide (EtG) and ethyl-sulfate (EtS), percent carbohydrate deficient transferrin (CDT), and phosphatidyl-ethanol (PEth). GGT, ALT, AST, CDT, and PEth are tested in blood samples. EtG and EtS can be tested in urine or hair samples.

After hearing all the options, the patient tells you that she is interested in naltrexone. She is intrigued though and asks, "So why would an opioid blocker help with my alcohol problem? I have never used heroin before." You feel embarrassed when you cannot answer her question and decide to review your old textbooks and learn about the neurobiology of AUD.

### How does alcohol affect the brain?

In individuals with AUD, the effect of alcohol on the brain can be divided into three stages: binge intoxication, withdrawal negative affect, and preoccupation anticipation. The binge intoxication stage represents the positive reinforcement aspect of alcohol use and is controlled by the incentive salience aspect of alcohol. The ventral tegmental area (VTA) and the nucleus accumbens (NAc) play a major role in this stage. The withdrawal negative affect stage is marked by the reward deficit and stress surfeit that accompany the abrupt discontinuation of alcohol leading to withdrawal symptoms. The amygdala and thalamic nuclei play a major role in this stage. The third stage, preoccupation anticipation, represents the cognitive and executive aspects of control over alcohol consumption. The prefrontal cortex, the orbitofrontal cortex, hippocampus, and insula play a major role in this stage.

The acute consumption of alcohol leads to a reduction in glutamate N-nitrosodimethylamine (NMDA) activity and an increase in gamma-aminobutyric acid (GABA) activity. This renders the VTA hyperexcitable, and dopaminergic neurons in the VTA release dopamine in the NAc. This is called the *brain reward pathway*. When alcohol consumption becomes chronic, GABA receptor function is reduced while NMDA receptor function is increased to compensate for the exogenous alcohol effects. Similarly, the VTA becomes less excitable in the absence of alcohol and more alcohol is needed to achieve the same effect on the reward pathway. If alcohol use is discontinued abruptly, the imbalance between NMDA and GABA activity favors NMDA in the absence of alcohol. This leads to an adrenergic surge in the locus ceruleus, resulting in the alcohol withdrawal symptoms.

The patient calls you within hours of leaving your office. Soon after taking the first naltrexone tablet, she starts feeling achy, has severe abdominal pain and generalized fatigue, is throwing up, is very sweaty, and complains of light sensitivity.

### What is the most likely explanation for her symptoms and how do you manage them?

The patient's symptoms are consistent with opioid withdrawal. It is possible that after the car accident, she was prescribed an opioid pain medication that she was still taking. Naltrexone, an opioid antagonist, would have displaced the opioids from their receptors and resulted in sudden onset of precipitated withdrawal. The treatment of precipitated withdrawal is supportive in nature. Aggressive oral hydration should be combined with antiemetics for nausea, loperamide for severe diarrhea, nonsteroidal antiinflammatories for muscle aches and pains, and clonidine to curb the adrenergic hyperactivity.

The patient decides that she does not need the opioid pain medication anymore and wants to give the naltrexone another try. She also remembers that you told her about motivational interviewing as a form of psychotherapy that is effective for AUD.

### What is motivational interviewing, and how does it differ from other psychotherapeutic modalities?

Motivational interviewing aims to help patients change problem behavior by increasing their motivation to change by identifying and resolving ambivalence. The premise of motivational interviewing is that people with substance use disorders are conflicted by their substance use. In treatment, the health care provider meets the patients where they are, seeks an understanding of the patients' perspective, and draws the patients' attention to the discrepancy between who they currently are and who they would like to be. The key is empowering patients to shift their perspective and to accept that the possibility to change exists. The basic communication style in motivational interviewing is reflected by the mnemonic ORAS—open-ended questions, reflections, affirmations, and summaries. A nonjudgmental approach allows the clinician to build rapport with the patient and understand the patient's feelings about his or her own behaviors. The patient and the clinician engage in "change talk" and identify reasons for possible changes that the patient is considering making. The clinician uses this opportunity to understand the patient's experience with alcohol, their concerns about alcohol use, and the benefits they reap from using alcohol. The clinician can also explore what the patient's wishes are for the future, including whether the patient wants to reduce or stop the use of alcohol. The clinician should maintain a patient-centered approach to treatment and avoid evoking resistance in the patient by eliciting patient readiness to change. Motivational interviewing involves expressing empathy, developing discrepancy, rolling with resistance, and supporting self-efficacy. The clinician empathically engages the patient, focuses the patient on potential change that he or she can realistically make, evokes change talk in the patient, and finally guides the patient in planning for change.

---

You recall what the patient told you about the car accident that led to excessive drinking and that when talking about her sleep problems, she reported having nightmares. You suspect co-occurring posttraumatic stress disorder (PTSD).

---

### *What treatment modality has been shown to be effective for individuals with co-occurring AUD and PTSD?*

*Dual diagnosis,* also referred to as *co-occurring disorders,* is a term for when someone simultaneously experiences a nonaddictive psychiatric disorder and a substance use disorder such as AUD. Comorbid PTSD/AUD is prevalent, and these patients are generally more difficult to treat than patients with either disorder alone. These patients have more physical problems, poor social functioning, more legal issues, are at higher risk for suicide and violence, are more resistant to treatment, and have more difficulty adhering to treatment. It is important to tailor treatment choices to particular patients, and understanding the reasons why patients use substances and how those reasons relate to their PTSD symptoms is important when choosing a treatment modality. There is a significant interplay between PTSD and AUD symptoms, and the integrated model of treatment has the same clinician targeting both disorders at the same time. Treating AUD reduces the negative effect associated with PTSD, and working on the trauma early in treatment reduces the risk of relapse and improves AUD outcomes. Seeking Safety is a therapy model that was found to be effective for the treatment of co-occurring PTSD and AUD. This model emphasizes the initial treatment goal of establishing physical and psychological safety.

---

With treatment for both conditions, the patient was able to feel in better control of her health, maintained her recovery with her cravings well under control, and her PTSD symptoms improved significantly.

---

**BEYOND THE PEARLS:**

- Patients with AUD often resist admitting to maladaptive drinking. They frequently present to health care providers reporting symptoms caused by their drinking, such as insomnia, anxiety, or mood disturbances. The astute clinician needs to assess whether substance use is contributing to such symptoms.
- There are several screening instruments that can be used to help identify patients with at-risk substance use, such as the Alcohol Use Disorder Identification Test (AUDIT) for maladaptive alcohol use and the Drug Abuse Screening Test (DAST) for illicit drug use.
- According to the *Diagnostic and Statistical Manual of Mental Disorders*, Fifth Edition (DSM-5), severity of AUD is based on the number of symptoms present rather than the relative severity of presenting symptoms.
- AUD is more common among men, but women may be more sensitive to the effects of alcohol.
- Persons with AUD often have imbalanced dietary intake and impaired gastrointestinal nutrient absorption. They may present with hypoglycemia, hypokalemia, hypophosphatemia, and hypomagnesemia, as well as thiamine, folate, and vitamin $B_{12}$ deficiencies. Repleting these nutrients can help prevent or reverse complications.
- Laboratory evidence of alcohol use comes from direct biomarkers, including ethyl-glucuronide (EtG), ethyl-sulfate (EtS), percent carbohydrate deficient transferrin (CDT), and phosphatidyl-ethanol (PEth), as well as indirect biomarkers reflecting alcohol-mediated organ damage, including complete blood count (CBC), AST, ALT, and gamma-glutamyltransferase (GGT).
- Three medications are approved by the U.S. Food and Drug Administration (FDA) for the treatment of AUD—naltrexone, acamprosate, and disulfiram.
- Naltrexone is metabolized through the liver. As such, patients with elevated liver enzymes who are prescribed naltrexone should be monitored carefully.
- Naltrexone is an opioid antagonist and will displace the opioids from their receptors, resulting in sudden opioid withdrawal. Therefore it should also not be used in patients taking opioid analgesics.
- The basic communication style in motivational interviewing is reflected by the mnemonic ORAS—open-ended questions, reflections, affirmations, and summaries.

## References

41st Annual Scientific Meeting of the Research Society on Alcoholism, June 16–20—San Diego, California. (2018). *Alcoholism Clinical and Experimental Research, 42*(Suppl 1), 5A.

Anton, R. F., Moak, D. H., Latham, P., Waid, L. R., Myrick, H., Voronin, K., ... Woolson, R. (2005). Naltrexone combined with either cognitive behavioral or motivational enhancement therapy for alcohol dependence. *Journal of Clinical Psychopharmacology, 25,* 349.

Donoghue, K., Elzerbi, C., Saunders, R., Whittington, C., Pilling, S., & Durmmond, C. (2015). The efficacy of acamprosate and naltrexone in the treatment of alcohol dependence, Europe versus the rest of the world: A meta-analysis. *Addiction, 110,* 920.

Grant, B. F., Goldstein, R. B., Saha, T. D., Chou, S. P., Jung, J., Zhang, H., ... Hasin, D. S. (2015). Epidemiology of DSM-5 alcohol use disorder: Results From the National Epidemiologic Survey on Alcohol and Related Conditions III. *JAMA Psychiatry, 72,* 757.

Laaksonen, E., Koski-Jännes, A., Salaspuro, M., Ahtinen, H., & Alho, H. (2008). A randomized, multicentre, open-label, comparative trial of disulfiram, naltrexone and acamprosate in the treatment of alcohol dependence. *Alcohol and Alcoholism, 43,* 53.

Matsumoto, C., Miedema, M. D., Ofman, P., Gaziano, J. M., Sesso, H. D. (2014). An expanding knowledge of the mechanisms and effects of alcohol consumption on cardiovascular disease. *Journal of Cardiopulmonary Rehabilitation and Prevention, 34*(3),159–171.

Oslin, D. W., Leong, S. H., Lynch, K. G., Berrettini, W., O'Brien, C. P., Gordon, A. J., & Rukstalis, M. (2015). Naltrexone vs placebo for the treatment of alcohol dependence: A randomized clinical trial. *JAMA Psychiatry*, *72*, 430.

Smedslund, G., Berg, R. C., Hammerstrøm, K. T., Steiro, A., Leiknes, K. A., Dahl, H. M., & Karlsen, K. (2011). Motivational interviewing for substance abuse. *Cochrane Database of Systemic Reviews*, CD008063.

# CHAPTER 16

# Substance Use Disorders

Stefana Morgan ■ Tammy Duong

A 71-year-old divorced male with a history of childhood chickenpox presents to the primary care office with an exquisitely painful unilateral vesicular rash on his trunk. The patient is an attorney but winding down his practice in preparation to retire. He indicates no past psychiatric history other than "feeling blue after my first divorce 30 years ago." He is diagnosed with shingles and is prescribed acyclovir to prevent post-herpetic neuralgia. The patient expresses concern that pain will interfere with work on an important litigation case. He is given a 1-month prescription of hydrocodone.

---

**BASIC SCIENCE PEARL**                                            **STEP 1**

The three main opioid receptors are mu, kappa, and delta. They are transmembrane G-coupled proteins.

---

**BASIC SCIENCE PEARL**                                            **STEP 1**

*Opioid* is a broad term for any compound that acts on opioid receptors. Opioids have analgesic effects by binding at the mu receptor.

---

Two weeks later, the patient misses his follow-up appointment, and the provider receives an electronic refill request for hydrocodone. The busy provider refills the script for another month. He receives another refill request 20 days later, ahead of the next scheduled refill. He denies the request and tells the patient to present for a follow-up appointment.

---

The patient returns to the clinic and reports continued pain. He requests another refill of hydrocodone for post-herpetic neuralgia. He denies feeling depressed or anxious. On physical examination, blood pressure is 180/90 mm Hg, pulse rate is 99/min, respiration rate is 14/min, and oxygen saturation is 98% on room air. Physical examination is significant for a scar on his trunk, but no rash is present. Ecchymosis is apparent on his left forearm and there is a superficial abrasion on his left knee. On mental status examination, the patient appears slightly disheveled, his eyes are injected with periorbital dark circles, he is not closely shaven, and his blazer is wrinkled. The patient's affect is anxious and slightly irritable. He explains his injuries by reporting that he recently fell.

His primary care provider suspects that the patient is misusing his opioid prescription.

*What is the prevalence of substance use disorders in older adults?*
The prevalence of older adults experiencing substance use disorders (SUDs) is expected to increase substantially as the baby-boomer generation continues to age. In contrast to prior generations of older adults who traditionally have had relatively low rates of substance use, baby boomers came of age during the 1960s and 1970s at a time of evolving attitudes toward alcohol and drug use.

Alcohol and marijuana are the most commonly used substances in the United States. On an average day 6 million older adults use alcohol and 132,000 older adults use marijuana. In 2012, among adults who were 50 years and older, 4.6 million adults reported using marijuana and close to one million reported past-year use of cocaine, inhalants, hallucinogens, methamphetamine, or heroin. Older adults also account for a quarter of all prescription drugs sold in the United States, including benzodiazepines, opiate analgesics, and muscle relaxants prescribed to treat anxiety, pain, and insomnia.

Benzodiazepines and opioids are the drugs that are most commonly misused among older adults. Half of adults over 65 years old who misuse prescription opioids obtained them through a prescription from their own providers. Chronic pain and opioid use disorders are often comorbid, causing complicated doctor–patient relationships, difficulties in down-titrating opioid medications, and even leading some patients to resort to illegal sources of opioids.

| CLINICAL PEARL | STEP 1/2/3 |
|---|---|
| Different opioids have similar side effect profiles. They differ by their potencies and half-lives. Convert one opioid to another by using morphine as the standard equivalent. | |

*Why are SUDs underdiagnosed in older adults?*
Providers may have a lower index of suspicion of substance abuse disorders in older adults because of a variety of reasons, including (1) stereotypes of SUD presentations based on younger populations; (2) stereotypes of older patients based on geriatric cohorts before the baby boomer generation; (3) provider discomfort in bringing up substance use with older patients; (4) heightened stigma against mental health problems including SUDs in older patients, which may cause them and their families to deny the substance use; or (5) diminished societal roles and worsening social isolation, allowing patients to hide their substance use.

*In general, when should you consider substance use disorders as a diagnosis?*
In younger patients, SUDs are comorbid with poverty, homelessness, and antisocial behaviors. However, geriatric populations are more likely to suffer neglect of their medical needs due to substance use. These patients are also far more likely to present with physical symptoms rather than psychiatric symptoms, such as injuries, falls, memory disturbance, cognitive impairment, executive dysfunction, increased tolerance to prescription drugs, and requiring multiple early refills on medications. Other psychosocial factors that should trigger providers to include SUDs in their differential diagnosis include insomnia, depression, anxiety, mood lability, irritability, distress surrounding new medical diagnoses, loss of spouse or friends, family conflict, and financial or legal problems. Table 16.1 lists risk factors related to problematic substance use in late life.

On further interview with the patient, the patient reveals that his law practice owes money for back taxes and that his wife is threatening to divorce him. He has psychological distress and poor sleep habits. He also admits to difficulties in completing complex tasks that previously came easily to him—such as accounting, billing, and planning.

*How do you screen for substance use disorders in the older adult?*
Once the clinician has considered substance use as a part of the differential, the provider should consider further clinical interviewing and obtaining collateral information from the

TABLE 16.1 ■ **Risk Factors Related to Substance Use in Late Life**

| Type of Risk Factor | Risk Factors |
| --- | --- |
| Physical | Gender: male for alcohol, female for prescription drugs |
| | Caucasian ethnicity |
| | Chronic pain |
| | Physical disabilities or reduced mobility |
| | Poor functional status |
| | Medical comorbidities |
| | Polypharmacy |
| Psychiatric | Avoidant coping style |
| | History of alcohol or substance use disorders |
| | History of psychiatric illness |
| Social | Affluence |
| | Bereavement |
| | Unexpected retirement |
| | Social isolation (not living with family) |
| | Transitions in care/living situations |

chart, family, friends, and other clinicians. Additionally, the patient should be screened for at-risk substance use.

Validated screening tools used to screen patients for alcohol and substance use disorders in older adults include the CAGE questionnaire, the Alcohol Use Disorders Identification Test-C (AUDIT-C), the Michigan Alcoholism Screening Test—Geriatric Version (MAST-G), and the Drug Abuse Screening Test (DAST). The CAGE questionnaire has been modified to evaluate for both alcohol and substance use disorders.

---

The patient admits that to cope with his stress he has been using increasing amounts of opioids, beyond what he needs for pain control. He screens positively for substance use and is at elevated risk for negative consequences from substance use.

---

### *What is a brief intervention that can be performed in the office to reduce patient risk?*
Most patients who screen positive for at-risk substance use do not meet full criteria for a substance use disorder but still are at an elevated risk of suffering consequences and developing the full disorder. This risk can be ameliorated by a brief intervention as an initial treatment approach. Brief interventions use a nonjudgmental attitude to express concern for the high-risk behavior and provide psychoeducation on the deleterious effects of drinking and substance use on the patient's health and well-being. It is also important to provide information on the dangers of combining alcohol and other sedatives (opioids, benzodiazepines, muscle relaxants, gabapentin, and pregabalin). Brief interventions, such as those based on motivational interviewing (MI) or motivational enhancement treatment (MET), can be as short as one 15-minute interaction. Table 16.2 summarizes the components of a brief office intervention for at-risk substance use.

---

TABLE 16.2 ■ **Brief Office Intervention**

- Express nonjudgmental concern for the patient's drinking compared with peers
- Advise (to stop or decrease substance use)
- Educate on the links between substance use and health
- Offer referral to addiction treatment, if appropriate

| CLINICAL PEARL | STEP 2/3 |
|---|---|

Normative feedback is the most common type of brief interventions and has been found to be most effective for older adults. In this interaction, the patient's alcohol or substance use is compared with that of other older adults, and the patient is given brief advice.

---

The provider determines the patient is at a high risk for developing hazardous consequences of substance use. The provider does a brief intervention and provides psychoeducation and advice to abstain or decrease opiate use. The patient agrees with this plan to taper hydrocodone over the next few weeks.

On the follow-up visit, the patient has used all of his supply of hydrocodone and reports he has borrowed extra tablets from a friend. He is unable to complete his duties at work, skips social occasions such as his granddaughter's birthday, and he misses the filing deadline for his tax returns. His wife is fed up with his behavior and is now staying at their daughter's home.

---

### *How is a diagnosis of substance use disorder established?*

*The Diagnostic and Statistical Manual of Mental Disorders*, Fifth Edition (DSM-5) outlines the diagnostic criteria for substance use disorders. However, some older adults may not report certain features described by the DSM-5, such as cravings, guilt about using, or persistent desire to stop or cut down. This might be especially true for older adults that are regularly using opioids for chronic pain or benzodiazepines for sleep or anxiety. In such instances, the provider needs a comprehensive understanding of the clinical picture, which includes chart review and collateral information from loved ones. Additionally, the patient's response to decreasing or stopping the medication is also informative. Some patients will begin to experience psychological symptoms of addiction, such as cravings, as well as physiologic symptoms, such as withdrawal. Others will engage in concerning behaviors, such as frequent presentations at the primary care office exhibiting pain or other somatic symptoms, inability to reduce the dose and frequency of the prescription drug, interpersonal conflict with providers, and attempts to obtain prescription drugs illegally or via doctor-shopping.

After diagnosis, the next steps include informing the patient of the diagnosis, describing their symptoms of SUD, and explaining that treatment can be very effective.

| BASIC SCIENCE/CLINICAL PEARL | STEP 1/2/3 |
|---|---|

Signs and symptoms of opioid intoxication include sedation, euphoria, miosis, slurred speech, depressed respiratory rate, lowered heart rate, and constipation.

---

This patient meets DSM-5 criteria opioid use disorder, including (1) increasing and unplanned time periods being intoxicated from opiates or recovering from the aftereffects; (2) failure to fulfill important work and social obligations; (3) being unable to stop use despite attempting to; (4) increased tolerance; and (5) using drugs despite negative consequences to his health, such as having falls and cognitive impairment. The "moderate" modifier would be added, because the patient meets five criteria for the DSM-5 definition of opiate use disorder.

| CLINICAL PEARL | STEP 2/3 |
|---|---|

To meet criteria for a substance use disorder, a patient must meet at least two of eleven symptom criteria. Mild disorders meet two to three criteria, moderate disorders meet four to five symptoms, and severe disorders have at least six symptoms present.

The diagnosis is opiate use disorder, moderate.

The provider shares the diagnosis with the patient and explains the DSM-5 criteria that are met. The patient seems resistant to the diagnosis and cites that he does not have the subjective psychological symptoms, such as cravings or guilt regarding use. Physiologic signs of addiction including tolerance and withdrawal are explained to him. He reports understanding the diagnosis but still claims, "I can stop using the hydrocodone anytime I want."

### What complications of opioid use should be screened for in this patient?

Patients with opioid use disorder who use combination formulations of opioids plus acetaminophen (APAP) are at risk of APAP toxicity and should be warned that for older adults the maximum safe dose for APAP is 2 grams per 24 hours. Additionally, APAP toxicity may be cumulative with alcohol-related hepatocellular injury.

The patient reports headache, nausea, diarrhea, and anxiety. His blood pressure is 180/90 mm Hg, pulse rate is 120/min, respiration rate is 14/min, and oxygen saturation is 98% on room air. His skin is clammy and with piloerection.

### How do you recognize and treat withdrawal?

**BASIC SCIENCE/CLINICAL PEARL**                                          **STEP 1/2/3**

Signs and symptoms of opioid withdrawal include restlessness, dysphoria, mydriasis, rhinorrhea, lacrimation, myalgias, yawning, piloerection, increased heart rate, abdominal pain, nausea, and diarrhea.

The opioid withdrawal scale can be used to quantify and track severity of opioid withdrawal symptoms and is outlined in Table 16.3.

Withdrawal is the constellation of symptoms that occurs once a substance has been eliminated from the body after the body has become accustomed to the drug. Withdrawal treatment is sometimes referred to as *medical detoxification* or *detox*. It is the medical treatment of withdrawal symptoms and is clinically and physiologically necessary for the safe transition from intoxication to sobriety. However, withdrawal treatment is only the first stage of substance use treatment and alone has not been shown to lead to long-term changes in behavior (i.e., relapse prevention).

Low acuity and motivated patients with mild-to-moderate opioid use disorders may be tapered off opioids in primary care clinics with minimal complications. Withdrawal symptoms from opioids are not medically dangerous but are highly unpleasant and should be treated symptomatically. For example, anxiety or hypertension can be treated with clonidine and lorazepam, but anticholinergic medications should be avoided because of their deliriogenic nature in older adults. More advanced opioid use disorders should be treated in specialty clinics with buprenorphine.

**CLINICAL PEARL**                                                        **STEP 1/2/3**

Buprenorphine is a high-affinity partial mu receptor agonist and a weak kappa receptor antagonist. As it is a partial receptor agonist, the analgesic and euphoric effects plateau. It can help prevent relapse because of its high-affinity to the mu receptor; other opioids cannot displace it.

## TABLE 16.3 ▪ Opioid Withdrawal Scale

**Resting Pulse Rate**
0  pulse rate 80 or below
1  pulse rate 81–100
2  pulse rate 101–120
4  pulse rate greater than 100

**Restlessness**
0  able to sit still
1  reports difficult sitting still but is able to do so
3  frequent shifting or extraneous movements of legs/arms
5  unable to sit still for more than a few seconds

**Bone or Joint Aches**
0  not present
1  mild diffuse discomfort
2  severe diffuse aching of joints/muscles
4  patient rubbing joints or muscles and unable to sit still because of discomfort

**GI Upset**
0  no GI symptoms
1  stomach cramps
2  nausea or loose stools
3  vomiting or diarrhea
5  multiple episodes of diarrhea or vomiting

**Anxiety or Irritability**
0  none
1  patient reports increasing irritability or anxiousness
2  patient obviously irritable or anxious
4  patient so irritable or anxious that participation in assessment is difficult

**Gooseflesh Skin**
0  skin is smooth
3  piloerection of skin can be felt or hairs standing up on arms
5  prominent piloerection

**Sweating**
0  no report of chills or flushing
1  subjective report of chills or flushing
2  flushed or observable moistness on face
3  beads of sweat on brow or face
4  sweat streaming off face

**Pupil Size**
0  pupils pinned or normal size for room light
1  pupils possibly larger than normal for room light
2  pupils moderately dilated
5  pupils so dilated that only the rim of the iris is visible

**Runny Nose or Tearing**
0  not present
1  nasal stuffiness or unusually moist eyes
2  nose running or tearing
4  constantly running or tears streaming

**Tremor**
0  no tremor
1  tremor can be felt but not observed
3  slight tremor observable
4  gross tremor or muscle twitching

**Yawning**
0  no yawning
1  yawning once or twice during assessment
3  yawning three or more times during assessment
4  yawning several times/minute

**Score:**
5–12 = mild; 13–24 = moderate; 25–36 = moderately severe; more than 36 = severe withdrawal

*GI*, Gastrointestinal.
Reproduced from: Wesson, D.R., Ling, W. (2003). The Clinical Opiate Withdrawal Scale (COWS). *J Psychoactive Drugs*, 35, 253.

---

The patient is in mild opioid withdrawal. He asks for medical treatment for his withdrawal.

---

***What are the different settings for treatment of substance use disorders in older adults?***
A breadth of SUD treatment settings and approaches is available to older adults. These options include brief intervention in the primary care office; self-help, 12-step programs; weekly outpatient visits with mental health professionals; day or evening programs, including classes and groups; residential treatment ranging from several weeks to 6 to 12 months; and medical detoxification inpatient settings. It is important that providers know and discuss this continuum of care

TABLE 16.4 ■ **Psychosocial Modalities Available for Substance Use Disorder Treatment**

| Intervention | Goals for Treatment |
| --- | --- |
| Harm reduction:<br>• Legal diversion programs<br>• Community outreach<br>• Clean-needle and naloxone distribution<br>• Advocacy | • Reduce negative consequences associated with drug use<br>• Advocate for social justice in protecting the dignity and rights of people who use drugs<br>• Acknowledge the interplay of substance use and poverty, discrimination, and social inequalities<br>• Improve the quality of life of individual drug users and advance the well-being of their community as a whole |
| Self-help programs:<br>• Alcoholics anonymous<br>• Narcotics anonymous<br>• Life ring<br>• Self-management and recovery training | • Help patients find a community<br>• Peer-mentoring |
| Therapy:<br>• Motivational enhancement therapy<br>• Cognitive behavioral therapy<br>• Supportive therapy models | • Address ambivalence about change<br>• Develop coping skills<br>• Address cognitive distortions<br>• Offers guidance and encouragement |
| Case management | • Improve access to transportation and health care<br>• Address basic needs: shelter, nutrition, safety |

with patients. This education can help address patient fears that treatment will lead to loss of autonomy, which prevents patients from engaging in care.

### What psychosocial treatments are available?

There are a number of models and psychosocial approaches to SUD treatment that are outlined in Table 16.4. It is important for providers to recognize their own bias toward people who use drugs and the stigma or shame that patients experience if they relapse. Attention to addressing stigma and dispelling the notion of addiction as a moral failing is especially important in geriatric populations, who are more likely to experience or imagine SUD treatment as dehumanizing or degrading.

### What is medication-assisted therapy (MAT)?

Although patients and providers may only be familiar with psychosocial interventions, evidence shows that psychosocial treatment alone is less effective than combination treatment, which includes both psychosocial interventions and pharmacologic treatment.

Pharmacotherapy or medication-assisted therapy (MAT) can reduce cravings; improve relapse rates; reduce mortality from overdoses; and increase likelihood of abstinence, alone or in combination with psychosocial interventions. MAT is the first line in moderate and severe use disorders. Effective pharmacotherapy for opioid use disorders includes opioid replacement therapy, such methadone and buprenorphine.

---

**CLINICAL PEARL**                                                                      **STEP 1/2/3**

As a high-affinity partial mu receptor agonist, buprenorphine can induce opioid withdrawal symptoms if it is administered in patients who have recently taken alternative opioid drugs. Buprenorphine displaces these drugs off the mu receptor but induces less receptor activity.

| CLINICAL PEARL | STEP 2/3 |
|---|---|

Naloxone is an opioid receptor antagonist. It can be used to reverse opioid overdose.

Buprenorphine can be combined with naloxone in a sublingual formulation. When absorbed through the oral mucosa, very little of naloxone exhibits it mu-antagonistic effects. However, when the medication is crushed and taken via parenteral routes, then naloxone is activated and induces opioid withdrawal. This combination is meant to prevent diversion and drug abuse. It only can be prescribed by providers with a special license issued by the federal Drug Enforcement Administration.

Methadone is a full mu-receptor agonist with a long half-life, which can prevent withdrawal symptoms for 24 hours and provide steady control of cravings throughout the day. It is only administered in methadone clinics—that is, federally regulated opioid treatment programs (OTP). Methadone clinics incorporate psychosocial interventions and require daily attendance for the first several months, which leads to an excellent retention rate of 80% at 6 months.

Naltrexone is a mu-receptor opioid antagonist that decreases cravings, reducing relapse rates. Long-acting injectable naltrexone, but not oral naltrexone, has been shown to be better than placebo to treat opioid use disorder. However, naltrexone is less effective than buprenorphine or methadone. Patients who require opioid analgesia cannot use naltrexone.

All patients with an opioid use disorder should receive a home naloxone rescue kit, which can be administered by family members in case of an overdose.

---

The patient seeks residential SUD treatment given his moderate opioid use disorder. He starts oral naltrexone for the first few weeks of treatment; however, he has trouble remembering to take the medication every day and opts for a monthly long-acting naltrexone injection. After 30 days in residential treatment, the patient is discharged to the community where he remains sober from opioids. He continues his treatment with daily narcotics anonymous meetings, weekly visits with a therapist, and monthly meetings with a psychiatrist who continues to prescribe naltrexone.

---

## BEYOND THE PEARLS:

- Substance intoxication differs from substance-induced disorders in that with the latter, the substance has long been metabolized out of the patient's system and the patient is developing a new mental health diagnosis they did not have before.
- Fentanyl and carfentanyl are frequent impurities found in opioids sold on the street. They are thousands of times more potent than morphine and account for many overdoses.
- Naloxone can be intranasal or injectable, and harm reduction programs distribute it freely in many states.
- Methadone extends survival; when patients stop it, they have a high likelihood of relapsing, even 10 years after starting treatment.

## References

Kuerbis, A., Sacco, P., Blazer, D. G., & Moore, A. A. (2014). Substance abuse among older adults. *Clinics in Geriatric Medicine, 30*(3), 629–654.

Le Roux, C., Tang, Y. & Drexler, K. (2016). Alcohol and opioid use disorder in older adults: Neglected treatable illnesses. *Current Psychiatry Reports, 18*(9), 87.

Mattson, M., Lipari, R. N., Hays, C., & Van Horn, S. L. (2011). A day in the life of older adults: Substance use facts. *The CBHSQ Report:* May 11, 2017. Rockville, MD: Center for Behavioral Health Statistics and Quality, Substance Abuse and Mental Health Services Administration.

Schepis, T. S., McCabe, S. E., & Teter, C. J. (2018). Sources of opioid medication for misuse in older adults: results from a nationally representative survey. *Pain, 159*(8), 1543–1549.

Schepis, T. S., Simoni-Wastila, L., & McCabe, S. E. (2019). Prescription opioid and benzodiazepine misuse is associated with suicidal ideation in older adults. *International Journal of Geriatric Psychiatry, 34*(1), 122–129.

# CHAPTER 17

# Cluster A Personality Disorders

Meredith E. Harewood

A 26-year-old man presents to the psychiatry outpatient clinic for an evaluation. He is persuaded to go to the clinic by his older sister, who accompanies him. The sister is concerned because the patient has only a couple of friends whom he does not see very often, he has never had a girlfriend, and he seems uninterested in dating or expanding his social circle. She is worried that he is depressed or anxious, or worse. His sister notes that he has an "unhealthy obsession" with science fiction and has created intricate stories since he was young. She thinks that sometimes his characters are more real to him than people in the real world. Family history is pertinent for a maternal uncle with schizophrenia and a paternal cousin with social anxiety.

### What is the initial differential diagnosis based on this information?

Major depressive disorder or persistent depressive disorder can cause social withdrawal and lack of motivation. Anxiety disorders can also cause a person to become socially isolated, particularly with social anxiety disorder, which interferes with creating new friendships. Several aspects of an emerging psychotic disorder, such as schizophrenia or schizoaffective disorder, can cause social withdrawal, including paranoia, and lack of motivation to participate in activities (avolition), as well as a decreased desire to socialize (asociality). Individuals with autism spectrum disorder (ASD) often have deficits in social reciprocity that make it difficult to form close friendships. Many people with ASD are also uninterested in friendships. Avoidant personality disorder and schizoid personality disorder also feature a lack of close relationships.

### Is taking a developmental history appropriate?

Even in adult patients a developmental history can be illuminating in terms of early neurodevelopmental and social development, as well as for biologically based temperament, which tends to be relatively stable across a person's lifetime. Information about premorbid functioning—functioning before symptom onset—can be helpful in narrowing the differential diagnosis. In this patient it is of particular interest to discover if he had any developmental delays and if his social disinterest has existed since he was a small child.

The patient's sister does not recall their parents remarking on any delays in motor or language milestones. As a baby and toddler he seemed much the same as his two older siblings. Neither the sister nor the patient recall anything resembling odd, repetitive mannerisms or extremely restricted interests. He is the youngest of four children. Although he is very intelligent, the sister states her brother has been "clueless" about social interactions since he was a child, and he has always had difficulty making friends. The patient had a reputation for being "weird" in middle school and high school because of his odd style of dressing and poor attention to grooming. He is not particularly close with any of his siblings. He has always earned good grades in school and in college, and he is currently a graduate student in computer science at the local university.

*What questions should this patient be asked?*

Clinicians should screen for the major categories of anxiety, depression, and psychotic disorders. Because his sister is particularly concerned about social isolation, clinicians should ask the patient his view of social relationships and assess his social functioning in personal and occupational situations. Clinicians should assess his ability to perceive, interpret accurately, and respond to social cues, which are impaired in ASD. They should also assess his desire for social connectedness.

---

Alone, the patient confides that he only came here because his sister kept pestering him. He does not see that there is anything wrong with him and is content with his life. The patient did not volunteer any other information, so clinicians must follow up on the topics his sister mentioned. He has two friends with whom he plays board games and talks about programming and hard science. He is not interested in making more friends. He is also not interested in dating and does not really see himself getting married. He admits to some anxiety when speaking with people, but he does not think this impedes him in any way. He dislikes being in groups of people. Some of his colleagues complain he is too blunt, and his siblings say he is "socially inept." Although the patient respects the other people in his graduate program, he prefers to keep to himself because people generally want to "get into his business." He expresses distrust of large technology companies and the police; however, he thinks everyone in today's society has reason to fear and that he is not being singled out. He denies depression and derives enjoyment from his activities, especially his research and his extensive writing of science-fiction stories. He knows the characters in his writings are a product of his imagination, is not into the occult or paranormal phenomena, is not superstitious, and denies hallucinations. He lives alone in a studio apartment and handles his own finances.

On mental status examination, the patient is dressed in clothes that are clearly several years out of date, his jacket bears a large coffee stain, his socks are mismatched and his clothes are faintly malodorous. No abnormal movements are observed. He is reserved but talkative when addressing a topic he is passionate about. Eye contact is intermittent. His affect is restricted but not flat or blunted and mood is "good." His thought process is linear, and he answers all questions appropriately. He correctly states the day, date, time, location, and purpose of this visit. He is able to answer questions of abstraction (e.g., train and bicycle are both modes of transportation) correctly and accurately interprets a few proverbs. He does not display magical thinking and adds that these are silly questions to ask a graduate student.

---

*How has the differential diagnosis changed?*

His reality testing is intact; he denies hallucinations; and his speech is clear, organized, and linear. His affect is restricted, but it is somewhat reactive to the topic of conservation. His distrust of technology companies and the police is not because he thinks they are specifically targeting him and does not seem bizarre, therefore the distrust does not constitute persecutory or paranoid delusions. This eliminates a psychotic disorder. The patient is also a successful graduate student, which would be difficult if suffering from psychosis. He does not report sad moods or anhedonia (a reduction or lack of interest in pleasurable activities or an inability to derive enjoyment from previously pleasurable activities), which rules out depression, and he does not report significant anxiety. ASD, specifically high-functioning autism without intellectual or language impairment, remains on the differential, as does avoidant personality disorder. Clinicians should also consider the other cluster A personality disorders: paranoid personality disorder and schizotypal personality disorder.

---

The patient says that he is content to immerse himself in his studies, his research, online computer games, and his writing. He does not want his family to worry about him or his sister to keep pestering him to make friends and get a girlfriend; he likes being alone and this is just the way he is.

---

*What is the diagnosis, and what are the deciding factors?*

This young man is uninterested in close social relationships, appears odd and eccentric, and spends most of his time alone. Persons with avoidant personality disorder are socially inhibited

TABLE 17.1 ■ Characteristics of Schizoid Personality Disorder

- Pervasive pattern of detachment from social relationships
- Little or no desire for or enjoyment from close relationships, including being part of a family
- A restricted, or narrow, range of emotional expression (affect) in interpersonal settings, appearing cold, aloof, or detached
- Little or no desire for sexual experiences
- Typically chooses solitary activities and engages in few activities
- Lacks close friends or confidants other than first-degree relatives
- Appears indifferent to the opinions of others
- The symptoms do not occur exclusively during a psychotic disorder, a mood disorder, or autism spectrum disorder, or during another medical condition

because they are extremely self-critical and hypersensitive to rejection and criticism. However, they typically yearn for closer relationships.

This patient has schizoid personality disorder. These individuals lack a desire for social connectedness and intimacy, therefore they usually lack close friends or confidants and typically rarely have romantic or sexual relationships. These individuals may be seen as "loners," eccentric, or socially awkward. They appear unconcerned about or indifferent to what others think of them, including praise or criticism; consequently, they can appear aloof and are often indifferent to their appearance in terms of fashion or grooming. They prefer activities and employment that are mechanical, involve numbers, or are abstract, such as mathematics or computer games. They also choose jobs that do not involve competition or much social interaction, such as positions where they work night shifts. These individuals have a narrow range of emotional expression, and their facial expressions can appear "bland." They often do not reciprocate social gestures and exchanges, such as waves, nods, and smiles. Some persons with schizoid personality can have rich fantasy lives. Table 17.1 summarizes the characteristics of schizoid personality disorder.

| BASIC SCIENCE PEARL | STEP 1 |
| --- | --- |

In order to diagnose a personality disorder, a person's pattern of relating to the world and inner experience must be pervasive, begin by early adulthood, be stable over time and inflexible, and be present in a variety of contexts.

### Why is it important to ask his sister additional questions?

The patient's statement that he does not perceive a problem illustrates the importance of obtaining collateral information from a family member, spouse, or someone else who knows the patient well when the clinician expects a personality disorder. Although these patterns of traits seem maladaptive, problematic, or distressing to those around them, individuals with personality disorders often find these traits ego-syntonic and therefore do not portray them as problems. Oftentimes, personality-disordered individuals do not present for treatment at all.

### What is the development, course, and prognosis of schizoid personality disorder?

Schizoid personality disorder usually begins in early childhood and typically persists throughout a person's life. Most individuals function fairly well in terms of their work and activities of daily living, and therefore do not have many problems that require psychiatric attention. Indeed, like the patient who only came in at the behest of his sister, most people with schizoid personality do not seek mental health treatment and do not engage in therapy. Therapy is the treatment of choice, typically supportive therapy and sometimes group therapy aimed at modeling or actively building social skills. Family therapy may also be helpful to enhance understanding

---

### TABLE 17.2 ■ Characteristics of Paranoid Personality Disorder

- Pervasive pattern of distrust and suspiciousness of others.
- Suspects with little basis that others are exploiting, deceiving, or undermining them.
- Constantly doubts the loyalty or trustworthiness of friends or associates such as coworkers.
- Perceives personal slights or malevolent intentions in benign comments, motives, or events.
- Reluctant to confide in others for fear the information will be used against him or her.
- Recurrent suspiciousness about a significant other's or sexual partner's fidelity.
- The symptoms do not occur exclusively during a psychotic disorder, a mood disorder, or autism spectrum disorder, or during another medical condition.

---

among family members and reduce any intrusiveness and intolerance that may exacerbate the patient's withdrawal.

*How does schizoid personality disorder compare to paranoid personality disorder?*
In contrast with schizoid personality disorder, persons with paranoid personality disorder have more social involvement, they care greatly what others think about them, and are chronically and pervasively suspicious of other people.

Individuals with paranoid personality disorder are extremely sensitive to slights and often misperceive benign interactions as malicious, deceptive, or exploitative. They perceive attacks on their reputation or character that are not intended or apparent and can lash out angrily if challenged or stressed. They interpret "hidden meanings" in interactions and hold grudges. They frequently display intense jealousy in romantic relationships and question the loyalty of friends, associates, and significant others. They can appear to others as cold and unemotional; consequently, they are often socially isolated and avoid intimacy. Like schizoid personality disorder, persons with paranoid personality disorder can seem unemotional or affectively restricted and socially isolated and have few close friends. However, individuals with schizoid personality disorder usually do not have prominent paranoid ideation. Inherent mistrust of others means that patients with paranoid personality disorder usually do not initiate treatment. Table 17.2 summarizes the characteristics of paranoid personality disorder. Cognitive-behavioral interventions may be useful.

---

| BASIC SCIENCE/CLINICAL PEARL | STEP 1/2/3 |
|---|---|

If paranoia, hypervigilance, and suspiciousness appear only after a traumatic event, consider posttraumatic stress disorder.

---

*How does schizoid personality compare to schizotypal personality disorder?*
Individuals with schizotypal personality disorder have social and interpersonal deficits because of marked anxiety in social situations; discomfort in relating to others; peculiar beliefs, thinking, and behavior; and perceptual distortions.

Magical thinking, perceptual distortions, and strange beliefs in phenomena, such as the occult, telepathy, and the paranormal, that is outside of cultural norms are the hallmarks of this disorder. Individuals with schizotypal personality disorder may have odd thinking and speech patterns (e.g., vague, convoluted). They can also have few close relationships outside of first-degree relatives, as in schizoid individuals. In contrast to individuals with schizoid personality disorder, individuals with schizotypal personality disorder can have impaired reality testing and strange thought processes. Unlike schizophrenia, complaints of depression and anxiety are high in individuals with schizotypal, which is often the presenting complaint. Table 17.3 summarizes the characteristics of schizotypal personality disorder.

#### TABLE 17.3 ■ Characteristics of Schizotypal Personality Disorder

- Pervasive pattern of cognitive or perceptual distortions and eccentric or odd behavior
- Odd beliefs or magical thinking that influences behavior
- Unusual perceptual experiences
- Odd thinking and speech
- Ideas of reference, suspiciousness, or paranoid ideation
- Excessive social anxiety or discomfort in social settings that is associated with paranoia rather than the fear of social judgment
- Inappropriate or constricted affect
- The symptoms do not occur exclusively during a psychotic disorder, a mood disorder, or autism spectrum disorder, or during another medical condition

Low-dose antipsychotic medications have been shown to be effective for the cognitive and perceptual aspects of this disorder in placebo-controlled trials. Useful therapy modalities include supportive therapy, cognitive-behavioral interventions, and group therapy focused on social skills. The course of the disorder is fairly stable, with only a small percentage of patients eventually developing schizophrenia.

***What are some other commonalities between the cluster A personality disorders?***
As children and adolescents, all groups have poor peer relationships, social anxiety, underachievement in school, and can appear odd and therefore attract teasing by peers. Individuals with any cluster A disorder can have temporary, brief psychotic states if overly stressed. There is a higher incidence of psychotic disorders in relatives of people with cluster A personality disorders. It is highest in schizotypal personality disorder.

***Are there any other nonpersonality disorder psychiatric disorders to consider?***
Autism spectrum disorder (ASD), without language or intellectual impairment—also referred to as *high-functioning* or *mild* autism—can be very difficult to distinguish from schizoid personality disorder. This includes many individuals formerly diagnosed with Asperger syndrome, which was removed from the *Diagnostic and Statistical Manual of Mental Disorders*, Fifth edition (DSM-5). Individuals with Asperger are now typically diagnosed with ASD or another developmental disorder. This is when an early developmental history from a parent, caregiver, or an older sibling can be very helpful. Generally, in ASD, individuals are more socially impaired, may have strange or idiosyncratic language or speech, and have more severely restricted interests. Adolescents and adults with high-functioning autism may have had more severe impairment and more symptoms and stereotyped behaviors (repetitive, typically purposeless movements, also referred to as *self-stimulatory* or *stimming* behaviors, such as hand flapping) as children, which resolved with maturity or therapeutic intervention.

---

**BEYOND THE PEARLS:**

What else should I consider before diagnosing a personality disorder?
- **Culture and religion**: There are some accepted cultural beliefs and practices, such as shamanism, spirits, reincarnation, and magical beliefs, related to illness and health that can resemble schizotypal beliefs and behaviors.
- **Special populations**: Minority groups and certain oppressed populations often have historical reasons to be suspicious of members of the majority ethnic group, authority, or the medical establishment.
- **Age**: In elderly individuals, personality change can occur with dementias and phenotypically resemble a personality disorder.
- **Comorbid medical conditions**: Postictal states in epilepsy, personality change occurring after stroke or head injury.

The young man agrees to attend a social skills group so he can learn some techniques to improve his relationships with his graduate school professors and colleagues. He declines to start individual therapy.

## References

American Psychiatric Association. (2013). *Diagnostic and statistical manual of mental disorders* (5th ed.). Washington, DC: Author.

Maytal, G., & Smallwood, P. (2012). Personality disorders. In T. Stern, J. Herman, & T. Gorrindo (Eds.), *Massachusetts General Hospital psychiatry update and board preparation* (3rd ed., pp. 207–213). Boston, MA: Massachusetts General Hospital Psychiatry Academy Publishing.

Weissman, S. H. (2018). Personality disorders. In M. H. Ebert, J. F. Leckman, I. L. Petrakis (Eds.), *Current Diagnosis & Treatment: Psychiatry* (3rd ed.). New York, NY: McGraw-Hill.

# CHAPTER 18

# Cluster B Personality Disorders

Jessica Dotson ■ Christian Gerwe

A 21-year-old female presents to the emergency department with arm lacerations. She reports a long history of psychiatric illness and says she has been diagnosed with bipolar disorder, posttraumatic stress disorder, attention-deficit hyperactivity disorder (ADHD), depression, and anxiety. She has tried numerous psychotropic medications, all of which have been unsuccessful in treating her symptoms. She feels unable to function in society and recently dropped out of college and moved back home to live with her mother. She constantly worries about how others perceive her and worries that the people closest to her will abandon her or hurt her. She states, "People are always out to get me." She also experiences frequent nightmares and an increased startle response. The arm lacerations did not require suturing, routine laboratory studies are ordered, and a psychiatry consult is placed.

### What is the first step in evaluating this patient?

Initial steps of a full psychiatric evaluation include obtaining a thorough history from the patient, obtaining information from collateral individuals (such as family, friends, or outpatient providers), and review of basic laboratory studies to rule out medical causes for presenting symptoms. This patient's medical workup was within normal limits. Given the patient presented with concerns of people being out to get her, abandon her, or hurt her, it is important to determine whether she is acutely psychotic and responding to internal stimuli during the evaluation. Her mental status examination revealed a linear thought process, she was able to respond to questions appropriately, and she did not endorse auditory or visual hallucinations, illusions, or delusions. Given she is not demonstrating overt paranoia, it is likely that she is exhibiting a defense mechanism known as *projection*, which is common in patients with personality disorders (particularly borderline personality disorder and narcissistic personality disorder). Projection occurs when an individual's unwanted feelings, or characteristics that the individual finds unacceptable in his/herself, are displaced onto someone else. Patients with borderline personality disorder often fear abandonment from loved ones and project this fear by accusing those close to them of planning to abandon them or hurt them in some manner. Projection is often a component of paranoia in patients with psychotic disorders and contributes to the delusions associated with paranoia. Paranoia itself is composed of multiple other characteristics, including reality distortion and disorders of reasoning, which this patient does not demonstrate.

Upon further discussion with the patient, she reports a long history of interpersonal conflicts, most recently with her significant other and her mother's boyfriend. The patient has been feeling very alone and unable to care for herself, and she has felt depressed off and on for many years, which has worsened since going to college. During her first semester of college, she started cutting herself during periods of stress. This provided a sense of relief. She states, "I have mood swings all the time," elaborating that she feels sad one minute, angry the next, and then becomes hyperactive. She cycles through these emotions numerous times a day. She states further, "No one understands my bipolar disorder."

*What is the differential diagnosis?*
The differential diagnosis includes anxiety disorders, depressive disorders, psychotic disorders, posttraumatic stress disorder, substance use disorders, borderline personality disorder, and symptoms related to another medical condition. Patients with borderline personality disorder are frequently misdiagnosed with bipolar disorder. They often have a history of numerous psychiatric diagnoses, which is evident with this patient. They typically have symptoms that are characteristic of many psychiatric illnesses, but may not meet full diagnostic criteria for each individual condition. It is also common for patients to have other comorbid psychiatric illness.

The most likely diagnosis for this patient is borderline personality disorder. According to the *Diagnostic and Statistical Manual of Mental Disorders*, Fifth Edition (DSM-5), a person must have a long history of unstable interpersonal relationships, fluctuating self-image, and volatile changes in affect. These individuals are also impulsive. The symptoms start in early adulthood and occur in a variety of settings. For the diagnosis, the patient must experience five or more of the following:

- Extreme efforts to avoid feeling abandoned, whether real or imagined
- History of intense close relationships that are not stable, marked by alternations between extremes of idealizing the other person and devaluing them (splitting)
- Persistent instability of self-image or sense of self (identity disturbance)
- Being impulsive in at least two areas that are potentially harmful to self (e.g., sexual indiscretions, substance use, overspending)
- Recurrent suicidal behaviors and/or threatening suicide, which can also include self-harming behavior, such as cutting or burning
- Affective instability (severe mood swings)
- Feeling empty
- Trouble controlling anger (short-tempered)
- Brief paranoid ideation (caused by stressful situations) or severe dissociation (feeling disconnected from reality)

---

**CLINICAL PEARL**                                                                 **STEP 1/2/3**

It is important to distinguish mood lability, which is a characteristic of mood disorders (such as bipolar disorder), from affective instability, which is a trait often seen in personality disorders (particularly borderline personality disorder). Mood lability is described as a rapid oscillation of mood that fluctuates between euthymia (normal mood), depression, and elation. The mood states occur over a period of days to weeks. This mood shifting results in the characteristic depressive and/or manic episodes seen in bipolar disorder. Affective instability is defined as rapid (moment-to-moment) affect shifting with random patterns and dysregulation of emotions. These changes can occur multiple times per day, as seen in this case. Affective instability is often misattributed to the common sign of mood lability seen in bipolar disorder.

---

*What are additional considerations for this patient?*
It is imperative to discuss medical history and presenting symptoms as well as her current emotional state. There may be medical comorbidities that could be missed if the evaluation is too focused on the psychiatric presentation. In addition, medical illnesses or physical ailments may influence psychiatric symptoms and vice versa.

---

The patient's medical history includes migraines, heartburn, and vague diffuse muscle pain. Current medications are topiramate, venlafaxine, aripiprazole, trazodone, prazosin, omeprazole, and ibuprofen. Prior medications included hydroxyzine, buspirone, clonazepam, melatonin, fluoxetine, citalopram, quetiapine, and an unspecified stimulant.

In addition to having numerous psychiatric diagnoses, patients with borderline personality disorder will often have numerous medical conditions as well. At times the conditions will interfere with seeking treatment or with adhering to a psychiatric treatment regimen. This can often lead to polypharmacy. As seen with this case, individuals with cluster B personality disorders are often prescribed psychotropic medications from a variety of classes (such as mood stabilizers, antidepressants, anxiolytics, or antipsychotics). The reasons for this are multifactorial in nature but in part arise from diagnostic uncertainty (particularly in the initial stages of treatment) and attempting to target the wide array of symptoms that a patient with borderline personality disorder will often present with. Pharmacotherapy is particularly useful in managing the features of the personality disorder that interfere with functioning.

The patient has had two inpatient psychiatric admissions (at age 16, after an overdose on Tylenol, and at age 18, after self-inflicted arm lacerations). She reports that these hospitalizations were not particularly helpful to her. She sees a psychiatrist every 1 to 2 months and does not have a current therapist. She tells you that psychotherapy has been of minimal benefit in the past and says, "I know you will be great, because I know you'll really be able to understand me and all that I've been through." She reports prior conflicts with every therapist she has met because "no one understands me." Family history reveals that her mother has migraines, fibromyalgia, anxiety, and a history of multiple suicide attempts. She does not know her biological father. She uses marijuana daily for her anxiety and denies other illicit substance use. She is an only child and reports that her mother drank alcohol a lot and had numerous boyfriends when she was growing up. One of her mother's boyfriends sexually abused the patient from ages 5 to 12. When she told her mother about the abuse, her mother blamed the patient. They have subsequently had a tumultuous relationship.

Ego defenses are conscious or unconscious mental processes used during periods of conflict to prevent unwanted emotions. Individuals with personality disorders typically exhibit maladaptive or immature defenses. The patient in this case is using the defense mechanism known as *splitting* in an attempt to resolve the current conflict and unwanted thoughts and emotions. This defense mechanism is frequently used and is the belief that someone is either all good or all bad (that same person may vary between the two extremes depending on the circumstance). There is rarely a gray area or ambiguity. Another mechanism frequently used in those with borderline personality disorder is reaction formation. This occurs when a thought or emotion is replaced by the opposite thought or emotion and is an unconsciously derived process. Some of the other frequently used defense mechanisms include fantasy, dissociation, isolation, projection, passive aggression, acting out, and projective identification. Personality disorders are ego-syntonic (acceptable to the ego) and alloplastic (try to alter external factors instead of themselves; external locus of control).

The term *personality* refers to an individual's traits, both emotional and behavioral, that adapt to one's environment. Personality disorders develop when these traits become maladaptive. In general, personality disorders are inflexible and pervasive, lead to impairment or distress, are long-standing, have a pattern of behavior that deviates from cultural norms, and manifest in a variety of ways (cognition, affectivity, interpersonal functioning, and impulse control).

The personality disorders are divided into clusters, each with typical characteristics. Cluster A personality types are also known as *eccentric* or *weird*, whereas cluster C personality types are

TABLE 18.1 ■ Cluster B Personality Types

| Disorder | Key Features |
|---|---|
| Borderline personality disorder | Mood instability, unstable relationships, identity instability, impulsivity, feelings of emptiness, often a history of self-harm and suicidal ideation. Use splitting as defense mechanism. Females > males |
| Histrionic personality disorder | Attention seeking, emotional, sexual provocativeness, overly concerned with appearance. Females > males |
| Narcissistic personality disorder | Grandiosity, require admiration, lack empathy, sense of entitlement, react poorly to criticism |
| Antisocial personality disorder | Impulsive, lack remorse, violate rights of others. There must be evidence of conduct disorder symptoms before age 15. Males > females |

described as *worried*. Borderline personality disorder is within cluster B, which is considered the *wild* group. Other disorders within this cluster division include narcissistic personality disorder, histrionic personality disorder, and antisocial personality disorder. Collectively individuals with one of the cluster B personality disorders may be described as dramatic, emotional, or erratic (see Table 18.1).

The patient denies current suicidal ideation and denies that the self-inflicted arm lacerations were performed with intent to die. Rather, she elaborates that she cut herself after an argument with her significant other out of anger. She states that she has a job interview in 2 days and does not want to be admitted to the hospital. Her mother corroborates the patient's description of events leading up to admission and does not think the patient was attempting to kill herself. She does not think the patient needs to be admitted to the hospital. There are no firearms in the home. Voluntary psychiatric admission is offered, but she declines. A safety plan is discussed with both the patient and mother, and she is subsequently discharged from the emergency room with a follow-up appointment scheduled with her psychiatrist. She is encouraged to resume therapy.

Personality disorders are typically diagnosed in early adulthood, but traits may be seen as early as adolescence. If a diagnosis is made before age 18, the traits should be present for at least 1 year (with the exception of antisocial personality disorder, which can only be diagnosed after age 18). An individual with a personality disorder will typically have fluctuations in the level of impairment that will likely persist throughout life. In those with borderline personality disorder or antisocial personality disorder, the traits may be less evident (or even remit) with age if there are stabilizing factors that arise, such as a stable relationship or job stability. The personality traits should be persistent over time and be evident across different settings in order for a diagnosis of a personality disorder to be made. It may require many observations by a clinician to accurately make the diagnosis. The primary treatment approach is psychotherapy; however, pharmacotherapy is often used for comorbid mood, anxiety, or psychotic symptoms. Often patients will have comorbid psychiatric illnesses, and the personality disorder may interfere with appropriate treatment for them. There is a particularly high incidence of comorbid major depressive disorder. The mainstay of treatment for borderline personality disorder is dialectical behavior therapy (DBT). However, other forms of therapeutic interventions include transference-focused psychotherapy, psychodynamic psychotherapy, and supportive psychotherapy. These therapies show varying levels of success in this patient population.

Individuals with borderline personality disorder will often be evaluated in an emergency room setting in an acute crisis or as a result of an impulsive act. It is then imperative to perform a thorough risk assessment to determine an appropriate disposition. Both risk factors and protective factors should be considered. With the patient in the case, primary risk factors include impulsivity, a prior suicide attempt, family history of suicide attempt, and access to means of harm by knives or medications. Protective factors were lack of current suicidal ideation, future-oriented thought process with identifiable goals, presenting symptoms without potential lethality (did not require sutures), and a collateral person who felt the patient would be safe. Although this patient declined admission, it is common for patients with borderline personality disorder to be admitted to psychiatric units for crisis stabilization. The prevalence of borderline personality disorder is estimated to be 20% of all psychiatric hospitalized patients. Hospitalization can be beneficial, especially in the initial stages of observation and treatment, but can also evolve into a maladaptive coping strategy over time.

**BEYOND THE PEARLS:**

- Studies have evaluated the clinical benefit of lamotrigine for borderline personality disorder, with results that have not shown a significant benefit. However, more studies need to be performed.
- Some patients with borderline personality disorder may have shortened REM latency, disturbance of sleep maintenance, abnormal dexamethasone suppression test (DST), and abnormal thyrotropin-releasing hormone test results. Similar findings are found in depressive disorders.
- Mentalization-based treatment (MBT) focuses on an individual being attentive to his/her mental states and the states of others, which is a key component of interpersonal interactions. It is believed that if a patient with borderline personality disorder can improve mentalization, then the person will be better able to regulate thoughts and emotions. There have been randomized, controlled research trials that have shown this treatment to be effective for borderline personality disorder.
- Studies have demonstrated an association between cannabis use and borderline personality traits in young adults. In addition, it has been shown that cannabis use in adolescence is related to depressive and anxious symptom development and chronicity.

## References

American Psychiatric Association. (2013). Personality disorders. *Diagnostic and statistical manual of mental disorders,* (5th ed.). Washington, DC: Author.

Crawford, M. J., Sanatinia, R., Barrett, B., Cunningham, G., Dale, O., Ganguli, P., ... LABILE study team. (2018). The clinical effectiveness and cost-effectiveness of lamotrigine in borderline personality disorder: A randomized placebo-controlled trial. *American Journal of Psychiatry, 175*(8), 756–764.

Heilbrun, A. B., Diller, R. S., & Dodson, V. S. (1986). Defensive projection and paranoid delusions. *Journal of Psychiatric Research, 20*(3), 161–173.

Perry, J. C., Presniak, M. D., & Olson, T. R. (2013). Defense mechanisms in schizotypal, borderline, antisocial, and narcissistic personality disorders. *Psychiatry, 76*(1), 32–52.

Raynal, P., & Chabrol, H. (2016). Association between schizotypal and borderline personality disorder traits, and cannabis use in young adults. *Addictive Behaviors, 50,* 144.

Renaud, S. M., & Zacchia, C. (2012). Toward a definition of affective instability. *Harvard Review of Psychiatry, 20*(6), 298–308.

Sadock BJ, Sadock VA, Ruiz P. (2014). Personality disorders. In *Kaplan & Sadock's synopsis of psychiatry: Behavioral sciences/clinical psychiatry* (11th ed.) Philadelphia, PA: Wolters Kluwer.

Subramaniam, P., Rogowska, J., Dimuzio, J., Lopez-Larson, M., McGlade, E., & Yurgelun-Todd, D. (2018). Orbitofrontal connectivity is associated with depression and anxiety in marijuana-using adolescents. *Journal of Affective Disorders, 239,* 234–241.

Tao, L., Bhushan, V., Chen, V. L., & King, M. R. (2016). *First aid for the USMLE step 2 CK* (9th ed.). New York, NY: McGraw-Hill Education.

Tao, L., & Bhushan, V. (2017). *First aid for the USMLE step 1 2017.* New York, NY: McGraw-Hill Education.

# CHAPTER 19

# Cluster C Personality Disorders

Courtney Eaves

---

A 23-year-old graduate student, who is in her first semester of pharmacy school, presents to the student mental health clinic at the request of her parents. She complains of having consistent problems turning in assignments on time and is now failing several classes. This has caused more stress, which only seems to be worsening the problems she is having with school. She is spending an excessive amount of time on school at the expense of her interpersonal relationships.

---

*What other information is important to know?*

Obtaining more detailed information about the presenting complaint is the most important first step. Asking why the patient is having trouble turning in assignments is critical in determining the next steps in treatment for this patient. Additionally, you would want to gather a thorough psychiatric and medical history (as well as screening for both depression and anxiety).

---

When the patient starts an assignment, she has a very specific way of studying the information, which includes rewriting much of the information and then highlighting it in multiple colors. She explains this process to you in great detail. She has a few friends and is dating a fellow student but reports her primary focus is school, often at the expense of her social life. She speaks of her boyfriend in a formal and serious manner and her affect is constricted. She endorses some anxiety about her grades and school and also seems to worry about other aspects of her life. She reports no medical issues and no significant psychiatric history.

---

*You suspect the patient is suffering from obsessive-compulsive personality disorder; what other questions should be asked to confirm the diagnosis?*

The patient is presenting with several criteria for this diagnosis, including preoccupation with lists and organization, perfectionism interfering with task completion, and an excess devotion to work/school. Additional criteria to ask about, that may be interfering with her functioning, include being inflexible about morals and ethics, being very careful about spending money, having trouble throwing out items of insignificance, and having difficulty working in groups because others will not do things her way. She may come across as stubborn to others because of her rigidity in thinking.

TABLE 19.1 ■ **Distinguishing OCPD from OCD**

| Obsessive-Compulsive Personality Disorder | Obsessive-Compulsive Disorder |
| --- | --- |
| Preoccupation with order and perfectionism, inflexibility, difficulty working with others due to lack of control | Irrational thoughts and behaviors that are repeated over and over |
| Behaviors persistent and unchanged over time | Symptoms tend to fluctuate over time |
| Belief that their behaviors serve a positive purpose in their lives | Patients distressed by their obsessions and/or compulsions |
| Less likely to seek professional help | Often seek professional help |

*How is obsessive-compulsive personality disorder distinguished from obsessive-compulsive disorder (see Table 19.1)?*

---

**CLINICAL PEARL**                                                            STEP 2/3

OCPD is *ego-syntonic*, meaning the feelings and behaviors are in harmony with the patient's own goals and self-image, whereas OCD is *ego-dystonic*, meaning the accompanying obsessions and/or compulsions are in conflict with the person's needs or self-image. This explains why those with OCD often seek treatment on their own, whereas those with OCPD may take more time to realize the need for intervention by a physician or therapist.

---

You assess for the above-mentioned aspects of this disorder. The patient tells you that she was recently assigned a group project (due next week), and she is having significant difficulty working with the others because they have their own ideas and plans for the project. She feels unable to control the project or work with the other members. She would much prefer to complete the assignment alone. You discuss with the patient her preliminary diagnosis and go over the treatment options.

*What are the treatment options for OCPD?*

Psychotherapy is the mainstay of treatment for OCPD. Both cognitive-behavioral therapy (CBT) and psychodynamic therapy can be helpful. Increasing insight into behaviors, and how those behaviors affect the person, is one of the most important aspects of therapy. Because people with this disorder generally lack flexibility in daily routines and in expectations of others, therapy can be quite difficult at times. If there is comorbid depression or anxiety (because of how this disorder is negatively affecting life), an antidepressant medication may also be prescribed.

*What are the most common defense mechanisms used in obsessive-compulsive personality disorder that can be addressed in therapy (see Table 19.2)?*

---

Your patient starts going to psychotherapy and focuses on the relationship between her thoughts, feelings, and behaviors. She is able to gain more insight into why she has difficulty working with others in a group setting, as well as how to study more effectively (e.g., purposefully cutting out excessive list making and highlighting). She also begins to make a conscious effort at interpersonal relationships and reports to her therapist weekly on how this is going. The patient and her psychiatrist also agree on starting an SSRI for the patient's continued anxiety surrounding school.

TABLE 19.2 ■ Defense Mechanisms in OCPD

| Defense Mechanism | Definition | Example |
|---|---|---|
| Rationalization | Attempting to explain or justify behavior or an attitude with logical reasons, even if these are not appropriate | A college student constantly cancels plans with friends and blames it on having too much schoolwork to do |
| Intellectualization | Reasoning is used to block confrontation with an unconscious conflict and its associated emotional stress | A person told they have cancer asks for details on the probability of survival and the success rates of various drugs |
| Reaction formation | Acting in the opposite manner to disturbing or socially unacceptable thoughts or emotions | A young woman who feels she may be gay joins a very conservative church |
| Isolation of affect | Attempting to avoid a painful thought or feeling by objectifying and emotionally detaching oneself from the feeling | Someone fails a major test but shows minimal or no outward emotion of the disappointment |
| Undoing | Trying to reverse or "undo" a thought or feeling by performing an action that signifies an opposite feeling than the original thought or feeling | A person strongly dislikes someone and then buys the person a gift |

---

**CLINICAL PEARL** | **STEP 2/3**

OCPD is part of the cluster C personality disorders that are generally characterized as anxious and fearful disorders (or "worried"). People with any of the cluster C personality disorders all have an overwhelming level of anxiety.

---

*What are the other cluster C personality disorders and how would you diagnose and treat them?*

The three personality disorders in this cluster are avoidant, dependent, and obsessive-compulsive personality disorders. *Avoidant personality disorder* involves a patient being hypersensitive to rejection and often misinterpreting social cues because of low self-esteem. This leads to a lack of close friendships and feelings of loneliness. These patients often will not seek out new friendships or put themselves in social situations because of fear of not being liked. Those with *dependent personality disorder* feel that they must rely on others for help with decision-making and constantly worry about loss or abandonment from those they are close to. They may stay in abusive or neglectful relationships because of this fear. As with OCPD, avoidant and dependent personality disorders are treated with psychotherapy primarily. Often antidepressants, particularly SSRIs, are prescribed for associated anxiety or depression that accompanies the personality disorder.

*What is the cause of cluster C personality disorders?*

There is no known cause of cluster C disorders, but there appears to be a genetic association related to family members with anxiety disorders. It is common to find a first-degree relative with an anxiety disorder when conducting a thorough family history.

*How can you differentiate avoidant personality disorder from schizoid personality disorder?*

Those with schizoid personality disorder voluntarily choose to withdraw socially and maintain few friendships. Those with avoidant personality disorder have a desire for social relationships but find establishing and maintaining these relationships very difficult because of fear of rejection and feelings of inadequacy.

**CLINICAL PEARL**                                                                      **STEP 2/3**

Those with avoidant personality disorder want friends but are too anxious to make and keep relationships, whereas those with schizoid personality disorder are okay with not having friends and often appear indifferent and apathetic.

**BEYOND THE PEARLS:**

- OCPD is diagnosed twice as much in men versus women.
- OCPD is the most common personality disorder with a prevalence of 7% to 8% in the general population.
- Prevalence of avoidant personality disorder is about 2%.
- Prevalence of dependent personality disorder is about 0.5% to 1%.
- All personality disorders, including those in cluster C, must develop by early adulthood.

## References

American Psychiatric Association. (2013). *Diagnostic and statistical manual of mental disorders* (5th ed.). Washington, DC: Author.

Diedrich, A., & Voderholzer, U. (2015). Obsessive-compulsive personality disorder: A current review. *Current Psychiatry Reports, 17*(2), 2.

First, M. B., Williams, J. B. W., Karg, R. S., & Spitzer, R. L. (2015). *Structured clinical interview for DSM-5 disorders, clinician version (SCID-5-CV)*. Washington, DC: American Psychiatric Association.

Gordon, O. M., Salkovskis, P. M., Oldfield, V. B., & Carter, N. (2013). The association between obsessive compulsive disorder and obsessive compulsive personality disorder: Prevalence and clinical presentation. *British Journal of Clinical Psychology, 52*(3), 300–315.

Grant, J. E. (2014). Clinical practice: Obsessive-compulsive disorder. *New England Journal of Medicine, 371*(7), 646–653.

McMain, S., & Pos, A. E. (2007). Advances in psychotherapy of personality disorders: A research update. *Current Psychiatry Reports, 9*, 46–52.

Torgersen, S., Kringlen, E., & Cramer, V. (2001). The prevalence of personality disorders in a community sample. *Archives of General Psychology, 58*(6), 590–596.

# CHAPTER 20

# Eating Disorders

Olesya Pokorna

A 15-year-old-female is brought into a primary care clinic by her parents for amenorrhea. Her menstrual cycle has been regular until about 3 months ago, and she denies being sexually active. She is an aspiring ballet dancer and reports being under a lot of pressure to join a prestigious company after graduating from high school. She watches her weight closely and restricts her diet to green vegetables and small amounts of lean protein. Over the past several months, she has been reducing portion sizes because of fear of gaining weight before an upcoming ballet competition. Past medical history is unremarkable. On physical examination, her blood pressure is 98/50 mm Hg, pulse rate is 56 beats/min, respiration rate is 12/min, temperature is 95°F, and body mass index (BMI) is 17.5 kg/m2. She appears cachectic, and her skin is cold, dry, and covered with fine, downy hair. The rest of the examination is normal, and the pregnancy test is negative.

### How do you diagnose anorexia nervosa?

According to the *Diagnostic and Statistical Manual of Mental Disorders*, Fifth Edition (DSM-5), anorexia nervosa is diagnosed when a patient manifests restriction of food intake leading to abnormally low body weight, intense fear of gaining weight, and distorted body image. People suffering from this condition usually have low insight into severity of their condition and are resistant to treatment. The DSM-5 distinguishes two subtypes of anorexia nervosa: binge-eating/purging and restrictive. A BMI less than 18.5 kg/m2 serves as a cutoff for abnormally low weight in adults. Anorexia nervosa occurs in less than 1% of the general population, with female to male ratio of 10:1. The exact mechanism of illness is not known, but clustering of this eating behavior within families points toward genetic inheritance. There is a high prevalence of psychiatric comorbidities in anorexia nervosa, including major depression, anxiety, alcohol use disorder, personality disorders, and increased prevalence of suicidality. Anorexia nervosa usually starts in adolescence or early adulthood, can be insidious, and is sometimes triggered by a stressful life event. The disease has a chronic course and results in high rates of mortality. Personality traits, such as perfectionism, high levels of harm avoidance, competitiveness, and neuroticism, are commonly seen in patients with anorexia.

---

**CLINICAL PEARL**                                                    STEP 1/2/3

**Diagnostic criteria for anorexia nervosa**

- Persistent restriction of food intake leading to abnormally low body weight
- Intense fear of gaining weight
- Distorted body image
- Subtypes include restricting type and binge-eating/purging type

---

*What is on your differential diagnosis?*

Bulimia nervosa is characterized by binge-eating/purging behaviors consisting of episodic over-eating and compensatory behaviors such as self-induced vomiting, laxative or diuretic abuse, and excessive exercise. However, unlike anorexia nervosa, diagnosis of bulimia nervosa does not require abnormally low weight; in fact, people with this condition usually have normal or above normal BMIs. In contrast to bulimia nervosa, binge eating disorder is characterized by binging episodes without compensatory behaviors.

| CLINICAL PEARL | STEP 1/2/3 |
|---|---|

Although purging is thought of as a hallmark of bulimia nervosa, patients with anorexia frequently engage in this behavior as well. Below normal body mass index (BMI) distinguishes anorexia from bulimia. Patients with binge-eating disorder have episodes of binges without compensatory behaviors.

When evaluating an underweight patient with suspected anorexia, consider other psychiatric and medical disorders, which can present as weight loss, malnutrition, and fear of weight gain, such as malabsorption syndromes, neoplasms, chronic infections, hyperthyroidism, or delusional or psychotic disorder characterized by paranoia about food intake or fears of being poisoned.

*What are the common findings on a physical examination?*

Patients with anorexia nervosa may present with various degrees of cachexia. Vital sign changes include hypotension, bradycardia, and hypothermia. Other signs may include dry, scaly skin with bluish discoloration, bruising, lanugo hair, and brittle hair and nails. Fingers on the dominant hand may have calluses from self-induced vomiting, also called "Russel's sign." Patients with purging behaviors may have swollen parotid and submandibular glands, and dental examination may reveal enamel erosion and dental cavities. Muscle atrophy and peripheral edema may be present, and heart murmur from mitral valve prolapse may also be appreciated. Physical examination findings in anorexia nervosa are summarized in Table 20.1.

*What are the medical complications of anorexia nervosa?*

Anorexia nervosa carries a high burden of medical comorbidities and is linked to the highest rate of all-cause mortality among all psychiatric conditions. Self-starvation may cause nutrient

TABLE 20.1 ■ **Physical Examination Findings in Anorexia Nervosa**

**Vital signs:** hypotension, orthostatic hypotension, bradycardia, and hypothermia

| Organ | Manifestation |
|---|---|
| General | Cachexia, emaciation |
| Ear, Nose, and Throat | Dental erosion |
| Skin | Dry skin, lanugo, hair loss, brittle nails, bruising, loss of subcutaneous fat, pallor |
| | May have calluses on dorsal side of dominant hand from self-induced vomiting (Russell's sign) |
| | Look for signs of self-harm, such as cutting or burning |
| Lymph nodes | Enlarged submandibular and parotid lymph nodes |
| Cardiovascular | Bradycardia, arrhythmia, midsystolic click followed by a late systolic murmur from MVP |
| Extremities | Peripheral edema, acrocyanosis |
| Musculoskeletal | Muscle atrophy, muscle weakness |

*MVP,* Mitral valve prolapse.

deficiencies and induce a catabolic state, resulting in breakdown of fat and protein tissues for gluconeogenesis. This process leads to atrophy of multiple organs, including heart, brain, kidneys, gastrointestinal tract, and smooth and skeletal muscles. For example, cardiac effects can lead to structural abnormalities, such as mitral valve prolapse, decreased ventricular volume, and pericardial effusions. Associated functional abnormalities lead to bradycardia, hypotension, increased QT interval, and arrhythmias. Common gastrointestinal symptoms include constipation and gastroparesis. The reproductive system is frequently affected by weight loss. Disruption in hypothalamic-pituitary signaling may lead to secondary amenorrhea, anovulation, and infertility. Neuropsychiatric manifestations are caused by brain atrophy and can manifest as cognitive impairment, as is seen in vitamin $B_{12}$ deficiency. Wernicke encephalopathy and Korsakoff syndrome are sometimes seen in severe cases of vitamin $B_1$ deficiency. Dermatologic manifestations include dry skin, easy bruising, brittle hair and nails, and acrocyanosis. The following electrolyte abnormalities are frequently seen: hyponatremia, hypokalemia, hypoglycemia, hypochloremic metabolic alkalosis due to vomiting, and acidosis from laxative abuse. Colorless, downy hair, called lanugo, appears all over the body to conserve heat. Other common manifestations include osteoporosis, anemia, and thrombocytopenia. Symptom severity is directly related to the degree of weight loss and varies depending on the duration of the illness. Whereas some adverse sequelae, such as myocardial atrophy, amenorrhea, or gastroparesis, remit with weight restoration, others, including osteoporosis or brain atrophy, may remain irreversible. General medical sequelae of anorexia nervosa is summarized in Table 20.2.

### What laboratory workup should you order?

Anorexia nervosa is a clinical diagnosis; however, additional medical workup is necessary to evaluate for comorbid medical problems and rule out organic causes of weight loss. Consider ordering a complete blood count with differential, metabolic panel, thyroid panel, 25-hydroxyvitamin D, electrolyte panel, albumin and prealbumin, liver function tests, pregnancy test in females, and electrocardiogram. If there is a history of low impact bone fractures, consider ordering dual energy x-ray absorptiometry scan to evaluate bone density.

### How do you treat anorexia nervosa?

Anorexia nervosa is notoriously difficult to treat. After a period of acute psychiatric and medical stabilization, treatment is conducted in an outpatient setting or partial day programs. First-line treatment is nutritional rehabilitation, weight restoration, and psychotherapy; psychopharmacological options are generally ineffective. Antidepressants, particularly selective serotonin reuptake inhibitors (SSRIs), can be used to treat comorbid mood and anxiety disorders, but they do not

**TABLE 20.2 ■ General Medical Sequelae of Anorexia Nervosa**

| Organ | Manifestation |
| --- | --- |
| Heart | Structural abnormalities: loss of myometrium, mitral valve prolapse, decreased ventricular volume, pericardial effusions, myocardial fibrosis<br>Functional abnormalities: bradycardia, hypotension, ECG changes (QT interval and arrhythmias) |
| Reproductive system | Abnormalities in HPA axis, amenorrhea, infertility. Low testosterone and estrogen levels |
| Endocrine | Abnormalities in HPA axis. Euthyroid-sick syndrome, osteopenia |
| Gastrointestinal | Gastroparesis, constipation, diarrhea due to villous atrophy, acute pancreatitis, elevated liver enzymes |
| Hematologic | Neutropenia, leukopenia, thrombocytopenia |
| Neurologic | Brain atrophy, Wernicke encephalopathy, Korsakoff syndrome |

*ECG,* Electrocardiogram; *HPA,* hypothalamic-pituitary-adrenal.

facilitate weight restoration. Given significant medical comorbidities, a choice of an antidepressant should be guided by its side effect profile. For example, bupropion should not be used because of its propensity to lower seizure threshold; tricyclic antidepressants are known for their adverse cardiac effect profile and should be avoided in patients with anorexia. This patient does not require an acute medical or psychiatric stabilization and can be first managed in an outpatient setting.

---

**CLINICAL PEARL**                                                          **STEP 2/3**

Patients with unstable vital signs, BMI <15 kg/m2, or failure to improve in an outpatient setting should be hospitalized to restore nutritional and hydration status. Family and cognitive behavioral therapy is first line in outpatient setting. Medications are not effective.

---

The patient is referred to a dietitian and mental health services for counseling. She misses her scheduled appointment with her primary care physician. A month later she presents to a local emergency department (ED) after collapsing when exercising. According to history obtained in the ED, the patient continues restricting her caloric intake. She stays late to work out after the dance practices and had one episode of fainting during a ballet class. She saw a psychologist for an intake appointment but missed subsequent sessions because she was worried about gaining weight as a result of therapy. On physical examination, her blood pressure is 89/55 mm Hg, pulse rate is 53/min, respiration rate is 15/min, temperature is 97°F, and BMI is 14.9 kg/m2. Laboratory workup is remarkable for a potassium level of 1.7 milliequivalents per liter and glucose 1.5 mmol/L.

---

*When do you consider inpatient medical or psychiatric hospitalization?*
The patient has failed to improve in an outpatient setting and now presents with concerning low BMI and unstable vital signs, which warrants hospitalization. Indications for inpatient medical hospitalization are significant electrolyte abnormalities, arrhythmias, unstable vital signs, and persistent weight loss while in outpatient treatment. Patients with anorexia should be screened for comorbid psychiatric conditions, including depression and anxiety. Always perform a thorough suicide risk assessment to determine a need for psychiatric admission.

---

While in the ED, the patient's hypoglycemia and hypokalemia are corrected and she is given intravenous fluids. She reluctantly agrees to inpatient hospitalization for nutritional rehabilitation. Four days after starting the feeds, she develops lower extremity edema; the metabolic panel is remarkable for a potassium level of 1.7 milliequivalents per liter.

---

*What is your diagnosis?*
Refeeding syndrome is a potentially fatal complication of nutrition rehabilitation in patients who are severely malnourished and underweight. Clinical features include cardiac arrhythmias, seizures, electrolyte abnormalities, congestive heart failure, and rhabdomyolysis. During starvation, mineral reserves are depleted and metabolism shifts from carbohydrates to fat and amino acids as a primary source of energy production. This results in a decrease in insulin and an increase in glucagon levels. In response to higher carbohydrate intake during refeeding, insulin secretion rises, signaling a shift from catabolism toward anabolism. Glycogen, fat, and protein synthesis requires phosphates, magnesium, and potassium, which are already depleted due to malnutrition. In addition, higher levels of insulin drive these electrolytes inside the cells, further increasing their serum deficit. Hypophosphatemia and volume overload are the cardinal signs of refeeding syndrome. Phosphate, in the form of adenosine triphosphate, is required for various energy-dependent

processes, including glucose phosphorylation. If phosphate is not replenished, tissue hypoxia and cardiac and respiratory failure may ensue.

| BASIC SCIENCE PEARL | STEP 1 |
| --- | --- |

During starvation, metabolism is switched to a catabolic state characterized by decreased insulin and increased glucagon levels, low metabolic rate, and breakdown of tissues for energy, leading to shrinkage of adipose tissue and muscle and organ atrophy. Whole body depletion of vitamins and electrolytes develops.

| BASIC SCIENCE PEARL | STEP 1 |
| --- | --- |

During refeeding, metabolism switches to an anabolic state, relying on carbohydrate metabolism for energy production. Increased levels of insulin mediate glucose and microelement uptake into the cells and lead to hyponatremia, hypokalemia, and hypothosphatemia. Hypophosphatemia is a hallmark of refeeding syndrome.

| BASIC SCIENCE/CLINICAL PEARL | STEP 1/2/3 |
| --- | --- |

Fluid overload is classic sign of refeeding syndrome. Oliguria from increased sodium and water resorption in kidneys can produce volume overload, which in combination with cardiac impairment due to starvation, may lead to acute heart failure.

### How do you prevent and treat a refeeding syndrome?

To prevent refeeding syndrome, electrolyte and vitamin deficiencies should be corrected before starting the feeds. Caloric intake and fluids should be increased gradually and slowly, particularly in the early stages of refeeding. It is recommended that a feeding rate be started at 5 to 10 kcal/kg/day. Electrolytes should be monitored daily and replenished promptly. If refeeding syndrome develops, treatment involves aggressive correction of electrolyte abnormalities and slowing nutritional intake. Continuous telemetry monitoring and intravenous electrolytes may be indicated in some cases. If a patient is resistant to eating or is unable to tolerate oral intake then feeding tubes can be used.

---

By the time of discharge, the patient gains 10 pounds and her vital signs and electrolytes remain stable. She is discharged to a day program specializing in eating disorders.

---

### What are the basic principles of cognitive behavioral therapy (CBT) for eating disorders?

CBT for eating disorders focuses on the mechanisms that perpetuate anorexia. The first step is to help patients recognize maladaptive, automatic cognitions that contribute to disease maintenance. For example, a patient who equates thinness with achievement or effective self-control learns to incorporate other domains of self-evaluation. Treatment interventions target behavioral change through regular self-monitoring of food intake, thoughts, and feelings around eating, and help replace maladaptive habits with healthier behaviors. CBT also focuses on relapse prevention planning. This treatment modality emphasizes psychoeducation and involvement of family and significant others in a therapeutic process.

---

Over the next year, her condition continues to improve. She achieves a BMI >18 kg/m2 and starts menstruating again. As her weight normalizes, her insight and eating habits also improve.

---

**BEYOND THE PEARLS:**

- Adjunctive olanzapine use may help restore weight in patients who failed first-line treatment.
- Selective serotonin reuptake inhibitors (SSRIs) are not effective for treating depression or preventing relapse in severely underweight patients presumably because of low synaptic levels of serotonin. Tryptophan, an essential amino acid obtained from diet and a precursor for serotonin, is depleted in malnourished patients. With weight restoration, SSRIs may become beneficial for relapse prevention.
- Insight and eating habits tend to improve with weight restoration.
- To minimize the risk of refeeding syndrome, feeds should start slowly at 5 to 10 kcal/kg/day and increased slowly over 7 to 10 days. Vitamins and serum electrolytes should be replenished before feed initiation. Serum electrolytes should be monitored daily and aggressively corrected if indicated.
- If refeeding syndrome develops, feeding should be discontinued and restarted at a lower rate. Continuous cardiac monitoring may be necessary.

## References

American Psychiatric Association. (2006). Treatment of patients with eating disorders, third edition. American Psychiatric Association. *American Journal of Psychiatry, 163*, 4.

Mehanna, H. M., Moledina, J., & Travis, J. (2008). Refeeding syndrome: What it is, and how to prevent and treat it. *BMJ, 336*(7659), 1495–1498.

Mehler, P. S. (2001). Diagnosis and care of patients with anorexia nervosa in primary care settings. *Annals of Internal Medicine, 134*, 1048.

Mehler, P. S., & Brown, C. (2015). Anorexia nervosa - medical complications. *Journal of Eating Disorders, 3*, 11.

Murphy, R., Straebler, S., Cooper, Z., & Fairburn, C. G. (2010). Cognitive behavioral therapy for eating disorders. *Psychiatric Clinics of North America, 33*(3), 611–627.

# CHAPTER 21

# Schizophrenia vs Brief vs Schizophreniform

Timothy Yff ■ Eugenia Brikker ■ Mitesh Patel

A 20-year-old male presents to the psychiatric emergency service with a 1-month history of bizarre behavior. His family reports that during the last month the patient has become paranoid, religiously preoccupied, and has been walking around the house naked. The patient is a college student and was admitted to a psychiatric hospital 3 weeks ago with psychotic symptoms that were believed to be secondary to stress related to finals. He was hospitalized for 3 days, started on olanzapine, and discharged home after symptoms quickly resolved. Upon discharge from the hospital, the patient stopped taking medication. He did well for approximately 1 week but then became symptomatic again. For the past 2 days he has not been sleeping, has been constantly pacing the house, and has been very paranoid. The patient's father attempted to drive him to the emergency room, but the patient was uncooperative and tried to exit the vehicle multiple times, leading to a motor vehicle crash.

*What additional information would you like to know about this patient?*
A good history is essential when a patient is being evaluated for new onset psychosis. Collateral information obtained from family can be useful in reconstructing an accurate timeline related to the onset/emergence of symptoms. Consider the following information:

- The age and gender of the patient are important considerations when evaluating new onset psychosis. Schizophrenia equally affects men and women, but the age of presentation is different. Men typically present in the late teens to early 20s and women present in the mid-to-late 20s. New onset psychosis in an individual over the age of 50, with no previous psychiatric history, would be more concerning for psychosis secondary to a medical etiology and would warrant a complete medical workup.
- The timeframe or acuity of onset of symptoms is also important to consider. Schizophrenia typically begins with a prodromal period. Prodromal symptoms frequently begin in adolescence and precede onset of psychotic symptoms. They can last weeks to months. Prodromal symptoms are characterized by gradual onset and may initially appear as subtle changes in mood or personality. They can also include a decline in the ability to function. Prodromal symptoms may begin with increasing irritability or social withdrawal. Other characteristic behaviors may include peculiarity of thought or behavior, newfound interest in religion, and declining school/work performance.
- The duration of psychotic symptoms and a description of the behaviors that the family has observed. The active phase of psychosis includes delusions, hallucinations, and disorganized thinking and behavior.

TABLE 21.1 ■ Primary versus Secondary Psychosis

| Type | Differential Diagnosis |
| --- | --- |
| Primary psychosis | Schizotypal personality disorder<br>Delusional disorder<br>Brief psychotic disorder<br>Schizophreniform disorder<br>Schizophrenia<br>Schizoaffective disorder<br>Mood disorder with psychotic features<br>Neurocognitive disorders<br>Posttraumatic stress disorder |
| Secondary psychosis | Endocrine—thyrotoxicosis, steroid-producing tumors<br>Metabolic—acute intermittent porphyria<br>Autoimmune—lupus, Hashimoto encephalopathy, anti-N-methyl-D-aspartate receptor encephalitis<br>Infectious—neurosyphilis, human immunodeficiency virus<br>Neurologic—seizures, demyelinating disease, space-occupying lesions, cerebrovascular accidents, basal ganglia disorders<br>Head injury—chronic traumatic encephalopathy<br>Nutritional deficiencies—cobalamin deficiency, thiamine deficiency, pellagra<br>Substance/medication induced—drugs of abuse, pharmaceutical medications |

- Severe or prolonged trauma can precipitate psychotic symptoms. It is therefore useful to know if a patient has experienced trauma.
- Reproductive history must be reviewed with all females. Psychosis can frequently present in the postpartum period and puts both the mother and infant at increased risk for harm. Careful evaluation of symptoms and a risk assessment must be completed.
- Medical illness can also precipitate psychotic symptoms. It is vital to carefully review a patient's medical history, as well as medication list, to ensure that a secondary cause of psychosis is not overlooked.

A thorough physical examination and medical workup are needed when evaluating a patient with new onset psychosis (as it is important to rule out medical causes). Vital signs should be reviewed. Laboratory evaluation includes a complete blood count (CBC), complete metabolic panel (CMP), thyroid-stimulating hormone (TSH), and urine drug screen. Consider head imaging, such as computed tomography (CT), if focal neurologic deficits are present. Table 21.1 summarizes primary psychosis (psychosis caused by psychiatric disorders) and secondary psychosis (psychosis caused by medical problems or substance intoxications).

*If the patient's urine drug screen is positive for substance abuse, does that change your evaluation or treatment considerations?*

Substance abuse frequently co-occurs with mental illness. Although it can make diagnosis more difficult, it should not change treatment considerations. If there is a clear history of substance use with no prior psychiatric history, this is more suggestive of substance-induced psychosis (although this does not completely exclude primary psychosis). Both substance intoxication and withdrawal can present with psychotic symptoms. Table 21.2 summarizes various substances and the symptoms associated with their intoxication and/or withdrawal. Of particular importance is alcohol and benzodiazepine withdrawal, as these can be life-threatening if not rapidly diagnosed and properly treated.

**TABLE 21.2 ■ Symptoms of Intoxication and Withdrawal from Substances**

| Drug | Intoxication | Withdrawal |
|------|-------------|-----------|
| Stimulants (cocaine, amphetamines) | • Anxiety<br>• Paranoia<br>• Hallucinations<br>• Delusions of persecution<br>• Aggression/agitation | • Anxiety<br>• Depression<br>• Cravings<br>• Fatigue |
| Heroin | • Miosis<br>• Euphoria<br>• Depressed respiration<br>• Nodding | • Nausea/vomiting<br>• Anxiety<br>• Myalgias<br>• Chills |
| Marijuana | • Anxiety<br>• Paranoia<br>• Conjunctival injection<br>• Dry mouth<br>• Increased appetite | • Irritability<br>• Depression<br>• Insomnia<br>• Tremor<br>• Anorexia |
| Ecstasy/MDMA | • Depression<br>• Confusion<br>• Sweating<br>• Jaw muscle tension | • Depression<br>• Paranoia<br>• Insomnia<br>• Fatigue |
| Alcohol | • Impaired judgment<br>• Suicidal behavior<br>• Slurred speech<br>• Decreased attention span<br>• Ataxia | • Dysphoria/irritability<br>• Anxiety/tremulousness<br>• Insomnia<br>• Autonomic hyperactivity<br>• Seizure |
| Benzodiazepines | • Impaired attention/concentration<br>• Confusion<br>• Dizziness<br>• Ataxia | • Anxiety<br>• Insomnia<br>• Autonomic hyperactivity<br>• Disordered perceptions/psychosis<br>• Seizure |

On evaluation the patient states that he has been searching on the Internet how to become president. He believes that his parents have brought him to the hospital to prevent him from becoming president. He reports that he does not need to be in the hospital and that he does not have a mental illness. The patient is disheveled, agitated, and only partially cooperative. He appears to be very guarded and makes limited eye contact. On mental status examination, he is alert and oriented. Although he can answer simple questions with repeated questioning, his speech pattern is markedly disorganized and tangential. Although he denies auditory and visual hallucinations, he is noted to be internally preoccupied and responding to internal stimuli. His insight and judgment are both noted to be poor. He denies suicidal or homicidal ideation. He denies any history of substance or alcohol use. He does not have any known acute or chronic medical issues. Physical examination is unremarkable. CBC, CMP, TSH, and urine drug screen are negative for any significant findings.

### What symptoms does this patient have that suggest a psychotic condition?

Patients with psychotic conditions have the presence of positive, negative, and cognitive symptoms. Positive symptoms are feelings or behaviors that are not usually present in a person without psychosis. In this patient, we see paranoid thoughts (delusions), religious preoccupation, and bizarre/hallucinatory behavior. Negative symptoms are a lack of feelings and behaviors that are normally present in people without a psychotic illness. In this case we see poor hygiene and self-care. A very common negative symptom in patients with schizophrenia is an absence of emotion demonstrated by a flat affect. Cognitive symptoms interfere with a patient's normal thought process and ability to accurately interpret the environment. In this case we see a disorganized speech pattern and poor executive functioning demonstrated by poor insight and judgment.

***What about this patient's presentation would suggest a diagnosis of a primary psychiatric illness?***
The patient denies drug use, and a urine drug screen confirms this. Medical causes for this patient are less likely, as basic laboratory work and physical examination are unremarkable. Based on information obtained from family, the patient appears to have had persistent symptoms that have lasted about 1 month, which also makes acute causes (medical or toxic) less likely. The positive response to olanzapine and marked deterioration after discontinuing suggests that he has a primary psychotic condition (such as schizophrenia). The patient also fits the typical age range for a male with a primary psychotic condition.

---

**CLINICAL PEARL**                                        **STEP 1/2/3**

Antipsychotic medications work primarily as dopamine antagonists, lowering levels of dopamine.

---

### DSM-5 Diagnostic Criteria for Schizophrenia
Presence of at least one of the following symptoms: delusions, hallucinations, or disorganized speech, with or without the presence of: disorganized behavior, catatonia, or negative symptoms.

At least two of the symptoms listed previously must occur together for at least 1 month. The person's level of functioning at work/school, with interpersonal relationships, or self-care has fallen well below the level of functioning before the onset of symptoms. The problems are ongoing for at least 6 months, and other causes of psychosis have been ruled out. Table 21.3 lists the time course of symptoms for various diagnoses of primary psychotic disorders.

---

The patient has been raised by his mother and father who are married. He is an only child. Developmentally, he achieved all milestones on time. He has done well in school and is currently a junior in college studying business. He is employed part time at a package handling service. The family reports that for approximately 1 to 2 months before the onset of bizarre behavior, the patient had been more socially isolated. Family history is significant for an uncle with schizophrenia.

---

***If you suspect a diagnosis of schizophrenia, what elements of the history would be good versus poor prognostic indicators?***
This patient presents with a relatively rapid onset of symptoms that are predominantly positive. He had high premorbid functioning, is male, and has an age of onset that is on the younger side. There is also a family history of schizophrenia. Table 21.4 summarizes prognostic indicators for schizophrenia.

---

The patient is admitted to an inpatient psychiatric unit. After evaluation, he is started on aripiprazole. The patient initially refuses to take medication and makes several attempts to escape the unit. He is frequently agitated, requires seclusion many times, and receives chemical restraint for his protection. He continues to be paranoid and reports that the hospital is involved in an elaborate plot to prevent him from becoming president. He is refusing meals and is only eating packaged food because of a fear of being poisoned. After multiple seclusions and emergency treatments, the patient becomes compliant with scheduled medication. He has a quick improvement in symptoms. He is discharged home with his family and scheduled for follow-up with an outpatient psychiatrist.

TABLE 21.3 ■ Time Course of Symptoms in Psychotic Disorders

| Time Course of Symptoms | Diagnosis |
| --- | --- |
| Less than 1 month | Brief psychotic disorder |
| Greater than 1 month and less than 6 months | Schizophreniform disorder |
| Greater than 6 months | Schizophrenia |

TABLE 21.4 ■ Prognostic Indicators in Schizophrenia

| Good Prognostic Indicators | Poor Prognostic Indicators |
| --- | --- |
| • Later age of onset | • Early age of onset |
| • Female gender | • Male gender |
| • Predominance of positive symptoms | • Predominance of negative symptoms |
| • Good premorbid functioning | • Poor premorbid functioning |
| • Good social support | • Poor social support |
| • Acute onset of symptoms | • Gradual onset of symptoms |
| • No family history of schizophrenia | • Positive family history of schizophrenia |
| • Few relapses | • Frequent relapses |
| • Presence of mood symptoms | • Comorbid substance abuse |

*The patient had expressed that he did not want to be hospitalized. What about this patient's presentation allowed him to be hospitalized involuntarily?*

Although laws for involuntary psychiatric hospitalization for exacerbated illness vary by state, commonalities exist. These criteria include:

1. The patient reasonably represents an acute danger to self or others.
2. The dangerousness is due to a psychiatric illness.
3. The patient is likely to benefit from psychiatric hospitalization.

All states also have a system to allow civilians to petition for a psychiatric evaluation for a person that they believe to be psychiatrically disabled. This patient represents a risk to self and others because he caused a motor vehicle accident, exhibits poor self-care, and has agitated behavior. He demonstrates that he is impaired mentally by the presence of psychotic symptoms. His encouraging response to antipsychotics is evidence that he can be expected to benefit from hospitalization.

---

**CLINICAL PEARL**                                                                          **STEP 2/3**

Antipsychotic medications carry adverse risks such as parkinsonism, dystonia, akathisia, tardive dyskinesia, metabolic syndromes, and neuroleptic syndrome. These side effects contribute to the reasoning of why it is important to maintain autonomy if the patient possesses adequate judgment.

---

*What are some treatment challenges when treating a patient with a suspected diagnosis of schizophrenia?*

As in this patient, a high proportion of patients with schizophrenia have little insight into their own illness and behaviors. As many as 80% of patients with schizophrenia may deny having a mental illness. This presents challenges in treating this patient population, and noncompliance with treatment is high. Many studies predict medication nonadherence to be between 25%

to 50%. Even when involuntarily admitted to a psychiatric hospital, a patient retains the right to refuse treatment. In these cases, medications can be forcibly given only in emergency situations when the patient is demonstrating destructive, extremely disruptive, or immediate dangerous behavior (such as hitting their head against the wall or loudly threatening another patient).

If a patient continues to be a risk to self and others and refuses treatment, a practitioner may seek forced maintenance medication treatment. Laws regarding this vary by state, but generally, a reasonable effort must be made, over a reasonable length of time, to allow a patient to accept treatment before forced treatment can be pursued. There is evidence that insight into illness and judgment regarding future treatment improves after positive symptoms abate, which is why forced treatment can be beneficial even after discharge from the hospital. Many antipsychotic medications come in long-acting injectable forms, which can improve compliance by providing long-term treatment without a need to remember to take medication daily.

---

**CLINICAL PEARL**                                                                                      **STEP 2/3**

The treatment of choice for most cases of schizophrenia is an antipsychotic medication. However, if catatonia is present, the initial treatment is typically an antipsychotic with a benzodiazepine. Catatonia is a state exemplified by slowed rigid movements, bizarre posturing of muscles, occasional mutism or echolalia, and extreme negative symptoms.

---

**BEYOND THE PEARLS:**

- Based on current evidence, antipsychotic medications treat positive symptoms more effectively than negative symptoms. Negative symptoms can be persistent even when a patient is compliant with treatment and not having any positive symptoms. One antipsychotic medication, amisulpride, is suggested to provide greater improvement over negative symptoms than any other medications but is not available in the United States.
- Paliperidone comes in a long-acting injectable that is only given once every 3 months, the longest interval of any antipsychotic. In order to be eligible, a patient needs to be maintained on the month-long version for at least 4 months consecutively.
- There is evidence to suggest that schizophrenia and bipolar disorder are related based on genome-wide association studies that show a genetic relationship.
- Young patients (ages 16–30) with an episode of psychosis have a substantially greater 12-month mortality rate compared with patients without schizophrenia, up to 24 times as high. This argues for intensive clinical intervention for patients exhibiting the early stages of psychotic illness.

---

## References

Cardno, A. G., & Owen, M. J. (2014). Genetic relationships between schizophrenia, bipolar disorder, and schizoaffective disorder. *Schizophrenia Bulletin, 40*(3), 504–515.

Chue, P., & Lalonde, J. (2014). Addressing the unmet needs of patients with persistent negative symptoms of schizophrenia: Emerging pharmacological treatment options. *Neuropsychiatric Disease and Treatment, 10*, 777.

Gilleen, J., Greenwod, K., & David, A. S. (2010). Domains of awareness in schizophrenia. *Schizophrenia Bulletin, 37*(1), 61–72.

Kane, J. M., Kishimoto, T., & Correll, C. U. (2013). Non-adherence to medication in patients with psychotic disorders: Epidemiology, contributing factors and management strategies. *World Psychiatry, 12*(3), 216–226.

Schoenbaum, M., Sutherland, J. M., Chappel, A., Azrin, S., Goldstein, A. B., Rupp, A., & Heinssen, R. K. (2017). Twelve-month health care use and mortality in commercially insured young people with incident psychosis in the United States. *Schizophrenia Bulletin, 43*(6), 1262–1272.

# CHAPTER 22

# Schizoaffective, Delusional Disorder

Haley Wehder

A 24-year-old female patient presents to the emergency department because she is hearing male voices coming from inside the walls. She tells you that she has heard the voices every day for the past 5 months. She also claims that she has "special powers" and reports that the voices threaten to harm her or her family if she doesn't use these powers to obey their commands. Because of this, she has felt "empty and hopeless" almost constantly for the past 3 months. She feels guilt because of the danger to her family, as well as a decreased appetite that has led to a 20-pound weight loss. She admits that lately she has begun to consider suicide, and tearfully says, "I just don't know how else to make the voices stop. Even now they're telling me not to talk to you!" She has been sleeping more than usual and is not interested in leaving her house for any reason, which has led to the loss of her job. Before the voices began 5 months ago, the patient had no prior medical complaints. She reports smoking marijuana at a party once in high school but denies any current tobacco, alcohol, or drug use. She has had no recent falls or head injuries.

*What initial differential diagnoses would be important to consider given this patient's symptom history?*
This patient, who complains of hearing voices that others cannot hear, is experiencing a psychotic episode. Psychosis is generally defined as sensory experiences or beliefs that do not have a basis in reality. These typically take the form of auditory or visual hallucinations, complex delusions (fixed, false beliefs), and disorganization of speech or behavior. All of these symptoms can manifest in various ways. Cognitive ability may or may not be affected and should be assessed on presentation.

In order to appropriately treat a patient who is suffering with symptoms such as these, it is critical to begin with a broad differential diagnosis list. Causes of psychosis can be most easily subdivided into two groups: primary psychosis (which is due to a psychiatric condition) and secondary psychosis (which is caused by some other underlying medical condition). Typical nonpsychiatric medical causes of psychosis include substance use (most common), severe infection, vitamin or electrolyte abnormalities, certain hormone irregularities, and head trauma (e.g. intracranial bleeding). Of note, it is important to differentiate between delirium and psychosis in patients, because both can have very similar presentations but may differ in their underlying etiologies. Delirium is a form of altered mental status that typically has a more acute onset and is usually completely reversible once the causative agent is identified and treated.

*What diagnostic tests will you need to order to determine the etiology of this patient's psychosis?*
Laboratory testing can be critical in distinguishing between secondary causes of psychosis. Basic workup considerations are listed below:
- The most common cause of secondary psychosis is substance use, which can make it very difficult to differentiate between causes of altered mentation if multiple causes exist; therefore it is necessary to rule this out in all patients with a **urine toxicology screen** and a **thorough social history**. This patient denies any recent history of drug use.

- Infectious agents are another common cause of confusion, particularly once a patient reaches a state of sepsis, so clinicians should monitor **vital signs** and assess white blood cell counts with a **complete blood count (CBC)**. These tests can also help you rule out hypoxia and anemia as potential etiologies. Sexually transmitted infections, such as syphilis and human immunodeficiency virus (HIV), are well known causative agents of altered mentation. Clinicians should consider testing for these, particularly in high-risk populations.
- Many vitamins and electrolytes (e.g., calcium, $B_{12}$, folate, glucose) can lead to symptoms such as those seen in this patient. Obtaining a **complete metabolic panel (CMP)** would assess these potential abnormalities, as well as indicate liver disease, which can cause encephalopathy (another common cause of confusion).
- Hyperthyroid crisis (thyrotoxicosis) can lead to psychosis in patients with overproduction of thyroid hormone. Hyperthyroidism is also a cause of weight loss, which this patient has experienced. Investigation of thyroid hormone production can include measurements of **triiodothyronine (T3), thyroxine (T4), and thyroid-stimulating hormone (TSH)**.
- Head injury, particularly resulting in intracranial bleeding, can cause compression of brain structures that eventually gives rise to altered sensorium. Although this patient reports no history of injury, workup with **computed tomography (CT) of head without contrast** could be performed to assure there is no acute change.

| BASIC SCIENCE PEARL | STEP 1 |
|---|---|

Other identifiers of infection, known as *acute phase reactants,* can also be ordered during a laboratory workup. These include markers such as the erythrocyte sedimentation rate, C-reactive protein, and procalcitonin levels. However, these values do not help identify a particular infectious agent and instead serve as general indicators of an inflammatory response.

---

On examination, the patient's temperature is 37.1 °C (98.8 °F), pulse is 78/min, blood pressure is 127/72 mm Hg, and oxygen saturation is 98% on room air. She is tearful throughout the interaction and occasionally answers questions as if there are multiple interviewers in the room. She is alert and oriented to person, place, time, and situation. Auscultation of the heart and lungs reveals no abnormalities. Laboratory workup includes a CBC and CMP, both of which are within normal limits. Rapid Plasma Reagin (RPR) is nonreactive, and urine drug screen is negative. Urinalysis (UA) does not show signs of leukocyte esterase, nitrites, or ketones in the urine. TSH, $B_{12}$, folate, and calcium are all within range of their reference values. CT of head without contrast shows no acute sources of bleeding.

*Based on the results of the laboratory workup, how has the differential diagnosis changed?*
This patient is afebrile with a normal white blood cell count and negative urinalysis, making infection unlikely. Her urine toxicology screen showed no signs of acute intoxication from illicit substances. Liver function tests were normal, ruling out hepatic encephalopathy. Patient also did not have any electrolyte abnormalities (hypercalcemia, hyperglycemia leading to diabetic ketoacidosis, etc.) that would typically cause altered mental status, and she was found not to have hyperthyroidism. Given all of this and the negative head imaging, secondary causes of psychosis seem unlikely at this time. Therefore it is more reasonable to suspect that this patient is experiencing primary psychosis as a result of an underlying psychiatric disorder.

*If this patient has a suspected psychiatric disorder, what elements from the history will be critical in establishing a more definitive diagnosis?*
There are many psychotic disorders to consider in a patient who presents with auditory hallucinations (in the form of male voices for this patient) and delusions (manifested here as belief in a

### TABLE 22.1 ■ First Criterion (Criterion A) for Schizophrenia

Presence of at least one of the following symptoms: delusions, hallucinations, or disorganized speech. With or without the presence of: disorganized behavior, catatonia, or negative symptoms. ≥2 of the symptoms listed above must occur together for at least 1 month.

### TABLE 22.2 ■ Psychotic Disorders

| | |
|---|---|
| Brief psychotic disorder | Delusions, hallucinations, or disorganized speech lasting >1 day but <1 month; patient returns to baseline independently |
| Delusional disorder | Delusions present at least 1 month, otherwise patient is functionally unimpaired |
| Schizophrenia | Delusions, hallucinations, and/or disorganized speech in addition to disorganized or catatonic behavior and/or negative symptoms; episode must last at least 6 months |
| Schizoaffective disorder | Schizophrenia symptoms concurrent with a major mood episode (bipolar or depressive type); must have at least 2 weeks of psychotic symptoms without the accompanying mood symptoms |
| Schizophreniform disorder | Schizophrenia symptoms lasting >1 month but <6 months |

"special power"). Other key features of these conditions can include disorganization of thought and speech, abnormal motor movements, and negative symptoms, (e.g., blunt affect, anhedonia, poverty of speech or thought), although these are not seen in this patient example (Table 22.1).

One of the most critical aspects to obtain from the patient history is a timeline of symptoms. Many psychotic disorders are considered to be a spectrum of disease and can only be differentiated by the symptom time course. The schizophrenia spectrum includes: brief psychotic disorder (when episodes of disturbance last at least 1 day but less than 1 month), schizophreniform disorder (episodes last anywhere from 1 month to 6 months), and schizophrenia (episodes of at least 6 months duration, with at least 1 month of symptoms that meet the *Diagnostic and Statistical Manual of Mental Disorders* (DSM 5) Criterion A. All of these have largely the same symptomatology and rely heavily on duration of symptoms to differentiate between them (Table 22.1).

Another important consideration when looking at this patient history is endorsement of mood symptoms that correspond with the episode of psychosis. Typically, mood symptoms that overlap with psychotic disorders can be grouped as either depressive type or bipolar type. Just as with the symptoms of psychosis, timeline of the depressive symptoms is critical for diagnosis. Patients who experience symptoms consistent with a major depressive mood disturbance with psychosis (that lasts for most, but not all, of the duration of the mood disturbance) would be given a diagnosis of major depressive disorder (MDD) with psychotic features. Conversely, patients who exhibit psychosis and experience symptoms that qualify as a mood disturbance independent of the psychotic episode would qualify for a diagnosis of schizoaffective disorder. These patients must have at least 2 weeks of psychotic symptoms that are not accompanied by mood disturbance; this clarifies that the depressed mood is not the cause of the psychosis (Table 22.2).

In patients who suffer from one or more delusions for longer than 1 month, delusional disorder should also be considered. Patients who qualify for this diagnosis may experience hallucinations, but these are related to the theme of the delusion (which is the predominant symptom); furthermore, they must not meet Criterion A of schizophrenia. Whereas mood disturbances may coincide in this condition, they must be brief in comparison to the duration of the delusion. Finally, patients with delusional disorder are typically not impaired functionally.

Their ideas and behavior may likely be considered "normal" when the delusional theme is not taken into account.

*Considering the broad differential for psychiatric disorders, what is the most appropriate diagnosis for this patient?*

This patient has been experiencing delusions and auditory hallucinations for 5 months, meeting the criteria for schizophrenia. However, she also describes major depressive symptoms (guilt, loss of appetite associated with significant weight loss, increased sleep, loss of interest in daily activities, and suicidal ideation), as well as depressed moods that she describes as "empty and hopeless" (which meets the criteria for MDD diagnosis). She says these mood symptoms have gone on for 3 months, meaning they have lasted for the majority (but not entire) duration of her psychotic episode. This qualifies her for a diagnosis of schizoaffective disorder.

---

**CLINICAL PEARL**                                                        **STEP 1/2/3**

The SIG E CAPS mnemonic is an effective way to remember that a patient must exhibit changes in at least five of the following to qualify for a major depressive episode: Sleep, Interest, Guilt, Energy, Concentration, Appetite, Psychomotor activity, and Suicidal ideation.

---

Based on symptom duration and history of overlapping mood disturbance, it is determined that this patient has schizoaffective disorder. She is admitted to the inpatient psychiatric unit for acute crisis stabilization with medication, as well as evaluation for suicidal ideation.

---

*What are the ethical and legal factors involved in hospitalizing a patient with a psychiatric condition?*

One of the four guiding ethical principles in medicine is autonomy—the patients' right to make their own decisions in regard to the care they receive. This becomes an even more critical factor for patients with psychiatric conditions, who may or may not be in a state of mind to make appropriate choices for themselves at the moment of evaluation. Psychiatric illness does not automatically preclude patients from being considered capable of making such decisions; in these cases, issues of competency and capacity play a major role.

Competency is a legal determination of patients' overarching ability to play a role in their own care and, as such, is usually left for courts to decide. Capacity, on the other hand, is used in a clinical setting when a physician evaluates the capability of patients to make judgments about the management of their health. It is based on the idea that patients are able to process information given to them, understand the risks and benefits of all treatment options presented, and ultimately reach a decision that is rational in terms of their beliefs and values. Capacity is in constant flux and may change for the same patient on a case-by-case basis. It is part of the physician's responsibility to ensure that capacity is assessed and taken into account at all times.

For patients with psychiatric disorders, their ability to make decisions regarding their health can be even more variable and requires continuous reassessment by medical professionals. Physicians have the ability to involuntarily hospitalize patients who they believe lack capacity, particularly if they present a threat to their own safety or the safety of others. This could be employed in the current case because the patient in question is experiencing acute psychosis and has endorsed a desire to end her own life. However, if this method were chosen, it would be critical to allow the patient to resume decision making as soon as it was safe to do so; this would be the best way to ensure patient autonomy was maintained and respected.

*What are common pharmacologic and therapeutic options for treatment of schizoaffective disorder?*
Schizoaffective disorder is a complex combination of psychotic and mood disturbances. As such, it is common for patients to receive multiple treatment therapies at once, in order to minimize all symptoms as quickly and effectively as possible. The following therapeutic options have been shown to provide benefits to patients with schizoaffective disorder:

- **Antipsychotic medications**—as many as 93% of patients being treated for this disorder will receive an antipsychotic medication. These medications are broken into two large classes, the typical and atypical antipsychotics. Both types work through modulation of dopamine receptors in the brain. Typical antipsychotics (e.g., haloperidol) are effective in treating the positive symptoms (and to a limited extent negative symptoms) of patients with psychotic disorders but are well known for causing extrapyramidal symptoms as side effects of their use. Atypical antipsychotics (e.g., clozapine) have a better side effect profile but are even less effective in treating negative symptoms of schizophrenia. The only antipsychotic currently approved by the Federal Drug Administration (FDA) specifically for the treatment of schizoaffective disorder is paliperidone.
- **Mood stabilizers and antidepressants**–these medications are used in patients with bipolar-type and depressive-type schizoaffective disorder, respectively. Mood stabilizers (e.g., lithium, valproic acid) are primarily used for the treatment of mania. Many of the antiepileptic medications have been shown to be effective for mood stabilization.
  Antidepressants include the selective serotonin reuptake inhibitors (SSRIs; e.g., fluoxetine), serotonin norepinephrine reuptake inhibitors (SNRIs; e.g., venlafaxine), and tricyclic antidepressants (TCAs; e.g., amitriptyline). These are useful in patients who experience major depressive episodes but should be used with caution if there is any history of mania or hypomania symptoms.
- **Cognitive behavior therapy (CBT)**—this form of therapy can be a useful adjunct for patients, as it helps the patient identify and modify negative thoughts that can lead to negative feelings. Although individualized therapy is useful, patients may also benefit from group and family therapy.
- **Electroconvulsive therapy (ECT)**—this is not a first line treatment for schizoaffective disorder but may be used in patients who are refractory to other forms of treatment, particularly those suffering from severe depressive symptoms.

---

The patient spends 4 days on the inpatient psychiatric unit, where she participates in daily group therapy sessions that help her better understand and manage her disorder. She is started on a combination of paliperidone and fluoxetine for her psychotic and depressive symptoms. She is discharged after it is determined that she is stable and no longer suicidal. At a follow-up appointment in the outpatient psychiatry clinic 4 weeks later, she reports vast improvements in mood and psychotic symptoms since the initiation of her medications. She is no longer hearing voices and feels her quality of life has improved dramatically.

---

**BEYOND THE PEARLS:**

- Prognosis for patients with schizoaffective disorder is usually better than the prognosis for patients with schizophrenia; however, these patients typically do not do as well as patients who have a mood disorder only.
- The lifetime risk of suicide in these patients is 5%, and this is higher in patients who experience depressive symptoms.
- Although the exact cause of schizoaffective disorder is not understood, it is hypothesized that impaired glucose tolerance and insulin resistance may have some role. Recently two case studies showed that a ketogenic diet may be helpful in ameliorating symptoms in schizoaffective disorder.

## References

American Psychiatric Association. (2013). *Diagnostic and statistical manual of mental disorders* (5th ed.). Washington, DC: Author.

Cascade, E., Kalali, A., & Buckley, P. (2009). Treatment of schizoaffective disorder. *Psychiatry (Edgmont)*, *6*(3), 15–17.

First, M., Frances, A., & Pincus, H. A. (2014). *DSM-5 handbook of differential diagnosis.* Washington, DC: American Psychiatric Publishing.

Griswold, K. S., Del Regno, P. A., & Berger, R. C. (2015). Recognition and Differential Diagnosis of Psychosis in Primary Care. *American Family Physician, 91*(12), 856–863.

Gross, G., & Geyer, M. *Current antipsychotics.* Handbook of Experimental Pharmacology, v. 212. Berlin, Germany: Springer-Verlag.

Johnson, J. M., & Stern, T. A. (2014). Involuntary hospitalization of primary care patients. *Primary Care Companion for CNS Disorders, 16*(3).

Markanday, A. (2015). Acute phase reactants in infections: Evidence-based review and a guide for clinicians. *Open Forum Infectious Diseases, 2*(3).

Orr, R. D. (2004). Competence, capacity, and surrogate decision-making. Retrieved from https://cbhd.org/content/competence-capacity-and-surrogate-decision-making

Palmer, C. (2017). Ketogenic diet in the treatment of schizoaffective disorder: Two case studies. *Schizophrenia Research, 189,* 208–209.

Varelius, J. (2006). The value of autonomy in medical ethics. *Medicine, Health Care, and Philosophy, 9*(3), 377–388.

# CHAPTER 23

# Attention Deficit Hyperactivity Disorder

Alison Duncan  ■  Peter Ureste

A 7-year-old girl is brought in to the clinic by her parents because she is having problems at home and school. Parents describe her as "not a minute of rest." For at least the last 2 years, they notice that she cannot play quietly by herself. She is unable to follow directions and only follows through with tasks if her parents are "on her." She often gets in trouble and becomes upset when her electronics are taken away. The girl frequently loses her school supplies and misplaces notices from her teacher. At school, she cannot stay in her seat for more than a few minutes and is often in trouble with the teacher for wandering around the classroom. She has difficulty finishing assignments and often gets low marks for making careless mistakes. The girl loves to read cartoons or social media, but she struggles to finish a chapter book. Parents enroll the girl in soccer to help her "burn off some excess energy." She has a lot of fun kicking the ball around the field, but she is easily distracted and frequently leaves the field during actual games, which earns her ridicule from her peers.

## *What is attention deficit hyperactivity disorder (ADHD)?*

ADHD is a neurodevelopmental disorder that is most commonly identified in childhood. Diagnostic criteria include inattentive and hyperactive symptoms, which must be present before the age of 12 years. Symptoms must be present for at least 6 months, must be present in two or more settings, and must cause problems in daily functioning. There are three subtypes consisting of inattentive type, hyperactivity-impulsivity type, and mixed type. Symptoms of each subtype are summarized in Table 23.1.

| CLINICAL PEARL | STEP 2/3 |
|---|---|

Inattention, hyperactivity, or impulsivity are also found in other psychiatric conditions. These include major depressive disorder (poor concentration or psychomotor agitation), bipolar disorder (impulsivity, hyperverbal speech, flight of ideas, distractibility), substance use disorder (inattention, hyperactive, or impulsivity symptoms can occur depending on ingested substance), generalized anxiety disorders (difficulties with concentration, restlessness), and sleep–wake disorders, among others. For this reason, a thorough assessment with additional collateral history obtained from an informant should be pursued.

| BASIC SCIENCE | STEP 1 |
|---|---|

Hypoactivity of dopamine and norepinephrine in frontal-subcortical circuits underlie the dysfunction in ADHD.

TABLE 23.1 ■ **Symptoms of ADHD Subtypes**

| Inattention | Hyperactivity-Impulsivity |
|---|---|
| • Fails to give close attention to details | • Fidgets, taps hands or feet, or squirms in seat |
| • Difficulty sustaining attention in tasks | • Leaves seat when remaining seated is expected |
| • Does not seem to listen when directly spoken to | (such as leaves classroom) |
| • Does not follow through on instructions and | • Runs about or climbs in inappropriate situations |
|   fails to finish work | • Is unable to play or engage in leisure activities |
| • Has difficulty organizing tasks and activities | • Is often "on the go" as if "driven by a motor" |
| • Avoids, dislikes, or is reluctant to engage in | • Talks excessively |
|   tasks that require sustained mental effort | • Blurts out answers before a question is com- |
| • Often loses things | pleted |
| • Is easily distracted | • Has difficulty waiting his or her turn |
| • Is forgetful in daily activities | • Interrupts or intrudes on others |

*ADHD,* Attention deficit hyperactivity disorder.

The girl was born full term and without any complications during pregnancy, except for in utero exposure to tobacco. She has no significant medical history other than breaking her arm at age five after falling off a playground gym. Her family history is significant for ADHD (mother), major depression (both mother and father), and Wolf-Parkinson-White syndrome (father, who was treated with ablation).

### *What is relevant to a diagnosis of ADHD from this history?*
Heritability of ADHD has been estimated at as high as 76%. A number of genes have been associated with ADHD, including DAT1, DRD4, DRD5, 5HTT, HTR1B, and SNAP25. Other risk factors for ADHD include tobacco exposure in utero, low birth weight, and prematurity. As for this patient, her mother's prior history of ADHD and her prior exposure to tobacco in utero are all significant risk factors for developing ADHD herself.

### *The girl's mother has both ADHD and major depressive disorder. How common are comorbidities in ADHD?*
Comorbidity is very common in ADHD. The most common comorbid diagnoses are oppositional defiant disorder, conduct disorder, and specific learning disorder. Other disorders that may co-occur with ADHD include anxiety disorders, depressive and bipolar disorders, tic disorders, obsessive-compulsive disorders, and autism spectrum disorder. Adult ADHD has less of the typical motor symptoms seen in children. As many as 80% of adults with ADHD have at least one coexisting psychiatric disorder, including anxiety disorders, affective disorders, substance use disorders, and personality disorders.

During the appointment, the girl takes out nearly all of the toys from their baskets, despite frequent redirection from her parents to only play with one toy at a time. She takes delight in using two game pieces to bang on an empty metal shelf. She answers questions only after several attempts to get and maintain her attention.

Parents deny that she has had any history of trauma—she recovered from the broken arm just fine and loved having people decorate her cast. They describe her as "tough to get to bed" but say that she sleeps through the night once she has settled down. They describe her appetite as normal. She denies feeling sad and states that she's happy most of the time.

## What is your diagnosis?

The diagnosis of ADHD is made clinically. At this point, the patient meets all criteria for the disorder, and the diagnosis can be made. There is no standard "test" for ADHD, but there are several screening tools that can provide helpful information—especially in gathering information from school or afterschool activities. ADHD-specific rating scales focus directly on the symptoms of ADHD and have a sensitivity and specificity of greater than 90% when used in the appropriate population. The Connors Comprehensive Rating Scales and the ADHD Rating Scale IV have been validated in preschool-aged children. Other scales include the Vanderbilt Assessment Scale and Strengths and Difficulties Questionnaire. For assessing adults for ADHD, the Adult ADHD Self-Report Scale is a brief and practical choice.

---

The girl is evaluated with an electrocardiogram (ECG) that was read by pediatric cardiology. The results are normal.

---

An ECG is not required in the evaluation of ADHD. The exception is in cases where the patient is being considered for psychostimulant medications and a first-degree family member has a history of cardiac disease, such as arrhythmia or sudden cardiac death. The girl in this case has a family history significant for Wolf-Parkinson-White Syndrome.

---

She is started on an extended release formulation of methylphenidate 10 mg daily. During a follow-up visit 1 week later, her symptoms slightly improve in the morning but get worse as the day goes on. Over the next several visits, methylphenidate is titrated up to 40 mg daily. During the next follow-up appointment, she and her parents report that her ability to pay attention and participate in class and at home dramatically improve at this dose.

---

## What medications are used to treat ADHD?

Approximately 70% of patients will have a positive clinical response to a trial of psychostimulants. The two main classes of psychostimulants are methylphenidate and amphetamine. Both are available in multiple formulations with different delivery mechanisms and durations of action. Extended release forms are generally preferred over immediate release forms because of improved medication adherence with one pill a day, avoidance of the need for dosing while at school, and a steadier state of medication throughout the day with a gradual taper off by the afternoon/evening. Immediate-release forms are effective as an adjunct to an extended release formulation to extend the duration of treatment as needed. Table 23.2 summarizes many of the medications used for treating ADHD. It is important to note that studies suggest children treated with psychostimulants have a reduced risk of using illicit substances later in life.

| BASIC SCIENCE/CLINICAL PEARL | STEP 1/2 |
|---|---|

Methylphenidate's mechanism of action is reuptake inhibition of norepinephrine and dopamine into presynaptic neurons, which stimulates the cerebral cortex and subcortical structures similar to amphetamines.

Nonstimulant medications are considered second-line treatment for ADHD. They can be used in the case of adverse effects of stimulants, contraindications to stimulants, or treatment failure of stimulants. There is evidence for atomoxetine, extended-release guanfacine, and extended-release clonidine, though none of these have the robust effects of psychostimulants. The most frequent adverse effects for atomoxetine are transient gastrointestinal distress.

TABLE 23.2 ■ Psychostimulant Medications for Treating ADHD

| Stimulant | Duration of Action | Formulation | Dose Range (mg) | Dosage Schedule |
|---|---|---|---|---|
| **Methylphenidate** | | | | |
| Metabolized by de-esterification by carboxylesterase CES1A1 | | | | |
| Methylphenidate immediate release | 3–5 hours | Tablet, chewable, oral solution | 5–60 | Twice daily to three times daily |
| Methylphenidate hydrochloride extended release tablet | 3–8 hours | Wax matrix | 10–60 | Once daily to three times daily |
| Methylphenidate hydrochloride extended-release capsule | 6–8 hours | Capsule with beads | 10–60 | Once daily |
| Methylphenidate hydrochloride extended release tablets with osmotic-controlled release oral delivery system | 8–12 hours | Oros osmotic controlled-release tablet | 18–72 | Once daily |
| Methylphenidate transdermal | 11–12 hours | Transdermal system (skin patch) | 10–30 | Patch worn for up to 9 hours |
| Methylphenidate hydrochloride extended-release oral suspension | 10–12 hours | Oral suspension (banana) | 20–60 | Once daily |
| **Dexmethylphenidate** | | | | |
| Metabolized by CYP2D6, dopamine hydroxylase, flavin-containing monooxygenase | | | | |
| Dexmethylphenidate immediate release tablet | 3–4 hours | Tablet | 2.5–20 | Twice daily to three times daily |
| Dexmethylphenidate extended release capsule | 8–10 hours | Capsule with beads | 5–30 | Once daily |
| **Dextroamphetamine** | | | | |
| Metabolized by CYP2D6, dopamine beta-hydroxylase, flavin-containing monooxygenase | | | | |
| Dextroamphetamine immediate release tablet | 3–5 hours | Tablet | 5–30 | Twice daily to three times daily |
| Dextroamphetamine spansule | 6–8 hours | Capsule with particles | 5–40 | Once daily to twice daily |
| Dextroamphetamine extended release capsule | 6–8 hours | Capsule | 5–40 | Once daily to twice daily |
| Dextroamphetamine immediate release oral solution | 3–5 hours | Oral solution | 5–40 | Twice daily to three times daily |
| **Lisdexamfetamine** | | | | |
| Metabolized in the blood by hydrolytic activity of red blood cells to dextro-amphetamine and l-lysine | | | | |
| Lisdexamfetamine | 10–13 hours | Capsule or chewable tablet | 30–70 | Once daily |
| **Mixed amphetamine salts** | | | | |
| Metabolism involves CYP2D6 | | | | |
| Mixed amphetamine salts IR tablet | 3–5 hours | Tablet | 5–40 | Once daily to twice daily |

TABLE 23.2 ■ **Psychostimulant Medications for Treating ADHD (*Cont.*)**

| Stimulant | Duration of Action | Formulation | Dose Range (mg) | Dosage Schedule |
|---|---|---|---|---|
| Mixed amphetamine salts XR capsule | 10–12 hours | Capsule with beads | 10–30 | Once daily |

*ADHD,* Attention deficit hyperactivity disorder; *CYP,* cytochrome P450 enzyme; *IR,* immediate release; *XR,* extended release.

---

**BASIC SCIENCE/CLINICAL PEARL** **STEP 1/2**

Clonidine stimulates alpha2-adrenoceptors in the brainstem, thus activating an inhibitory neuron, resulting in reduced sympathetic outflow from the central nervous system. It is also used as an antihypertensive agent, and sudden discontinuation can cause rebound hypertension. Use of an extended release formulation can help mitigate this.

---

The girl is started on an individualized education program (IEP), which allows her to do quizzes and challenging assignments in a room with few distractions. Her teachers are guided to break assignments down into smaller, sequential parts for her. Her parents enrolled in a parenting skills class to help them better gain strategies for managing her behavior at home.

### What are the nonpharmacological treatments for ADHD?

Nonpharmacological treatments for ADHD include behavioral interventions, such as rewarding positive behavior, maintaining a daily schedule, and keeping distractions to a minimum. School-based interventions may also be helpful and include sitting nearest the teacher, taking tests in a less distracting environment, receiving a daily report card, and tutoring services. As for the patient discussed previously, she underwent an IEP, which may also be helpful. A less restrictive school plan known as a 504 may also be helpful. Social skills training can help with deficits affecting socializing with peers. Psychotherapy is most useful for treating the comorbidities of ADHD. Table 23.3

---

TABLE 23.3 ■ **Nonpharmacological Treatment Modalities for ADHD**

| | |
|---|---|
| Behavioral interventions | • Maintaining a family schedule |
| | • Keeping distractions to a minimum |
| | • Rewarding positive behavior |
| | • Using charts and checklists to help stay on task |
| | • Using calm discipline (for children), such as time out |
| School-based interventions | • Tutoring |
| | • Sitting near the teacher |
| | • Having extended time to complete tasks |
| | • Taking tests in a less distracting environment |
| | • Daily report cards |
| Social skills training | • To help with deficits in social skills and problems with peers |
| Psychotherapy | • Executive function training |
| | • Standard therapies for those with comorbidities, such as depression or anxiety |

*ADHD,* Attention deficit hyperactivity disorder.

TABLE 23.4 ■ Individualized Educational Program and 504 Plans

*Individualized education program (IEP)*
- Established under the Individuals with Disabilities Education Act (IDEA) for students who qualify for special education services.
- The IEP committee consists of one of the child's special education teachers; one of the child's regular education teachers; someone who can interpret the educational implications of the child's evaluations (usually the school psychologist); parents; a representative of the school district; a representative of transition service agencies; individuals with other relevant knowledge of the student (such as speech therapists or occupational therapists); and, as appropriate, the student.
- The IEP committee must review the plan at least annually, and more frequently if requested by the parent.
- The child must be reevaluated every 3 years.

*The IEP must:*
- State how the child is currently doing in school.
- Include annual, measurable goals for the student.
- Include special education and related services to be provided to the child or on behalf of the child.
- Include an explanation of the extent (if any) to which the child will not participate with nondisabled children in the regular class and other school activities.
- State what modifications in the administration of state and district-wide tests the child will need.
- State when services will begin, how often they will be provided, where they will be provided, and how long they will last.
- State what transition services needs must also be included for children 14 and up.
- State what transition services are needed to help the child prepare for leaving school, for children 16 and up.
- Beginning at least 1 year before the child reaches the age of majority, the IEP must state that the student has been told of any rights that will transfer to him or her at the age of majority.
- State how the child's progress will be measured and how parents will be informed of that progress.
- IEP plans are enforceable by law under IDEA.

*504 Plans*
- Established under Section 504 of the Rehabilitation Act of 1973.
- Applies to students who have a physical or mental impairment that substantially limits one or more major life activities but who do not qualify for an IEP.
- Has less stringent requirements for the team that develops the plan and what must be included in the plan.
- Appropriate for children who do not require specialized instruction but do require accommodations for a disability, no matter the severity of the disability.

summarizes these nonpharmacological treatment modalities for ADHD. Table 23.4 describes IEP and 504 plans.

She starts finishing her work and her marks in class improve. Parents report less conflict, and relationships at home improve. The combination of medication, educational support, parent training, and therapy improve the girl's ADHD symptoms.

**BEYOND THE PEARLS:**

- A majority of people diagnosed with ADHD in childhood continue to meet criteria for the disorder as adults.
- Weight and height should be closely monitored when patients are taking psychostimulant medications. Parents should be advised to make sure that children taking psychostimulant medications eat before they take the medication and have a substantial snack in the after-noon after the appetite-suppressant effects of the medications wear off.
- As many as 80% of adults with ADHD have at least one coexisting psychiatric disorder, including anxiety disorders, mood disorders, substance use disorders, and personality disorders. Therefore it is important to screen for these comorbid conditions in adults with ADHD.
- A useful screening question in adults with ADHD is to ask about their driving record. Adults with untreated ADHD will often have multiple moving violations.
- Some studies suggest that the antidepressant bupropion, a dopamine and norepinephrine reuptake inhibitor, may be efficacious in treating adult ADHD. Psychotherapy may be useful for treating the comorbidities of ADHD.

## References

Bowers, R. T., Weston, C. D., Mast, R. C., Nelson, S. C., & Jackson, J. C. (2019). *Green's child and adolescent clinical psychopharmacology* (6th ed.). Philadelphia: Wolters Kluwer.

Katzman, M. A., Bilkey, T. S., Chokka, P. R., Fallu, A., & Klassen, L. J. (2017). Adult ADHD and comorbid disorders: Clinical implications of a dimensional approach. *BMC Psychiatry, 17,* 302.

Rey, J., & International Association for Child and Adolescent Psychiatry and Allied Professions. (2012). *IACAPAP textbook of child and adolescent mental health.* Geneva: International Association for Child and Adolescent Psychiatry and Allied Professions.

# CHAPTER 24

# Autism Spectrum Disorder

Alison Duncan ■ Meredith E. Harewood

A 2-year-old boy is brought in by his parents because they are concerned about his delay in language and speech. He only uses about 10 words independently and does not yet speak in two-word sentences. Sometimes he will repeat what his parents say. The boy's parents report that he learned to walk on time. He does not engage in pretend play, nor is he interactive in his playing. The boy mostly plays with toy key rings. He likes to hold them and shake his forearms up and down in a flapping movement. He hates loud noises and will cry if the vacuum cleaner or blender is turned on. His daycare provider has noticed similar behaviors.

### What are the developmental milestones?

Developmental milestones are a set of behaviors, skills, or abilities that are demonstrated by an infant or young child by specified ages. There are four general domains of developmental milestones: gross motor, fine motor, language, and social skills. Many of these milestones are listed in Table 24.1 for the first 36 months of life. When a child does not meet a milestone, it is referred to as a *developmental delay*. Two-year-old children are expected to speak in two- and three-word sentences; however, this child does neither. By age 2, most children have a median vocabulary of 300 words, but the patient knows 10 words; therefore he has a language delay.

### So far, what is your differential diagnosis?

Language delay in a toddler could be secondary to intellectual disability, impaired hearing, a neurologic condition such as cerebral palsy or epilepsy, a neurodevelopmental disorder such as speech sound disorder or developmental verbal dyspraxia (an inability to use motor planning to perform the movements necessary to produce speech), or autism spectrum disorder (ASD).

| CLINICAL PEARL | STEP 2/3 |
|---|---|
| Assessment, diagnosis, and treatment of autism spectrum disorder (ASD) is best done by a multidisciplinary team. | |

The pediatrician reports that the boy received a score of 12 on his Modified Checklist for Autism in Toddlers (M-CHAT) screening questionnaire.

### What is the M-CHAT?

Developmental surveillance is the process through which children who have a developmental delay or are at risk of a developmental delay are recognized. This is done at routine health care visits by assessing for appropriate milestone acquisition, asking parents about any concerns for their child's development, and identifying risk factors. Developmental screening refers to using a

**TABLE 24.1** ■ **Developmental Milestones for First 36 Months**

| Age (Months) | Adaptive/Fine | Language | Gross Motor | Social |
|---|---|---|---|---|
| 1 | Grasp reflex, watches person | Responds to sound | Tonic neck posture, head lag | Begins to smile |
| 2 | Follow to 180 degrees | Coos, listens to voice | Lifts head to 45 degrees | Smiles on social contact |
| 3 | Moro reflex disappears | Vocalizations, listens to music | Lifts head and chest, reaches toward objects | Sustained social contact |
| 4 | Sees pellet, brings object to mouth | Laughs out loud | Grasps objects, no head lag, pushes feet when erect | Shows displeasure if loss of contact with caregiver |
| 7 | Transfers objects, radial palm grasp, rakes pellet | Polysyllabic vowel sounds | Rolls over, pivots, crawls/creep-crawls, sits briefly, bounces on own | Prefers mother, recognizes strangers, enjoys mirror |
| 10 | Thumb and forefinger grasp, pokes with forefinger, pincer picking, retrieves dropped object | Repetitive consonants (mama, dada) | Sits alone, pulls to stand, creeps/crawls | Responds to name, plays peek-a-boo or pat-a-cake, waves bye-bye |
| 12 | Picks up pellet without assistance | Says few words besides mama/dada | Walks holding one hand, rises independently | Plays simple ball game |
| 15 | Builds tower of three blocks, draws in a line | Jargon, follows simple commands, names familiar objects | Walks alone, crawls up stairs | Indicates wants, hugs parents |
| 18 | Builds tower of four blocks, scribbles a line | Says 10 words, names pictures, knows 1+ body parts | Runs stiffly, walks up stairs holding one hand | Feeds self, gets medical attention, seeks help, kisses parents |
| 24 | Builds tower of seven blocks, scribbles circle, folds paper | Uses two or three words together in a sentence | Runs well, walks up/down stairs, opens doors, climbs on furniture, jumps | Handles spoon, helps to undress, listens to story, pretend play, parallel play |
| 30 | Builds tower of nine blocks, scribbles horizontal/vertical line | Refers to self by "I," knows full name | Climbs stairs using alternating feet | Sociodramatic play, parallel |
| 36 | Builds tower of 10 blocks, makes bridge with three cubes, copies circle | Knows age/sex, counts to 3 seconds | Tricycle, stands momentarily on one foot | Plays games, "parallel" with other kids, helps to dress, washes hands |

standardized test to identify children who are at risk of developmental delay. The M-CHAT is a freely available two-stage parent report screening tool to assess risk for ASD. This questionnaire can be administered and scored by a pediatrician as part of a well-child visit, or by child psychiatrists, pediatric neurologists, and child psychologists. The total score is divided into three tiers of risk: low risk (0–2 points), medium risk (3–6 points), and high risk (7–23 points).

| CLINICAL PEARL | STEP 2/3 |
|---|---|

Hearing impairment, such as deafness or frequent ear infections, should be ruled out in the differential diagnosis of developmental delay or ASD.

### What is autism spectrum disorder?

ASD is a neurodevelopmental disorder that is characterized by two core symptoms, which are problems with reciprocal social interactions and communication, and behaviors that are restricted and repetitive. According to the Autism and Developmental Disabilities Monitoring Network, the estimated prevalence of ASD in 2014 was 16.8 per 1000. ASD is three to four times more common in boys than girls. The term *spectrum* refers to the fact that some people have a few mild symptoms whereas others have severe, disabling symptoms. In order to meet diagnostic criteria, symptoms must be present from early childhood and cause significant impairment in functioning. Additionally, the symptoms cannot be better explained by intellectual disability or global developmental delay. Symptoms of ASD are summarized in Table 24.2, and a comparison of a neurodevelopmentally appropriate toddler and a toddler with ASD can be found in Table 24.3. One should specify if an individual has accompanying

### TABLE 24.2 ■ Symptoms of Autism Spectrum Disorder

| A | Persistent deficits in social communication and social interaction manifested by one of the following: |
|---|---|
| | • Deficits in social-emotional reciprocity |
| | • Deficits in nonverbal communicative behaviors used for social interaction |
| | • Deficits in developing, maintaining, and understanding relationships |
| And | |
| B | Restricted, repetitive patterns of behavior, interests, or activities manifested by at least two of the following: |
| | • Stereotyped or repetitive motor movements, use of objects, or speech |
| | • Insistence on sameness, inflexible adherence to routines, or ritualized patterns of verbal or nonverbal behavior |
| | • Highly restricted, fixated interests that are abnormal in intensity or focus |
| | • Hyper- or hypo-reactivity to sensory input or unusual interest in sensory aspects of the environment |

### TABLE 24.3 ■ Comparison of a Neurodevelopmentally Appropriate Toddler Versus Signs of Autism Spectrum Disorder

| Behavior | Neurotypical Toddler | Signs of ASD |
|---|---|---|
| Communication by pointing | • Follows parent's pointing finger to see where the parent is pointing | • Ignores parent's pointing gesture, or gaze does not follow line of the point |
| | • Points to indicate wants (i.e., out-of-reach toy) | • Does not point to communicate wants |
| Pretend play | • Uses toys in pretend play (i.e. eats play food, pretends to talk on play phone) | • Uses toys, but not to act out interactive, pretend play |
| Sharing enjoyment | • Looks at parents to share interest or engage in play | • Enjoys toys but does not look to share the experience with eye contact, smiles, or engaging with others |
| Responding to name | • Responds to parents when name is called | • Does not respond to one's name |

*ASD,* Autism spectrum disorder.

intellectual impairment and/or language impairment. ASD is also further stratified into three severity levels: requiring support (Level One), requiring substantial support (Level Two), and requiring very substantial support (Level Three). The pathogenesis of ASD is not completely understood.

The boy's family history is significant for attention-deficit hyperactivity disorder (ADHD) in his mother, who is 43 years old. His father, who is 45 years old, has major depressive disorder. The boy's 50-year-old uncle has schizophrenia.

### What are the risk factors for ASD?
Risk factors for ASD include:

Neonatal
- Male gender
- Birth weight less than 2500 g
- Prematurity (under 35 weeks)
- Admission to a neonatal intensive care unit
- Perinatal or neonatal illness—such as encephalitis or sepsis
- Genetic disorder associated with ASD

Parental
- Maternal age older than 40
- Paternal age older than 40

Family history
- Sibling with autism
- Familial history of psychosis, mood disorder, or other mental illness

| CLINICAL PEARL | STEP 2/3 |
|---|---|
| Intellectual disability is often comorbid with ASD but is not part of the diagnostic criteria for ASD. | |

| CLINICAL PEARL | STEP 2/3 |
|---|---|
| The measles-mumps-rubella (MMR) vaccine does not have a link to ASD. Emotionally cold ("refrigerator") mothers and gluten also do not have a link with ASD. | |

| CLINICAL PEARL | STEP 2/3 |
|---|---|
| Heritability of ASD is between 50% and 80%. | |

The boy is referred for psychological testing, including the Autism Diagnostic Observation Schedule (ADOS). The results are consistent with ASD with accompanying language impairment. The psychologist recommends early intervention services, occupational therapy evaluation, speech therapy evaluation, and behavioral therapy.

| CLINICAL PEARL | STEP 2/3 |
|---|---|
| Symptoms of ASD must be present from early childhood but may not be fully apparent until the social demands of the environment exceed a child's capacity. Consequently, many children with high functioning ASD are not identified until elementary school or later. Likewise, learned behavioral strategies may mask the deficits later in life. | |

Back in your clinic, you make these referrals and discuss the value of genetic testing to screen for the many genetic syndromes that are associated with autism. The parents consent to the screening. You also have the parents meet with a social worker who orients them to the resources for developmental disabilities in your state and connects them to a local support group for parents of children with ASD.

### How useful is genetic testing in ASD?

Genetic testing is considered the standard of care for individuals with ASD. Initial genetic evaluation includes a three-tiered genogram, physical examination with special attention to dysmorphic features, chromosomal microarray, DNA testing for fragile X syndrome in males and mitochondrial and/or metabolic testing if appropriate clinical indicators are present. Several genetic syndromes are associated with ASD. These syndromes often carry increased risk in other systems, such as heart disease or increased cancer risk, which can guide surveillance decisions over the lifespan.

Genetic syndromes that are associated with autism include 22q11.2 deletions (including velocardiofacial syndrome), Angelman syndrome, fragile X syndrome, Prader-Willi syndrome, Rett syndrome, tuberous sclerosis, and Williams syndrome, CHARGE syndrome, de Lange syndrome, MED12 disorders (including Lujan-Fryns syndrome), PTEN-associated disorders (Cowden syndrome, Bannayan-Riley-Ruvalcaba syndrome), Smith-Lemli-Opitz syndrome, Smith-Magenis syndrome, and Sotos syndrome.

---

**CLINICAL PEARL**                                                        **STEP 2/3**

Seizures, gastrointestinal disturbances, sleep disorders, and immune disorders are medical comorbidities with ASD.

---

The boy and his family enroll in 20 hours per week of early intervention services that employ a combination of applied behavioral analysis and play-based therapy. In addition, the boy receives weekly speech therapy. The parents report that his vocabulary is improving and that he is learning how to react appropriately in social situations with other children and adults.

---

Early intervention is both indicated and effective for ASD. The disorder is considered a lifelong disability, but treatment can significantly improve a child's functioning and the quality of his social interactions. The most common and well-studied early intervention for ASD is applied behavior analysis (ABA) therapy. In ABA therapy, a trained ABA therapist evaluates the child's behaviors, his abilities, and challenges, and helps the child and family identify goals for treatment. The therapist teaches and reinforces desired behaviors (e.g., compliance, social skills) and discourages undesired behaviors (e.g., tantrums, aggression, self-stimulatory behavior), typically by withholding attention from the undesired behaviors. ABA typically takes place in the home, often with the parents as cotherapists. ABA may also be conducted at school to target behaviors there.

Other therapies that have some evidence for efficacy in ASD include social skills programs, augmentative and alternative communication systems, treatment and education of autistic and communication-related handicapped children (TEACCH) program, and cognitive behavioral therapy.

---

**BEYOND THE PEARLS:**

- Standard of care for the diagnosis of ASD includes obtaining a clinical history, developmental surveillance, psychological screening tests (e.g., the M-CHAT), neuropsychological testing to confirm the diagnosis, and genetic testing for associated genetic syndromes.
- The Autism Diagnostic Observation Schedule (ADOS) is often considered the gold standard in ASD diagnosis. Different versions, or modules, of the examination are given based on an individual's age. The Autism Diagnosis Interview-Revised (ADI-R) is the other most universally recognized, comprehensive diagnostic tool for ASD.

### References

Aites, J., & Schonwald, A. (2018). Developmental-behavioral surveillance and screening in primary care. In C. Bridgemohan (Ed.), *UpToDate*. Retrieved November 28, 2018, from https://www-uptodate-com.ucsf.idm.oclc.org/contents/developmental-behavioral-surveillance-and-screening-in-prima-ry-care?search=developmental%20surveillance&source=search_result&selectedTitle=1~34&usage_type=default&display_rank=1

American Psychiatric Association. (2013). *Diagnostic and statistical manual of mental disorders* (5th ed.). Washington, DC: American Psychiatric Association.

Davies, D. (2011). *Child development: A practioner's guide* (3rd ed.). New York, NY: The Guilford Press.

Moreno De Luca, D., & Ross, D. A. (2016). Autism spectrum disorder. *National Neuroscience Curriculum Initiative*. Retrieved from www.nncionline.org/course/autism-spectrum-disorder/.

Schaefer, G. B., & Medelsohn, N. J. and Professional Practice and Guidelines Committee. (2013). Clinical genetic evaluation in identifying the etiology of Autism Spectrum Disorders: 2013 guideline revisions. *Genetics in Medicine, 15*, 399–407.

Tanguay, P. (2010). Autism spectrum disorders. In M. Dulcan, (Ed.), *Dulcan's textbook of child and adolescent psychiatry*. Washington, DC: American Psychiatric Publishing.

# CHAPTER 25

# Impulse Control and Conduct Disorders

Alison Duncan ■ Peter Ureste

A 10-year-old boy presents to the clinic with his parents. He initially refuses to come into the office. After some cajoling, threatening, and then bribery with fast food, his parents convince him to join. They describe how he refuses to accept adult authority. The boy is sometimes motivated by rewards, but improvements in behavior are never sustained. He is easily annoyed and often loses his temper over small disappointments. The boy has already been suspended from school after hitting a teacher who was trying to restrain him when he refused to take a test and then ran out of the classroom and toward a busy street. His parents report that school was better last year because the boy got along well with his teacher, who gave him a lot of individual attention and special tasks. The boy has always been very hyperactive and has "no focus at all," and the teacher's attention helped him to keep his behavior under control. They explain that, "The teacher this year is too weak and cannot control the classroom."

### What are disruptive, impulse-control, and conduct disorders?

It is normal for toddlers to have temper tantrums and for adolescents to display irritability and risk-taking behavior within a mild to moderate range without severely disrupting basic functions like going to school or being part of a family. Disruptive, impulse-control, and conduct disorders are a group of disorders that are characterized by more severe and longer-lasting disruptive behaviors that interfere with the ability to function. This group of disorders includes oppositional defiant disorder, intermittent explosive disorder, conduct disorder, antisocial personality disorder, pyromania, and kleptomania. These conditions are unique in that their associated symptoms are often in conflict with societal norms and violate the rights of others. Table 25.1 lists the different disruptive, impulse-control, and conduct disorders according to the *Diagnostic and Statistical Manual of Mental Disorders*, Fifth Edition (DSM-5).

### What are the symptoms of oppositional defiant disorder (ODD)?

The diagnostic criteria for ODD include at least four symptoms in the areas of angry or irritable mood, argumentative or defiant behavior, or vindictiveness. Angry or irritable mood can manifest as being often angry and resentful, easily annoyed, or quick to lose one's temper. Argumentative or defiant behavior can be seen as arguing with authority figures, actively defying requests from authority figures or rules, deliberately annoying others, and often blaming others for his or her misbehavior. These symptoms last at least 6 months and occur in interaction with at least one individual who is not a sibling.

TABLE 25.1 ■ **Disruptive, Impulse-Control, and Conduct Disorders in the DMS-5**

Oppositional defiant disorder
Intermittent explosive disorder
Conduct disorder
Antisocial personality disorder
Pyromania
Kleptomania

DSM, *Diagnostic and Statistical Manual of Mental Disorders*, Fifth Edition.

---

**CLINICAL PEARL**                                                    **STEP 2/3**

Oppositional defiant disorder (ODD) is categorized as a disruptive, impulse-control, and conduct disorder. Diagnostic criteria include at least four symptoms in the areas of angry/irritable
mood and argumentative/defiant behavior or vindictiveness, lasting at least 6 months and
occurring in interaction with at least one individual who is not a sibling.

### How common is ODD?

The prevalence of ODD is 1% to 11%, with a greater proportion seen in preadolescent boys as
opposed to preadolescent girls (1.4:1). Onset is usually between preschool to early adolescence.
The disorder is frequently comorbid with attention-deficit hyperactivity disorder (ADHD), depression, anxiety, and conduct disorder.

---

**CLINICAL PEARL**                                                    **STEP 2/3**

Unlike attention-deficit hyperactivity disorder (ADHD), which requires symptoms to be present
in two or more settings, it is not uncommon for ODD symptoms to be limited to the home
setting and limited to interactions with family members. ODD with symptoms that are only
evident at home is considered mild; if symptoms are present in two settings then the disorder
is considered moderate; if present in three or more settings then ODD is considered severe.

### What are the risk factors of ODD?

Several risk factors have been identified for ODD, in addition to genetic risk. Harsh, inconsistent,
or neglectful child-rearing practices are commonly associated with ODD. High levels of emotional reactivity and poor frustration tolerance increase the chances of developing ODD. Physiologic
factors that are more common in children with ODD and conduct disorder (CD) include lower
heart rate, lower skin conductance response, reduced basal cortical reactivity, and abnormalities in
the amygdala and prefrontal cortex.

---

When the boy's parents take away his phone or television privileges, he sometimes deliberately
destroys their belongings.

---

### Does this boy have intermittent explosive disorder (IED)?

IED is a disorder consisting of recurrent, unpremeditated behavioral outbursts representing a failure to control aggressive impulses. Diagnosis requires manifestation of symptoms by one of two
ways. An individual must show verbal and physical aggression toward people, animals, or property
that occurs twice weekly, on average, for at least 3 months. However, the physical aggression does

**TABLE 25.2 ■ DSM-5 Diagnostic Criteria for Intermittent Explosive Disorder**

| A<br>(1 or 2) | (1) Verbal or physical aggression that does not result in property damage or injury to people or animals | Twice weekly, on average, for 3 months |
|---|---|---|
| | (2) Behavioral outbursts resulting in property destruction and/or physical assault against others or animals | Three outbursts within a 12-month period |
| B | Aggressiveness is out of proportion to the precipitating stressor | |
| C | Outbursts are not premeditated or committed to achieving a tangible goal | |
| D | Outbursts result in either marked distress or functional impairment | |
| E | Must be at least 6 years old | |

DSM, *Diagnostic and Statistical Manual of Mental Disorders*, Fifth Edition.

not result in property destruction or physical injury to people or animals. Or, within a 12-month period an individual has three behavioral outbursts resulting in destruction to property and/or physical assault that injures people or animals. Table 25.2 summarizes the DSM-5 diagnostic criteria for IED.

In the case of this patient, he likely does not have IED, as his property destruction is mediated—it is an aggressive response to his parents taking away his phone or television.

---

The boy was born full term and without complications during pregnancy. There were no adverse exposures during pregnancy. His medical history is significant for attention-deficit hyperactivity disorder (ADHD). Family history is significant for ADHD (mother), major depression (mother), posttraumatic stress disorder (mother and sister), alcohol and cannabis use disorders (biological father), and antisocial personality disorder (biological father).

He lives with his biological mother, stepfather and older sister. His mother is employed as an office manager and his stepfather is an electrician. His biological father is currently in prison on drug-related charges. Before his imprisonment, the boy's mother had a restraining order against his father because of domestic violence.

During an interview with the mother, she tearfully describes feeling terrified that her son will turn out like his biological father. She describes the father as charming and sweet when he was happy with her and cruel and abusive when he was not. After they divorced, she learned from her ex-mother-in-law that her ex-husband's problems had started in childhood. He was a bully in school and frequently initiated fights to maintain his control of the schoolyard. He smashed all the windows of an ex-girlfriend's car when he thought that his girlfriend had cheated on him. He sold drugs in high school. He manipulated an intellectually disabled cousin to perform the riskiest parts of selling drugs so that the cousin would get in trouble instead of him. He never showed remorse for this kind of behavior. She wants to do anything she can to make sure that her son does not follow this path and wonders if he should go to a "scared straight" program.

---

*What are the symptoms of conduct disorder (CD)?*

The boy's biological father was diagnosed with antisocial personality disorder and likely had CD in his youth. According to the DSM-5, CD is a "repetitive and persistent pattern of behavior in which the basic rights of others or major age-appropriate societal norms are violated." Symptoms include at least three in the areas of aggression to people and animals, destruction of property, deceitfulness or theft, and serious violations of rules. Some examples of symptoms include, but are not limited to, initiating physical fights, using weapons, cruelty to animals, deliberately engaging in fire setting with the intention of causing damage, or breaking into someone else's property. CD occurs in between 2% to 10% of the population, with a medical prevalence rate of 4%. Prevalence rates are higher in males than in females.

| CLINICAL PEARL | STEP 2/3 |
|---|---|

Adults with antisocial personality disorder typically show symptoms of conduct disorder (CD) before 15 years old.

| CLINICAL PEARL | STEP 2/3 |
|---|---|

The Macdonald triad is a set of three factors that may be associated with violent tendencies later in adulthood. These are cruelty to animals, obsession with fire-setting, and persistent bedwetting in childhood.

### What distinguishes CD from ODD?
Both, CD and ODD are related to conduct problems that bring the individual in conflict with adults and other authority figures, such as teachers and work supervisors. The behaviors of CD are typically more severe than those of ODD and often violate the rights of others. Children who are eventually diagnosed with CD are often initially diagnosed with ODD. Many children with ODD, however, will not develop CD.

---

Before the appointment, the boy's parents and teacher completed the Strengths and Difficulties Questionnaire (SDQ) regarding the boy. The boy was also given the SDQ but refused to fill it out. The results are summarized in Table 25.3.

---

### What are the suggested assessment tools for disruptive, impulse-control, and conduct disorders?
The SDQ is a freely available assessment tool that can be used to screen for (1) emotional symptoms, (2) hyperactivity/inattention, (3) conduct problems, (4) peer relationship problems, and (5) prosocial behavior (http://www.sdqinfo.org). Scores are generated in each of the categories and the scoring guide gives cut-points that were experimentally established, such that 80% of children are "average," 12% "slightly raised," 4% high, and 4% very high in each category except for the prosocial scale, where 80% of children are "average," 12% "slightly lowered," 4% low, and 4% very low. The SDQ has been translated into over 100 languages and normative data has been collected in 10 countries. There are versions for ages 2 to 4, 4 to 17 and 18 and older with data collected from parents, teachers, self, and other informants. The Swanson, Nolan and Pelham Questionnaire (SNAP) is a freely available screening tool for ADHD, which contains content relevant to ODD. Data is collected from parents, teachers and other caregivers. The Vanderbilt ADHD Diagnostic Parent Rating Scale is a freely available tool that screens for ADHD with additional scales that screen for ODD, CD, anxiety, and mood disorder. The Child Behavior Checklist is a

---

TABLE 25.3 ■ Results of the Strengths and Difficulties Questionnaire

|  | Mother | Stepfather | Teacher |
|---|---|---|---|
| Total difficulties score | Very high | High | Very high |
| Emotional problems score | Slightly raised | High | Slightly raised |
| Conduct problems score | Very high | High | Very high |
| Hyperactivity score | High | Slightly raised | Very high |
| Peer problems score | Very high | Slightly raised | Very high |
| Prosocial problems score | Slightly lowered | Slightly lowered | Average |
| Impact score | Very high | Very high | Very high |

tool available for purchase that screens for several psychiatric problems, including disruptive, impulse-control, and conduct disorders. The Conners-3 is a tool available for purchase that screens for ADHD and contains additional assessments for ODD and CD.

### What is your differential diagnosis for this patient?

This is an 11-year-old boy who is easily annoyed, loses his temper, and vindictive toward his parents. He is openly defiant toward authority figures, including his parents and teacher. His symptoms are present for at least 1 year. One might consider a diagnosis of conduct disorder, as he was previously suspended from school for hitting a teacher, but he has failed to demonstrate repeated violation of the rights of other people or animals. As such, a diagnosis of oppositional defiant disorder is more appropriate.

---

The boy is diagnosed with ODD and ADHD.

---

### What is the treatment for ODD?

Medications are generally not used to treat ODD or CD but may be useful for IED. However, medications may be used for comorbid conditions that frequently co-occur. For example, if a child or teen also has as ADHD or major depression then medication may be useful. Treatment may also involve training for the parents on how to respond to challenging behaviors. Two evidenced-based parent management training courses are "The Incredible Years (Webster-Stratton) and Triple P," or the "Positive Parenting Program." Both have been validated and found to be effective for externalizing disorders—characterized by maladaptive behaviors that are directed toward other people and the external environment—in a diversity of family types and backgrounds. Military-style "boot camps" for children with ODD and CD have been found to be ineffective. The "Scared Straight"–type programs have been found to be harmful, leading to overall worse outcomes.

---

The boy was started on a psychostimulant for ADHD, and his parents are enrolled in a parent management class. After completing the class, they report that the patient's behavior has improved substantially. They note that their parenting styles have become much more in tune with each other and consistent in their expectations and limit setting with their son.

---

### BEYOND THE PEARLS:

- Children with ODD often have parents with mood disorders, whereas children with CD often have parents with antisocial behavior. Parents of children with CD are more likely to be depressed, to have issues of substance use, and/or to have antisocial personality traits.
- A child with ODD may have symptoms in only one context—for example, they may have behavioral problems at home but not at school.
- The SDQ is a freely available screening tool that can be used to screen for emotional symptoms, hyperactivity/inattention, conduct problems, peer relationship problems, and prosocial behavior.
- Medication is not typically used to manage ODD or CD. It can be helpful in IEP or in common comorbid disorders, such as ADHD or depression.
- "The Incredible Years (Webster-Stratton) and Triple P," or the "Positive Parenting Program," are two evidenced-based parenting programs that have shown to be effective in reducing social, emotional, and behavioral problems in children.
- Military-style "boot camps" for children with ODD and CD have been found to be ineffective. The "Scared Straight"–type programs have been found to be harmful, leading to overall worse outcomes.

## References

American Psychiatric Association. (2013). *Diagnostic and statistical manual of mental disorders* (5th ed.). Washington, DC: Author.

Goodman, R., Ford, T., Simmons, H., Gatward, & Meltzer (2000). Using the Strengths and Difficulties Questionnaire (SDQ) to screen for child psychiatric disorders in a community sample. *British Journal of Psychiatry. 177*, 534–539.

Leijten, P., Raaijmakers, M., Orobio de Castro, B., van den Ban, E., & Matthys, W. (2017). Effectiveness of the Incredible Years Parenting Program for families with socioeconomically disadvantaged and ethnic minority backgrounds. *Journal of Clinical Child and Adolescent Psychology, 46*(1), 59–73.

Rey, J. & International Association for Child and Adolescent Psychiatry and Allied Professions. (2012). *IACAPAP textbook of child and adolescent mental health*. Geneva: International Association for Child and Adolescent Psychiatry and Allied Professions.

Riley, M., Ahmed, S., & Locke, A. (2016). Common questions about oppositional defiant disorder. *American Family Physician, 93*(7), 586–591.

Shatkin, J. P. (2015). *Child & adolescent mental health: A practical, all-in-one guide*. New York, NY: W. W. Norton & Company.

# CHAPTER 26

# Tic Disorders and Tourette Syndrome

Olesya Pokorna

J. is a 7-year-old boy who is brought in by his parents to an outpatient psychiatric clinic for an evaluation of repetitive eye blinking, sniffing, and head jerking.

### *What is a tic?*

Tics are sudden, rapid, nonrhythmic, repetitive movements, or vocalizations that can be voluntarily suppressed. Tics are preceded by a strong premonitory urge, subjectively described as an itch, pressure, tension, or tingling in an affected muscle group that is alleviated by performing a tic in a particular body part. Patients report significant relief and reduction of anxiety after a tic. Stress, anxiety, boredom, fatigue, and strong emotions can increase the severity and frequency of symptoms. Relaxation, focused concentration on a task, and engaging in a physical activity tend to be common alleviating factors. Tic frequency is markedly reduced during sleep. Severity and frequency of tics are highly variable and tend to wax and wane over time, with some tics going away while the new ones emerge.

---

**CLINICAL PEARL**                                           **STEP 1/2/3**

Tics are brief, nonrhythmic, repetitive movements or vocalizations that can be voluntarily suppressed. A tic starts with a premonitory urge sensation, whereas performance of a tic leads to significant relief and alleviation of anxiety.

---

### *How are tics categorized?*

Tics are usually categorized into motor versus vocal and simple versus complex. Motor tics can involve any body part and frequently affect the face, neck, and upper body. Common motor tics are eye blinking, grimacing, sniffing, neck turning, and shoulder shrugging. Simple motor tics involve a discrete muscle group, whereas complex tics are associated with a series of movements that look purposeful, such as self-hitting or gesturing. Vocal tics can range from utterances, such as grunting or throat clearing (vocal tics), to a repetition of words, phrases, or sentences (verbal tics). Coprolalia, or uttering of obscenities, is seen only in a minority of cases. Table 26.1 lists the categories of tics.

**TABLE 26.1 ■ Types of Tics**

| | |
|---|---|
| Simple motor | Eye blinking, nose twitching, shoulder shrugging, and head jerking |
| Complex motor | Facial grimacing, touching, self-hitting, bizarre gait, obscene gestures (copropraxia) |
| Simple vocal | Grunting, throat clearing, barking, sniffing, snorting |
| Complex vocal | Words, phrases, or sentences. Repetition of one's own words (palilalia), other people's words (echolalia), or usage of obscene language (coprolalia) |

TABLE 26.2 ■ Diagnostic Criteria of Tic Disorders

| Condition | Symptoms | Duration |
| --- | --- | --- |
| Provisional tic disorder | Single or multiple motor or vocal tics | Less than 1 year |
| Persistent tic disorder | Single or multiple motor and/or vocal tics | At least 1 year |
| Tourette syndrome | Multiple motor and at least one vocal tic | At least 1 year |

J.'s symptoms started about 9 months ago and have been waxing and waning over time, but he has never been symptom free for more than several days in a row. Although he can sometimes control the tics, he has not been successful all the time. He does not feel distressed by the symptoms, has been doing well in school, and has a lot of friends. He has no other medical problems, and his birth and developmental history are unremarkable. Family history is notable for anxiety and obsessive-compulsive disorder (OCD) in his older sister, and attention-deficit hyperactivity disorder (ADHD) in his father. Neurologic examination is unremarkable.

### What is your differential diagnosis?

Although both motor and vocal tics are present, symptom duration of less than 1 year calls for a diagnosis of provisional tic disorder (Table 26.2). Other diagnostic considerations include Tourette syndrome and persistent tic disorder. In contrast to Tourette syndrome, which requires the presence of multiple motor and at least one vocal tic, persistent tic disorder requires either motor or vocal tic(s). Provisional tic disorder is diagnosed when tics are present for less than 1 year. Of note, up to 25% of healthy elementary school children can develop transient tics, which spontaneously resolve within 1 year. Other diagnostic considerations include obsessive-compulsive disorder (OCD), chorea, seizures, akathisia, athetosis, dystonia, myoclonus, and stereotypies associated with developmental disorders. Tics can be differentiated from other abnormal movements by premonitory urges, suppressibility, a sense of relief after performing a movement, and a history of waxing and waning over time.

### The family asks for additional testing or imaging. What do you tell them?

Tic disorder is a clinical diagnosis and is based on symptoms, signs, and medical history rather than laboratory tests or imaging. Brain imaging, such as magnetic resonance imaging or computed tomography, are usually unremarkable and do not substantively contribute to establishing a diagnosis. However, imaging is indicated when neurologic examination is abnormal.

---

**CLINICAL PEARL**                                                        **STEP 2/3**

Tourette syndrome is a clinical diagnosis and does not require additional laboratory testing or imaging in the presence of normal neurologic examination.

---

### What are your initial treatment considerations?

Pharmacologic treatment is indicated when symptoms interfere with functioning—such as school performance, social interactions, and activities of daily living—or cause pain or injury. If symptoms are mild and are not bothersome to a patient, watchful waiting approach is appropriate as symptoms tend to wax and wane over time. Psychotherapy and psychoeducation are often sufficient to relieve mild symptoms and can be offered as a first step of treatment.

*What psychotherapy modalities are effective for Tourette syndrome?*
A type of cognitive behavioral therapy, called *habit reversal training* (HRT), is an effective behavioral treatment for tics. The first step is identifying a premonitory urge, followed by performing a competing response, such as an action that is not compatible with the tic behavior. For example, a patient who repeatedly shrugs the shoulders can use a competing response of pushing the shoulders downward and tensing the neck muscles until the urge dissipates. In addition to awareness and competing response training, patients learn relaxation techniques and get better understanding of situations that worsen tics.

---

The family are reassured by the psychoeducation you provide but wish to delay behavioral therapy. They come back for a 3-month follow-up and J.'s tics are more frequent and troublesome. The head jerking is more forceful and causes neck pain and headaches. In addition to existing symptoms, he blurts out phrases, such as "shut up" and "get out," and makes self-hitting motions with his arms directed toward his face. He has been concentrating very hard on controlling these tics in class and, as a result, is having difficulty paying attention and completing his work on time. J. is self-conscious about his symptoms, has been minimizing social interactions, and is tearful and irritable at home.

---

*What is your diagnosis?*
J. has had both motor and vocal tics for more than a year and now meets criteria for Tourette syndrome. The *Diagnostic and Statistical Manual of Mental Disorders*, Fifth Edition (DSM-5), criteria for Tourette syndrome specify that the symptoms should start before the age of 18 and have a history of both multiple motor and at least one vocal tic, which do not need to occur simultaneously. Symptoms should be present nearly every day for more than 1 year, and any symptom-free period should be no longer than 3 months. Although his current symptoms clearly cause distress, unlike most DSM-5 diagnoses, the criteria for Tourette syndrome does not require presence of functional impairment.

---

**CLINICAL PEARL**                                              **STEP 1/2/3**

The diagnosis of Tourette syndrome requires both motor and vocal tics at some point during the illness, but not necessarily at the same time. Symptoms should occur nearly every day, with no tic-free period exceeding 3 months, for at least 1 year, and start before age 18. The disorder must not be due to another medical condition or drug use.

---

*What is the pathophysiology of Tourette syndrome?*
Neurobiologic causes of tics are not well understood. Abnormalities in striatal-thalamic-cortical pathways produce abnormal movements. Heightened dopaminergic activity in these brain regions triggers tics, whereas medications that lower dopamine levels in the central nervous system (CNS) alleviate symptoms.

---

**BASIC SCIENCE PEARL**                                          **STEP 1**

Tics result from dysregulation in striatal-thalamic-cortical (mesolimbic) system. Abnormally high levels of dopaminergic activity in these brain areas trigger tics.

---

*What is the natural course and prognosis of Tourette disorder?*
Tourette disorder has a prevalence of less than 1% in the general population. Tics usually appear between 5 and 8 years of age, peak around 11 years of age, and subside during adolescence. By

early adulthood, a majority of patients have significant reduction in tics and about 30% are symptom free. However, many patients have residual mild tics throughout lifetime.

*What are the common psychiatric comorbidities of Tourette syndrome?*
Tourette syndrome is associated with various psychiatric conditions, including ADHD, OCD, learning disorders, conduct disorder, oppositional defiant disorder, sleep difficulties, and anxiety and mood disorders. Anger outbursts and aggressive and self-injurious behaviors are often seen in patients with Tourette syndrome. These conditions often cause significant distress and further contribute to functional impairment. When evaluating patients with Tourette syndrome, it is important to assess for these frequently comorbid conditions and plan treatment accordingly.

| CLINICAL PEARL | STEP 1/2/3 |
| --- | --- |

Tourette syndrome is highly comorbid with ADHD and OCD, which also run in affected families. Always screen for personal and family history of ADHD and OCD symptoms when evaluating a child with a tic disorder.

The patient's parents are planning to have another child soon and are concerned about the risk to siblings.

*How do you counsel them?*
The cause of Tourette syndrome is unknown. Although no specific gene has been implicated, there is evidence for genetic basis of Tourette given familial transmission; children with Tourette syndrome have a family history in about half the cases. Siblings of an affected child have an 8% risk of developing this syndrome, compared with 1% in the general population. Males are more commonly affected than females, with a male-to-female ratio of 4:1. Of note, relatives of children with Tourette syndrome are also more likely to carry diagnosis of ADHD, OCD, and mood and anxiety disorders.

*What treatment options would you offer at this time?*
Because current symptoms interfere with school and social functioning, cause psychological distress, and produce physical pain, medication is an appropriate next step in management. Summary of pharmacological treatments for tic disorders are listed in Table 26.3. The goal of

TABLE 26.3 ■ Pharmacologic Treatments for Tic Disorders

| Alpha-blockers | Clonidine, guanfacine | First-line treatment due to more favorable side effect profile<br>Consider for patients with comorbid ADHD |
| --- | --- | --- |
| Antipsychotics | FGAs:<br>• haloperidol, pimozide, fluphenazine<br>SGAs:<br>• risperidone, olanzapine, ziprasidone | Very effective but have significant side effect profile, including extrapyramidal side effects, tardive dyskinesia (FGAs), and metabolic syndrome (SGAs) hyperprolactinemia (risperidone) |
| Dopamine depleters | VMAT2 inhibitors<br>• Tetrabenazine<br>• Valbenazine | No risk of extrapyramidal side effects or tardive dyskinesia |

*ADHD,* Attention-deficit hyperactivity disorder; *FGAs,* first-generation antipsychotics; *SGAs,* second-generation antipsychotics; *VMAT2,* vesicular monoamine transporter 2.

treatment is reduction of tics to a tolerable level rather than complete elimination of symptoms, which is often difficult to achieve and can lead to overmedication and significant side effect burden. Alpha agonist blockers, such as clonidine and guanfacine, are first line for treating tics in the pediatric population. It is a particularly good choice for patients who have a diagnosis of comorbid ADHD, because alpha agonist blockers can also be used for controlling symptoms of impulsivity and inattention. Antidopaminergic agents such as antipsychotics (risperidone, fluphenazine) are considered second-line treatment because of unfavorable side effect profiles, particularly when taken long term. Compared to antipsychotics, tetrabenazine, a vesicular monoamine transporter inhibitor that acts by inhibiting dopamine release from presynaptic vesicles, is equally effective but does not cause tardive dyskinesia. Intramuscular botulinum toxin injections can be used for treating refractory motor and vocal tics and should be considered if motor tics cause muscle pain or injury.

---

Clonidine 0.05 mg twice a day is started. When J. presents for a follow-up appointment in 4 weeks, frequency and intensity of his motor and vocal tics are significantly improved, and he controls them more effectively using the skill he learned in therapy. His grades are improving, and he is calmer, less irritable, and less anxious.

The family read about pediatric autoimmune neuropsychiatric disorders associated with streptococcal infections (PANDAS) on the Internet and asks the psychiatrist for more information.

---

### What is PANDAS?

PANDAS remains a controversial diagnosis. It is postulated that streptococcal pharyngitis or skin infections can cause abrupt onset or worsening of preexisting tics and OCD symptoms in a small group of pediatric patients, presumably through autoimmune-mediated central nervous system injury. Diagnosis is established retrospectively and requires a confirmed history of streptococcal infection followed by acute worsening of neuropsychiatric symptoms. The benefit of prophylactic antibiotics has not been clearly demonstrated; standard treatments of OCD and tics remain a mainstream approach.

---

**BASIC SCIENCE PEARL**                                                      **STEP 1**

PANDAS is pediatric autoimmune neuropsychiatric disorder associated with streptococcal infections. The syndrome involves acute onset or worsening of tic and OCD symptoms following a streptococcal infection, particularly during winter–spring months. This diagnosis remains highly controversial.

---

### What are the complications of tic disorders?

Many patients with mild to moderate tics do not experience any distress or impairment associated with their symptoms. For others tics contribute to significant social, academic, and psychological difficulties. Although most children with Tourette syndrome have normal intellectual functioning, academic achievement is frequently suboptimal. Tics may interfere with the ability to focus, maintain a conversation or engage in social interactions, or attend public places that require people to stay still and quiet, such as school, office, places of worship, etc. People with tics may experience social stigma and isolation, peer rejection, criticism, and school and family conflicts, leading to overall lower quality of life and psychological distress. Comorbid psychiatric conditions, such as ADHD, OCD, and oppositional defiant disorder, further compound these problems. With regard to medical sequalae of tics, in rare cases repeated movements associated with motor tics can cause pain and injury; for example, tics involving repeated head jerking can cause spinal compression, disk herniation, myelopathy, or, in severe cases, cervical artery dissection. Self-hitting may lead to soft tissue injury or fractures; ocular trauma is particularly concerning with self-directed motor tics.

---

**BEYOND THE PEARLS:**

- Tourette syndrome patients with disabling refractory tics who failed psychopharmacological treatment may be candidates for deep brain stimulation (DBS), targeting subcortical areas of the brain. This treatment option remains new and, although it has demonstrated some clinical efficacy, more research is required. DBS is associated with a high rate of adverse outcomes, including infection, seizures, and stroke.
- Echophenomena, such as echolalia (repetition of another person's words) and echopraxia (repetition of another person's movements), can be a part of a tic repertoire. Imitation behaviors are a normal stage of early neurodevelopement that promotes learning and social interaction. Presence of echophenomena beyond the age of two or 3 years points toward an underlying neurologic pathology. Echophenomena is also seen in autism spectrum, developmental disorders, and dementia.

---

## References

Bagheri, M. M., Kerbeshian, J., & Burd, L. (1999). Recognition and management of Tourette's syndrome and tic disorders. *American Family Physicians, 59*, 2263.

Ganos, C., Ogrzal, T., Schnitzler, A., & Münchau, A. (2012). The pathophysiology of echopraxia/echolalia: Relevance to Gilles de la Tourette syndrome. *Movement Disorders, 27*(10), 1222–1229.

Gunduz, A., & Okun, M. S. (2016). A review and update on Tourette syndrome: Where is the field headed? *Current Neurology and Neuroscience Reports, 16*(4), 37.

Kurlan, R. M. (2014). Treatment of Tourette syndrome. *Neurotherapeutics, 11*(1), 161–165.

Shprecher, D., & Kurlan, R. (2009). The management of tics. *Movement Disorders, 24*(1), 15–24.

# CHAPTER 27

# Dissociative Disorders

Meredith E. Harewood

A call comes to the consultation-liaison service of a regional hospital to evaluate an 18-year-old woman in the emergency department (ED) who was found wandering the streets of a nearby suburb. A hurricane passed through the area yesterday, causing massive flooding, widespread damage, and prompting evacuations in several counties. It is still raining heavily. The first responder who found her said that at the scene, she appeared confused, she did not know where she was, and she was fixated on finding Nana Sophie. She could not state her name, her address, or her phone number, although she said she had been in a car and had "gotten out quickly." Furthermore, she told the first responder that "Nana Sophie is in trouble," and she knew this because she could hear Nana Sophie's voice. She has no identification and she does not have any possessions besides her clothes and raincoat. She has several scratches and bruises, mostly on her legs and hands, a fractured wrist, a bruise on her right forehead, and she complains of a headache.

### What is your initial differential diagnosis?

A medical cause must be thoroughly investigated before assuming a psychiatric cause. Delirium is chief on the list because of the patient's altered mental status, and one must order basic blood work, such as a complete blood count, comprehensive metabolic panel, thyroid panel, and blood culture. A clinician will want to consider neurologic etiologies, including amnesia or altered mental status due to head injury, postictal state from complex partial seizures, transient global amnesia, a central nervous system infection such as meningitis, or another organic brain disorder. If this patient were elderly, the clinician must also consider dementia, in which memory loss and wandering are common. Substance intoxication can also cause altered mental status. In terms of psychiatric etiologies, a primary dissociative disorder, amnesia or dissociation from a traumatic event—acute stress disorder or posttraumatic stress disorder (PTSD)—or a psychotic disorder are the most likely possibilities. An inability to provide basic demographic information can also be seen in intellectual disability. Lastly, a factitious disorder or malingering is also possible.

---

**CLINICAL PEARL**                                              **STEP 2/3**

Factitious disorder (formerly known as *Munchausen syndrome*) and malingering both involve fabricating symptoms. In factitious disorder, a person feigns or creates symptoms consciously without obvious rewards or gain for doing so. The motivation is thought to be to assume the sick role, which usually elicits sympathy, care giving, or attention. In malingering, a person fabricates symptoms for gain or reward, such as money, meals, or to avoid incarceration.

You speak to the emergency medicine physician, who gives you the pertinent positives and negatives of her examination. The patient appears well-developed and well-nourished. She is mildly hypothermic with a temperature of 96°F, suggesting that she had been out in the flood waters and rain for some time. Aside from one laceration on her lower left leg and a laceration on her right temple that required a few stitches, as well as a fractured wrist, her injuries are superficial lacerations, abrasions, and recent bruising. There are no old bruises or signs of assault. Neurologic examination is normal except for photophobia, phonophobia, and a mild headache, suggesting a concussion. There is no nuchal rigidity. The patient tends to doze when left alone but quickly becomes alert when wakened. Chest radiograph (CXR) is negative. A computed tomography (CT) scan of the brain and neurology consult are pending. Of note, the patient is unable to tell the ED physician anything about her identity or recent whereabouts, including the car or "Nana Sophie."

***What is important to include in your interview and to assess on mental status examination?***
One should assess for altered mental status, including most, if not all, of the questions included on the Mini-Mental State Examination. One should also assess for psychosis, paying attention to the linearity of thought process and speech. One should assess her autobiographical (memory of her personal history), remote, and recent memory and fund of knowledge. Assess for trauma and mood symptoms to the extent possible. Also, be alert for discrepancies in her presentation or her narrative, which may signal a factitious disorder or malingering. The latter two are diagnoses of exclusion.

The patient is awake and alert on interview. She does not know what circumstances led to her wandering in the storm. She does not recall anything before the emergency worker found her. Her memory since then is spotty; however, she can give a general description of her rescuer, and she remembers traveling in a small boat and arriving at this hospital. She is unable to give you her name, where she lives, or her family members' names. Her memory from the time she arrived in the hospital appears to be accurate and reasonably complete, including the diagnostic tests that have been performed. She provides the name of the hospital, her location as the ED, and the ED physician's name, as well as the month and year. She is 1 day off on the date. Clock drawing is accurate. Spontaneous three-word recall after 5 minutes is two out of three, and she recalls the third with a hint. Tests of attention are normal. Screening neurologic examination is identical to the ED physician's. Her thought process and speech are linear. She cannot recall ever hearing voices or experiencing visual hallucinations. Reality testing is intact. She appears to be of normal intellectual functioning. She is very worried about not being able to remember anything and cannot understand what could have caused this. She also thinks there is something else that she is anxious about, but she cannot recall what it is.

The complete blood count returns with only mildly elevated white blood cell count. All other labs are normal, including the preliminary results from the lumbar puncture. The blood culture is still pending. The brain CT scan is negative for pathology, including contusions, masses, or midline shifts. Her temperature returns to normal and she does not manifest a fever. Electroencephalogram (EEG) is normal. The patient is admitted to the internal medicine service for observation with psychiatry and neurology as consultants.

***How has your differential diagnosis changed based on your examination and these results?***
Since reaching the ED, the patient has been alert, she is oriented to place and time on examination, and she continues to be oriented when assessed. Additionally, short-term recall and attention are intact, which makes delirium unlikely. Lack of fever and nuchal rigidity (stiffness or reduced range of motion, with or without pain, when the neck is actively or passively flexed) and no signs of infection in her cerebral spinal fluid make meningitis unlikely. She does not have any obvious brain pathology that would explain the memory loss. She likely has a mild concussion (acute mild traumatic brain injury). In terms of psychiatric causes, she does not display signs of psychosis such as disorganized thoughts and speech or delusions.

TABLE 27.1 ■ **Characteristics of Dissociative Amnesia**

An inability to recall important autobiographical information, usually of a traumatic or stressful nature. This is inconsistent with ordinary forgetting.

- *Localized amnesia* is amnesia around a single event (e.g., a sexual assault) or discrete period of time (e.g., months or years of child abuse, war, or combat).
- *Selective amnesia* is the ability to recall some parts, but not all, or a traumatic or stressful event or period of time.
- *Generalized amnesia* is a complete loss of memory for one's personal life history (autobiographical memory). Sometimes this includes personal identity, such as one's name.
- A *dissociative fugue* consisting of confused wandering or purposeful travel may accompany generalized amnesia for important autobiographical information or identity.
- The symptoms cause significant distress or impairment in social, occupational, or other areas of functioning.
- The symptoms are not attributed to drug abuse, a medication, or a neurologic or medical condition.
- Symptoms are not better explained by another mental disorder or neurocognitive disorder.

### *What is your psychiatric differential diagnosis?*

Now that medical causes have been ruled out, it is likely this woman's condition has a psychiatric cause. Acute stress disorder, PTSD, schizophrenia, factitious disorder, borderline personality disorder, or malingering are on the differential.

---

**CLINICAL PEARL** $\qquad$ **STEP 2/3**

Acute stress disorder and post-traumatic stress disorder (PTSD) have the same basic symptoms. The time course distinguishes these two disorders. Acute stress disorder occurs up to 1 month after the traumatic event. Symptoms must last at least 3 days. After 1 month, a diagnosis of PTSD should be considered.

---

### *What is the diagnosis?*

This patient has *generalized amnesia*, an inability to recall any autobiographical details of one's life. Rarely, this may include a loss of memory of personal identity, as in this case. There are no concurrent cognitive, linguistic, or behavioral symptoms to indicate a neurocognitive disorder; therefore she is suffering from dissociative amnesia with dissociative fugue, one of the dissociative disorders. See Table 27.1.

A prerequisite of dissociative fugue is generalized amnesia. This may rarely include a loss of memory for personal identity, as in this case. Generalized amnesia is rare, the onset is usually sudden, and it is often precipitated by experiencing a traumatic event, such as war, natural disasters, childhood maltreatment, abuse, or other violent trauma.

---

**CLINICAL PEARL** $\qquad$ **STEP 2/3**

Dissociative fugue is purposeful travel or bewildered wandering associated with amnesia for identity or for other important autobiographical information. Fugue states are quite rare.

---

In those experiencing dissociative amnesia, one may progress in three stages to a fugue state. There is an initial stage of acute altered state of consciousness consisting of confusion, headache, and preoccupation with a single idea or emotion, and a second state characterized by loss of personal identity and memory for one's history. During this time, a person may experience transient hallucinations. If a person is found wandering and in this "bewildered" condition, it constitutes a fugue state, the second stage. Rarely, a person in a fugue state may progress to a third stage in which they travel purposefully to a new location and take on a new identity. The new identity is often less inhibited and more social than the person's previous personality.

### What are risk factors for dissociative amnesia and dissociative fugue?

Dissociative amnesia, like other dissociative disorders, is more likely to occur with childhood trauma, particularly sexual abuse, repeated trauma, interpersonal trauma, combat, and higher severity trauma. Mild traumatic brain injury can also precipitate dissociative amnesia.

---

The next day, the patient appears less anxious and certain aspects of her memory have spontaneously returned. She recalls her name and the names and phone numbers of her parents and boyfriend. Her parents confirm her identity and state they last heard from her about 30 hours before she was found. Their daughter told them that she and her boyfriend's first floor apartment was flooding and they decided to evacuate in their car. The patient cannot remember this, or how she came to be outside the car alone, but she becomes very agitated and is concerned about her boyfriend's safety and whereabouts. More details about her personal history, such as her schooling, friends, and hobbies, return over the course of her 3-day hospitalization. However, her memory of the events in the storm did not.

---

### What is the course and prognosis of dissociative amnesia?

Dissociative amnesia has been observed in all age groups. Episodes may be singular or repeated. Persons with dissociative amnesia are often not aware or only partially aware they have memory loss, especially with localized or selective amnesia. It is important to remove the person from the traumatic situation or source of stress, as in this case, and establish a safe environment. Amnestic-only episodes generally improve rapidly and completely. Fugue states of short duration often resolve spontaneously, as in this case. Prolonged fugue states may be permanent.

---

**CLINICAL PEARL**                                                        **STEP 2/3**

Transient global amnesia is a neurologic condition characterized by total or near-total anterograde amnesia (ability to form new memories) for a period of hours. During that time, the person may appear disoriented about time or the environment; however, they retain an awareness of who they are and they can perform complex tasks, such as driving or playing a musical instrument. Retrograde amnesia before the event may also occur but typically returns. Retention of self-awareness and intact autobiographical memory is what distinguishes this from dissociative amnesia.

---

### What distinguishes dissociative amnesia from dissociative identity disorder?

Dissociative identity disorder (DID), formerly known as *multiple personality disorder,* is characterized by at least two distinct personality states or "alters" or the experience of being possessed. The characteristics of DID are listed in Table 27.2.

Individuals with DID experience dissociative amnesia when alternative personalities are present. Dissociative fugues are common. The presence of the alternate personalities and length of episodes varies with many factors, including stress level. A personality typically has separate memories, attitudes, mannerisms, and speech patterns than the host personality. Personalities may exist at various levels of development (e.g., a young child, an adolescent) and have different genders and complexity. Individuals differ in their awareness of the other personalities (integration). The host personality may report hearing voices, presumably of the alters. Symptoms are thought to begin in childhood, although patients are usually not diagnosed until their late 20s.

TABLE 27.2 ■ **Characteristics of Dissociative Identity Disorder**

Disruption of identity characterized by two or more distinct personality states
- The disruption is a pronounced lack of continuity of the self and sense of control over one's action.
- There are accompanying changes in affect, memory, behavior, cognition, perception, and sensation.
- There are recurrent gaps in memory for everyday events, important personal events, or traumatic events.
- The disturbance is not an accepted part of the person's culture or religious practices.
- In children, the symptoms are not better explained by fantasy play.
- The symptoms cause significant distress or impairment in social, occupational, or other areas of functioning.
- The symptoms are not attributed to a substance, a neurologic, or a medical condition.

### What are associated features of individuals with DID?

Individuals with DID commonly experience comorbid depression, anxiety, substance abuse, self-harm, frequent and varied somatic complaints, conversion symptoms, and suicidality. Functional impairment ranges from minimal to severe. Multiple forms of interpersonal maltreatment and abuse in childhood and adulthood are an extremely common part of the history. Other overwhelming experiences, such as multiple medical procedures, or nonabuse trauma are also risk factors.

---

Two months later, the young woman appears in the psychiatry outpatient clinic. Her memory of the storm has mostly returned, although there were certain parts she could not recall. The car she and her boyfriend were driving became stuck in debris and started to fill with water. When they left the vehicle, they were swept away by the current and she watched him get pulled under the water. Her boyfriend was later found, although in serious condition. She is seeking treatment now for anxiety and intermittent episodes of feeling disconnected from herself, like she is watching herself go through the motions of daily life. At times, she feels like a robot that has no emotions. Sometimes she also feels like the world and other people exist in a fog or a dream, and she does not feel like she belongs to the world. She wonders if she is "going crazy."

---

### What is your differential diagnosis?

Possibilities for these new symptoms are additional dissociative amnestic episodes; PTSD; DID; depersonalization/derealization disorder; major depressive disorder; anxiety disorders, especially panic disorder; schizophrenia; and substance-induced symptoms.

Of note, the patient still has dissociative amnesia for what we now know was a traumatic event, although it is no longer localized amnesia like it was when she was discharged. She now has selective amnesia for certain parts of the event.

### What questions do you want to ask this patient?

It is crucial to assess for general mood symptoms, especially depressive symptoms, anxiety disorders, and symptoms of PTSD. With special regard to dissociative disorders, one should assess for "lost time," gaps in memory, level of functioning during the episodes, perceptual distortions of the objects or the environment, and visual or auditory distortions.

Also, do not assume that these symptoms started only after the traumatic events of the hurricane. A thorough psychiatric history is necessary, including asking all the same questions asked in the hospital—recall that the patient could not remember most of her autobiographical history—assessing for trauma in childhood and adolescence, and obtaining family psychiatric history, and social history.

The woman denies gaps in memory except for parts of the hurricane. She does not experience "lost time," but sometimes has the feeling that time is moving too slowly or too quickly, although she knows this is impossible. Sounds often feel muffled, and objects in the environment can appear momentarily abnormally sharp or blurry. This tends to happen more often when she is anxious and can last from minutes to a few days. She generally can attend to her tasks and work during the episodes, although she is not nearly as efficient. These episodes began when she was a child, although they have occurred more frequently since the hurricane. She had a few panic attacks in the weeks after she left the hospital, and she did not have them previously. She also reports mild depressive symptoms that started after the hospitalization. She denies hypervigilance, reexperiencing of the trauma, nightmares, or irritability beyond 2 weeks after the event. She volunteers in a shelter for those displaced by the hurricane. When asked about previous trauma, she revealed sexual abuse as a child by an older male neighbor who was a teenager at the time. The abuse started when she was 7 years old and continued for 5 years.

### What is your diagnosis?

This patient is also suffering from the dissociative disorder depersonalization/derealization disorder (DDD). The characteristics of Depersonalization/Derealization Disorder are summarized in Table 27.3.

Individuals with this disorder may have episodes of depersonalization, derealization, or both. During episodes of depersonalization, individuals may report feeling detached from their entire self, as if they do not exist during these episodes, or detached from parts of the self, including their emotions, thoughts ("My thoughts don't feel like they are coming from me"), physical sensations, or body parts. They often report feeling robotic or like they are lacking control of their actions. They may describe "out-of-body experiences." During episodes of derealization, individuals describe feeling like the environment, people, or inanimate objects are not real—artificial, dreamlike, and unfamiliar—or that they are detached from the world. They may describe auditory or perceptual distortions, such as sounds feeling too soft or loud and objects being blurred, flat, abnormally large or small (macropsia or micropsia), or sharpened. They may have an altered sense of time. Patients may report vague somatic symptoms during episodes, such as tingling or lightheadedness. They may have associated obsessional thinking about if they are "real" or if their surroundings are real. Comorbid anxiety and depression are common. Intact reality testing during and regarding these episodes and the absence of frank hallucinations distinguish this disorder from a psychotic disorder. Depersonalization and derealization are common in schizophrenia, occurring in 11% to 42% of individuals, and tends to become incorporated into their delusional system. Of note, an estimated 50% of the population has experienced an episode of depersonalization or derealization; persistent or recurrent episodes define the disorder.

It is important to distinguish PTSD in individuals who have a significant trauma history, because depersonalization, derealization, and dissociative amnesia commonly occur in PTSD.

---

TABLE 27.3 ■ **Characteristics of Depersonalization/Derealization Disorder**

- Depersonalization: experiences of unreality, detachment, or disconnection from one's body, thoughts, feelings, actions, or sensations AND/OR
- Derealization: experiences of unreality or detachment regarding one's surroundings
- Reality testing is intact during the episodes.
- The symptoms cause significant distress or impairment in social, occupational, or other areas of functioning.
- The symptoms are not attributed to a substance, a neurologic, or a medical condition.
- Symptoms are not better explained by another mental disorder.

This patient does not currently have avoidance (she volunteers in an environment with constant reminders of the hurricane) or intrusive symptoms associated with the traumatic event. The most important factor in diagnosis of DDD in this patient is the existence of symptoms before the traumatic events in the hurricane.

### What are the risk factors for dissociative disorders?
A history of trauma is the most prevalent risk factor for all dissociative disorders, especially childhood maltreatment. Childhood sexual abuse is a particularly strong risk factor, as in this patient. Repeated trauma increases the risk, although symptoms may develop after a single trauma. Certain temperaments and cognitive styles are a risk for DDD.

### What substances may cause dissociative symptoms and apparent memory loss?
Illicit substances that may cause dissociative amnesia or depersonalization/derealization include lysergic acid dimethylamide (LSD), phencyclidine (PCP), ketamine (also used as an anesthetic), or bath salts. Additional substances that are abused or misused that can cause depersonalization/derealization are other hallucinogens, alcohol, marijuana, cocaine, opiates, sedatives, and methamphetamine. Medications reported to cause depersonalization/derealization include haloperidol, certain general anesthetics, and indomethacin.

### What is the treatment for dissociative disorders?
Psychotherapy is the treatment of choice for all dissociative disorders. For dissociative amnesia, treatment also involves recovery of missing memories through therapy, free association, and sometimes with the aid of hypnosis. Therapy is often aimed at exploring the precipitating events or trauma. In all disorders, treating comorbid mental disorders may be beneficial in reducing the dissociative symptoms.

There is no evidence that medication is effective for directly treating dissociative disorders. Antipsychotics have no proven efficacy and are contraindicated because they can exacerbate dissociation. Anxiety is a common comorbid condition, and although benzodiazepines may decrease the accompanying anxiety, especially in the acute setting, they may also exacerbate dissociation. Medication can be helpful for comorbid psychiatric conditions. Antidepressants such as selective serotonin reuptake inhibitors can be helpful for comorbid depression, anxiety, or PTSD.

---

You prescribe sertraline for the woman's anxiety and refer her to a psychotherapist for trauma-focused cognitive behavioral therapy.

---

### BEYOND THE PEARLS:

In cultures with extremely restrictive social traditions, severe psychological stress or conflict often precipitate dissociative amnesia rather than trauma. Examples are family conflict, attachment issues, or conflict stemming from oppression.

### References

American Psychiatric Association. (2013). *Diagnostic and statistical manual of mental disorders* (5th ed.). Washington, DC: Author.

Fuehrlein, B., & Nurcombe, B. (2019). Dissociative disorders. In M. H. Ebert, J. F. Leckman, & I. L. Petrakis (Eds.), *Current diagnosis & treatment psychiatry*. (3rd ed.). New York, NY: McGraw-Hill Education.

Kremen, S. (2014). Transient global amnesia. In M. F. Mendez (Ed.), *UpToDate*. Retrieved October 28, 2018, from https://www.uptodate-com.ucsf.idm.oclc.org/contents/transient-global-amnesia?search=transient%20global%20amnesia&source=search_result&selectedTitle=1~17&usage_type=default&display_rank=1#.

Scholzman, S. C. (2012). Dissociative Disorders. In T. Stern, J. Herman, & T. Gorrindo (Eds.), *Massachusetts General Hospital psychiatry update and board preparation* (3rd ed.) (pp. 165–169). Boston, MA: MGH Psychiatry Academy Publishing.

Tunkel, A. R. (2018). Clinical features and diagnosis of acute bacterial meningitis in adults. In S. B. Calderwood (Ed.), *UpToDate*. Retrieved August 30, 2018, from https://www-uptodate-com.ucsf.idm.oclc.org/contents/clinical-features-and-diagnosis-of-acute-bacterial-meningitis-in-adults?search=bacterial%20meningitis&source=search_result&selectedTitle=1~150&usage_type=default&display_rank=1

# CHAPTER 28

# Narcolepsy

Peter Chung ■ Julie Flygare ■ Terese C. Hammond ■ Raj Dasgupta

A 23-year-old woman with no significant past medical history complains of excessive daytime sleepiness. She initially notices this symptom at age 22 as she struggles with her academics during law school. She reports having trouble staying alert and getting foggy during classes—despite caffeine intake and taking trips to the bathroom to wake herself up. She attributes her sleepiness to late night studying, irregular sleeping cycle, and lack of will power. Despite 7 to 9 hours of sleep on most nights, she still gets tired multiple times throughout the day and sometimes falls asleep for a few minutes in a cubicle at the library or while studying at night in bed. She reports feeling sleepy while driving with the most dramatic event occurring a few months ago. Most recently, while driving to school, she felt very tired just about a mile away from campus and the next thing she remembered, she woke up in the parking lot of law school with her car parked and her seat reclined. She was safe but could not recall any memories of arriving at school or choosing a parking spot. This scared her and motivated her to seek help. She reports no snoring, per her boyfriend.

The patient is otherwise healthy with no known medical issues. She takes no medications, nutraceuticals or over-the-counter products. She drinks two to four cups of caffeinated coffee on most days. She occasionally drinks one to three glasses of wine on the weekend, but does not smoke and has no history of illicit drug use. Her family history is significant only for a younger brother who is currently a third-year medical school student and has a similar issue with excessive daytime sleepiness that started during his junior year of high school. Her parents are both alive, well, and without similar complaints. Her vital signs in the office include blood pressure of 115/85, heart rate of 80 beats per minute, respiratory rate of 18 breaths per minute, and oxygen saturation of 99% on room air. She is alert and appears well, fluent, and cooperative. There are no significant physical examination findings.

*What is on the differential diagnosis?*
A detailed medical, psychiatric, medication, and sleep history is important in diagnosis. Chronic daytime sleepiness can be due to sleep deprivation, obstructive sleep apnea, central sleep apnea, circadian rhythm sleep–wake disorders such as rotating shift work, narcolepsy, periodic limb movements, mood disorders, depression, substance abuse, and idiopathic hypersomnia. Additional psychiatric and sleep history as well as a careful review of systems are necessary to further determine the etiology of her symptoms.

She denies any unintentional weight loss, depressed mood, suicidal or homicidal ideation, change in appetite, constipation, diarrhea, or changes in menstrual cycle. She is not sexually active and undergoes regular well-woman examinations, which have all been normal. In terms of sleep history, she reports a bedtime of 10 PM, although she often falls asleep earlier while reading a textbook or watching television. She reports having strange experiences where she thinks she wakes up to see a figure in her bedroom. She reports seeing a burglar rush at her with his arms stretched out to her neck. She also reports less frightening experiences like hearing her roommate coming home and feeling a cat scratching her arm. During these incidents, she feels awake but she cannot move her body to respond or speak. She reports feeling paralyzed. This sensation is often associated with fear or anxiety, especially after one night when she wakes up hearing a burglar break into her apartment and finding herself being choked in her bed, unable to move. She eventually concludes that these experiences did not happen after checking for signs of a break-in or asking her roommate if she came home. In addition, she reports symptoms that consist of buckling her knees and feeling heavy in her head while laughing and joking with her roommate in her apartment. She has never fallen or injured herself during these incidents but does need to sit or lean against the wall or table for support until the sensation passes. She also reports fumbling her glass of wine suddenly while carrying on a conversation and laughing with her friend at a party.

### How does this information change the differential diagnosis?

She discloses several new, distinctive symptoms. Hypnagogic hallucinations, such as the ones described by our patient, occur at sleep onset (versus hypnopompic hallucinations, which occur during transition from sleep to wake) and are thought to be associated with instability in the normal transition from wake to sleep. Sleep paralysis, the sensation of being aware but unable to move, is also indicative of some perturbation of the sleep–wake transition. It is unusual for normal sleepers to enter sleep through rapid eye movement (REM) sleep. A normal "REM latency" is at least 50 minutes after sleep onset. A sudden transition to REM sleep can lead to symptoms such as hypnagogic hallucinations or sleep paralysis, because REM is the predominate "dreaming stage" of sleep. Vivid images are common during REM and muscle atonia normally occurs as a protective mechanism to prevent injury by physically acting out dreams. Destabilized sleep–wake transitions may occur in the setting of anxiety disorder, substance or medication withdrawal (e.g., alcohol, amphetamines, antidepressants), schizophrenia, and other psychotic disorders, so hypnagogic and hypnopompic hallucinations and sleep paralysis are nonspecific. The sudden and transient episodes of muscle weakness associated with strong emotion that she describes are descriptive of cataplexy, which is highly sensitive for the diagnosis of type 1 narcolepsy but may also rarely occur in brain lesions involving the hypothalamus or brainstem.

### What features are suggestive of narcolepsy?

According to the *Diagnostic and Statistical Manual of Mental Disorders*, Fifth Edition (DSM-5) and *International Classification of Sleep Disorders*, Third Edition (ICSD-3), narcolepsy is a sleep disorder in which an individual experiences recurrent episodes of lapsing into sleep, napping within the same day, or an irrepressible need to sleep. These episodes must occur at least three times per week over the past 3 months. The classic clinical presentation consists of chronic daytime sleepiness, hypnagogic hallucinations, sleep paralysis, and cataplexy. Not all patients with narcolepsy have these symptoms, but only about one-third of patients experience all four symptoms. The following questions may be helpful in diagnosis (Table 28.1).

Onset of symptoms is most common among teenagers and young adults with a typical age of onset between 15 and 25. The presence of cataplexy is highly suggestive of narcolepsy. In the absence of cataplexy, alternative diagnoses must be investigated and excluded.

### What are diagnostic tests or evaluations that may be ordered?

Sleep logs and actigraphy may be helpful in getting a better assessment of excessive daytime sleepiness or in excluding other causes of hypersomnia, such as insufficient sleep, but are not diagnostic of narcolepsy. Polysomnography is helpful in evaluating other sleep disorders, such as sleep apnea, which need to be excluded in the work-up for narcolepsy. For patients in whom narcolepsy is strongly suspected (as in our patient), an overnight polysomnography to exclude concomitant sleep disorders followed by a multiple sleep latency test (MSLT) to evaluate for "sleep onset REM" is the recommended diagnostic approach. Narcolepsy with cataplexy is caused

TABLE 28.1 ■ Questions in the Evaluation of Suspected Narcolepsy

| Question | Implication |
|---|---|
| Are you sleepy most of the day? | Sleepiness present; caused by various conditions |
| Do you feel rested upon waking in the morning? Are your naps refreshing? | Sleepiness is not caused by quality of sleep but rather other condition (e.g., sleep apnea) |
| Do you have vivid dreams during daytime naps? | Possible REM sleep during naps |
| Do you ever have muscle weakness when you tell a joke or laugh? | Cataplexy |
| Do you ever see, hear, or feel things that you know are not there as you are falling asleep? | Hypnagogic hallucinations |
| Are you ever unable to move when you first awake or just before falling asleep? | Sleep paralysis |

by a decrease in central nervous system (CNS) orexin (hypocretin), which is produced by specialized cells in the lateral hypothalamus (Fig. 28.1). Most cases of narcolepsy with cataplexy are idiopathic, although these symptoms can be rarely mimicked by brainstem lesions in multiple sclerosis, head trauma, brain tumors, or degenerative disorders. Orexin/hypocretin level can be measured in CSF, but this assay is not widely available and is not part of the pathway for making the clinical diagnosis. In patients who have narcolepsy with cataplexy, human leukocyte antigen (HLA) DQB1*0602 is the most common and sensitive allele, and CSF orexin (when measured) is typically less than one-third of the normal values.

---

**BASIC SCIENCE PEARL**                                         **STEP 1/2/3**

Orexin, also known as *hypocretin,* is a neurotransmitter that regulates arousal, wakefulness, and appetite. It is low in narcolepsy.

---

The patient undergoes a sleep test with the following results.

---

**POLYSOMNOGRAPHY RESULT**

- Total sleep time: 460 minutes
- Sleep efficiency: 95%
- Sleep latency: 1 minute
- REM latency: 5 minutes
- Percent sleep stages:
  - Stage 1 (15%)
  - Stage 2 (55%)
  - Stage 3 (12%)
  - REM (18%)
- Total AHI: 1 event/hour
- PLM index: 3.2 events/hour
- Lowest oxygen saturation: 93%

*Does the sleep test result help in diagnosis?*
Polysomnography shows a total sleep time of 460 minutes with 95% sleep efficiency. The REM latency is 5 minutes. Sleep staging is normal, and there are no confounding sleep disorders such as obstructive or central sleep apnea, periodic limb movements, or parasomnias.

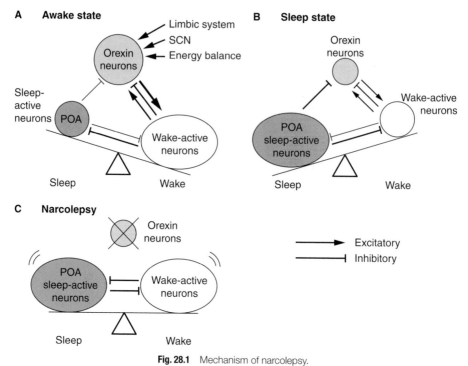

**Fig. 28.1** Mechanism of narcolepsy.

---

**BASIC SCIENCE PEARL**                                              **STEP 1/2**

Sleep consists of different stages with characteristic clinical features and electroencephalogram (EEG) waveform.

| Sleep Stage | Clinical Feature | EEG Waveform |
|---|---|---|
| Awake | Alert | Beta |
| Awake | Eyes closed | Alpha |
| Stage 1 | Light sleep | Theta |
| Stage 2 | Deep sleep | Sleep spindles and K complexes |
| Stage 3 | Deeper, non-REM sleep<br>Night terror, bedwetting, sleep walking | Delta |
| REM | Dreaming | Beta |

---

**CLINICAL SCIENCE PEARL**                                           **STEP 2/3**

Stimulants, psychoactive medications, or antidepressants can affect polysomnography results by rapid eye movement (REM) sleep rebound effects. Patients should discontinue stimulants and psychoactive medications 1 week prior, and antidepressants at least 3 to 4 weeks before testing.

Multiple sleep latency test (MSLT) is performed the next day. The MSLT consists of four or five 20-minute nap opportunities spaced 2 hours apart throughout the day. The patient slept on 4/4 of the nap opportunities and had an average sleep latency of 3 minutes. In three of the naps, sleep-on-set REM periods (SOREMPs) were noted. In the absence of sleep deprivation and sleep disorders as determined by polysomnography previously, an MSLT demonstrating two or more SOREMPs is diagnostic of narcolepsy. Her short REM latency on the diagnostic polysomnography and her overall MSLT sleep latency of 3 minutes are also supportive of the narcolepsy diagnosis.

### Is there an additional test that may be helpful?

Multiple sleep latency test (MSLT) is a follow-up sleep test to polysomnography after other sleep disorders have been ruled out. Patient's MSLT shows an average sleep latency of 3 minutes, and there were four sleep-onset REM periods. In the absence of sleep deprivation and sleep disorders as determined by polysomnography previously, an MSLT that shows an average sleep latency of less than 8 minutes and/or at least two sleep-onset REM periods (SOREMPs) is diagnostic of narcolepsy.

### What is the diagnostic criteria for narcolepsy?

Previous classification subdivided the disorder into narcolepsy with cataplexy and without cataplexy. Newer terminology classifies narcolepsy into two types, rather than on the basis of cataplexy alone. Although cataplexy remains the hallmark feature of narcolepsy type 1, it is absent in some patients who can still be diagnosed with narcolepsy type 1 based on low CSF orexin (hypocretin) levels. Narcolepsy type 2 is more difficult to diagnose as clinical symptoms of sleepiness, sleep paralysis, and hypnagogic or hypnapompic hallucinations can occur in various other conditions and exclusion of alternative etiologies is necessary. Tables 28.2 and 28.3 outline the diagnostic criteria for each type of narcolepsy.

**CLINICAL SCIENCE PEARL**                                              **STEP 2/3**

Narcolepsy consists of a tetrad of syndromes: daytime sleepiness, cataplexy, hypnagogic hallucination, and sleep paralysis. Diagnosis can be challenging, as patients have varying presentations. Cataplexy is a highly specific feature of narcolepsy. Other etiologies and conditions should be excluded before diagnosis of narcolepsy.

After reviewing all clinical history and diagnostic testing, you diagnose the patient with narcolepsy type 1. She was not surprised because once narcolepsy was suspected, she researched online and found her symptom experiences uncanny in similarities to those of other people living with narcolepsy. The only thing that surprises her now is how narcolepsy is portrayed in movies and the media, because those portrayals do not resonate with her experience. She is interested in interventions, both nonpharmacologic and pharmacologic.

### What are treatment options?

Most patients require pharmacologic treatment, especially if they experience cataplexy. Nonpharmacologic interventions include avoidance of drugs or medications that may worsen daytime sleepiness. They include alcohol, opiates, benzodiazepines, and antipsychotic medications. Behavioral intervention such as scheduled 20-to-30-minute napping sessions during the day is also helpful. Psychosocial support and routine screening for depression is necessary, as patients with narcolepsy are at increased risk for psychiatric comorbidities including anxiety and depression. The diagnosis of narcolepsy can be overwhelming, and some patients or family members are in

TABLE 28.2 ■ Diagnostic Criteria: Narcolepsy Type 1

Diagnostic Criteria: Narcolepsy Type 1
Criteria A and B must be met:
A. Patient has daily periods of irrepressible need to sleep or daytime lapses into sleep occurring for at least 3 months.
B. Presence of one or both of the following:
   1. Cataplexy and a mean sleep latency of <8 minutes and two or more SOREMPs on an MSLT. A SOREMP (within 15 minutes of sleep onset) on the proceeding nocturnal PSG may replace one of the SOREMPs on the MSLT.
   2. CSF hypocretin–1 concentration, measured by immunoreactivity, is either <110 pg/mL or less than one-third of normal value.

TABLE 28.3 ■ Diagnostic Criteria: Narcolepsy Type 2

Diagnostic Criteria: Narcolepsy Type 2
Criteria A through E must be met:
A. Patient has daily periods of irrepressible need to sleep or daytime lapses into sleep occurring for at least 3 months.
B. A mean sleep latency of <8 minutes and two or more SOREMPs on an MSLT. SOREMP (within 15 minutes of sleep onset) on the proceeding nocturnal PSG may replace one of the SOREMPs on the MSLT.
C. Cataplexy is absent.
D. Either CSF hypocretin concentration has not been measured or CSF hypocretin concentration measured by immunoreactivity is either >110 pg/mL or less than one-third of normal value.
E. The hypersomnolence and/or MSLT findings are not better explained by other causes, such as insufficient sleep, obstructive sleep apnea, delayed sleep phase disorder, or the effect of medication or substances or their withdrawal.

disbelief. Therefore it is important to have ongoing discussion and monitoring of treatment response by the patients, family members, and medical staff.

| MULTIPLE SLEEP LATENCY TEST (MSLT) | | |
|---|---|---|
| NAP | Sleep latency (min) | SOREM |
| 1 | 4.0 | (+) |
| 2 | 2.0 | (+) |
| 3 | 3.5 | (+) |
| 4 | 2.5 | (+) |
| Mean sleep latency: 3.0 minutes | | |

Common pharmacologic interventions include sodium oxybate, modafinil, methylphenidate, and amphetamine, which all treat daytime sleepiness. For symptoms of cataplexy, sodium oxybate or medications that suppress REM sleep are prescribed instead. Some REM-suppressant medications include venlafaxine, atomoxetine, and fluoxetine. They inhibit the reuptake of the neurotransmitters norepinephrine and serotonin. Abrupt withdrawal of these medications must be avoided as patients are at risk for developing uncontrolled rebound cataplexy ("status cataplecticus"). Of note, sodium oxybate (Xyrem) is highly effective at managing both

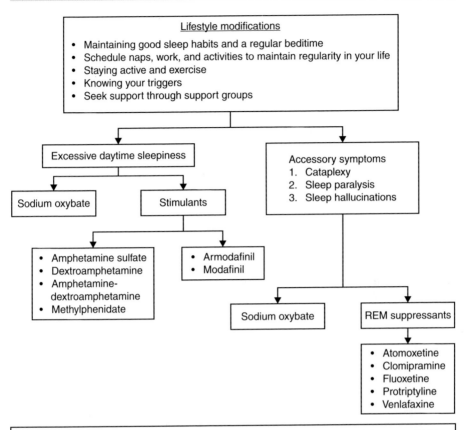

**Fig. 28.2** Treatment of narcolepsy.

hypersomnia and cataplexy in patients but has high diversion and misuse risk, so this medication is tightly controlled (Fig. 28.2).

After the clinic visit, the patient follows your treatment recommendations, both nonpharmacologic and pharmacologic for 3 months. She avoids alcohol, naps regularly, and takes modafinil 200mg initially once and then twice per day along with sodium oxybate 2.25 gram twice per day.

---

**CLINICAL SCIENCE PEARL**                                                         **STEP 2/3**

Sodium oxybate is a sodium salt of gamma hydroxybutyrate and acts through the gamma amino butyric acid (GABA) receptor. It targets symptoms of both sleepiness and cataplexy.

---

She returns to clinic for a follow-up visit after another 3 months. After titrating her sodium oxybate up to a current dose of 3 grams twice per night, she notices a significant decrease in her daytime sleepiness and improvement of her cataplexy. She experiences side effects from the modafinil in the form of heart racing and hands shaking. She experiences side effects of sodium oxybate in the form of nausea and stomach aches in the morning. She feels positive with the improvements and continues to work to adjust her treatment plan to manage her symptoms and side effects. She reports that a short 15-to-20-minute daily nap is a great relief for her remaining episodes of excessive daytime sleepiness, but faces logistical challenges at school. She works with her clinician and school to secure a private place to take her nap in the law school library. To manage the psychosocial impact and stigmas of the condition, she seeks the assistance of a trained therapist via weekly in-person appointments. She eventually also seeks social support through in-person and online support groups, patient organizations, and advocacy efforts. Connecting with other people with narcolepsy becomes a huge part of her journey to living well with narcolepsy.

---

**BEYOND THE PEARLS:**

- Suprachiasmatic nucleus of the hypothalamus is involved in circadian rhythm regulation.
- In young children, narcolepsy may sometimes present as excessively long night sleep or as resumption of previously discontinued daytime napping.
- Acetylcholine is the principal neurotransmitter during REM sleep.
- GABA (gamma-amino butyric acid) agonists such as alcohol, benzodiazepines, and barbiturates reduce REM and delta sleep.
- Norepinephrine, serotonin, and histamine suppress REM sleep. Therefore SSRI or SNRI antidepressants can suppress REM sleep.
- If narcolepsy type 1 is strongly suspected clinically, but the MSLT criteria is not met, a possible strategy is to repeat the MSLT.
- Narcolepsy is associated with higher rates of hypertension, which may be related only in part to stimulants or other medications. Patients with narcolepsy also have increased rates of obesity and diabetes.
- There is some genetic predisposition to developing narcolepsy if diagnosed among family members. First-degree relatives have increased risk for narcolepsy with cataplexy.
- DQB1*0602 haplotype (a subtype of DR2) is present in 95% of patients with cataplexy and in 96% of those with orexin deficiency.
- Sodium oxybate has high sodium load, which can have consequences in patients who are salt sensitive or have hypertension. Additionally, its effect on the central nervous system makes coadministration with any other medications, especially agents associated with respiratory depression such as hypnotics, dangerous and all medications should be carefully reviewed.
- Newer pharmacotherapy agents, including sodium oxybate, that have lower sodium content and medications that target different receptors, such as norepinephrine-dopamine reuptake inhibitor and histamine 3 inverse agonist, are soon to be available in the United States.

# References

American Academy of Sleep Medicine. (2014). *International classification of sleep disorders* (3rd ed.). Darien, IL: Author.

American Psychiatric Association (2013). *Diagnostic and statistical manual of mental disorders* (5th ed.). Washington, DC: Author.

Sateia, M. J. (2014). International classification of sleep disorders-third edition: Highlights and modifications. *Chest*, *146*(5), 1387–1394.

Tsujino, N., & Sakurai, T. (2013). Role of orexin in modulating arousal, feeding, and motivation. *Frontiers in Behavioral Neuroscience*, *7*(28), 1–14.

# CHAPTER 29

# Insomnia

Roya Noorishad ■ Lucas Cruz ■ Terese C. Hammond ■ Raj Dasgupta

A 53-year-old woman presents with difficulty falling asleep and excessive daytime sleepiness for the past 6 months. She had a well-woman examination approximately 8 months ago, which was significant for diet-controlled diabetes mellitus type II (DMII) and Graves' disease status post radioiodine ablative therapy. The remainder of her examination and all laboratory tests, including hemoglobin A1c and thyroid stimulating hormone, were normal. She denied any other health changes since her recent physical. However, she reports that on most nights of the week, she struggles to initiate sleep, usually laying in bed for up to an hour and a half "tossing and turning." After finally falling asleep, the patient reports that she wakes up "every 1 to 2 hours." Before 6 months ago, the patient had a very consistent sleep schedule, with a usual bedtime of 10 PM and wake up time of 6 AM. She explains that she lost her job as an office manager around the time her sleep difficulties began and she concedes that she often lays in bed worrying about her finances and her ongoing job search. She is out of bed at 7 AM but feels tired during the day and also reports poor concentration, excessive worry about her future, and lapses in memory. She tries not to nap but falls asleep in the afternoon for approximately 1 to 2 hours on most days. She often wakes from her nap feeling "completely groggy." Her bed time is irregular, usually between 11 PM and 1 AM, depending on what television show she is watching.

Besides her DMII and Graves' disease, her past medical history is significant for substance use disorder with alprazolam, in remission for 6 years, an incident of major depressive disorder (MDD) 4 years ago, and gastroesophageal reflux disease. On her current physical examination, her blood pressure is 130/80, heart rate is 85 bpm, respiratory rate is 18, and she is saturating at 97% on room air. Patient has a BMI of 26.2 kg/m$^2$ and is not a smoker. There are no other significant findings on physical examination. Family history is significant for an older brother with obstructive sleep apnea (OSA). On psychiatric review, patient endorses diminished interest in activities she used to enjoy, guilt about losing her job, and decreased energy.

### What is on the differential diagnosis?

Insomnia as defined in the *Diagnostic and Statistical Manual of Mental Disorders*, Fifth Edition (DSM-5), is a dissatisfaction with sleep quantity or quality due to difficulty falling asleep, maintaining sleep, or early morning awakenings. The disturbance must cause impairment in daytime functioning, occur at least three nights a week, and be present for at least 3 months. The dysfunction must occur with adequate opportunity for sleep. The disturbance cannot be due to another sleep-wake disorder or associated with the effects of substances or medication and cannot be explained by another medical or psychiatric disorder. Given this history, obstructive sleep apnea, thyroid dysfunction, major depressive disorder, generalized anxiety disorder, or substance use disorder may also be considered. Other causes of sleep-wake disorders are less likely in this patient, given her symptoms.

### What psychiatric disorders can present with sleep dysfunction?

Several psychiatric disorders include sleep impairment as a presenting symptom such as MDD, generalized anxiety disorder (GAD), bipolar disorder and psychotic disorders. MDD can present

## TABLE 29.1 ■ Psychiatric Disorders

Psychiatric Disorders That May Present with Sleep Disturbance

- Major depressive disorder
- Generalized anxiety disorder
- Bipolar disorder (e.g., mania)
- Schizophrenia, schizophreniform, brief psychotic disorder

- Substance use disorder (with benzodiazepines, alcohol, or cocaine)
- Post-traumatic stress disorder
- Adjustment disorder
- Dementia (neurologic)

with either insomnia or hypersomnia (sleeping greater than 9 hours per day). The latter is more common in atypical depression. GAD can also present with difficulty initiating or maintaining sleep, with rumination over daytime events usually a prominent complaint. Bipolar disorder in the acute manic episode frequently presents with a diminished need for sleep, although during a depressive episode, sleep may be disturbed similar to MDD. Psychosis in schizophrenia, schizoaffective disorder, schizophreniform, and brief psychotic disorder is often associated with impairments in sleep. Substance use disorder, especially with benzodiazepines or alcohol, can be a cause of insomnia and may persist through early sobriety. Finally, posttraumatic stress disorder (PTSD) must also be screened for as patients may have difficulty falling asleep secondary to hypervigilance or avoidance of nightmares. Though not a psychiatric disorder, dementia is frequently associated with behavioral disturbances and symptoms including insomnia. Table 29.1 summarizes some of the psychiatric and neurologic disorders that can present with sleep disturbance.

---

**CLINICAL PEARL**                                                      **STEP 2/3**

The symptoms of atypical depression or depression with atypical features (DMS-5) include mood reactivity (mood brightens temporarily), significant weight gain or increase in appetite, hypersomnia, leaden paralysis, or a longstanding pattern of interpersonal rejection sensitivity.

---

Given her history of GAD and previous incident of MDD, she did follow up with her internist approximately 4 months ago and was prescribed sertraline. She has been titrated up to a dose of 200 mg daily and since resuming the medication, she has noticed significant improvements in her mood. However, her difficulty falling and staying asleep has persisted. She denies any other substance use, specifically alprazolam or alcohol. On further questioning, she does report that her husband has recently commented about her snoring and she has gained 10 lbs in the last 6 months.

---

**CLINICAL PEARL**                                                      **STEP 2/3**

Selective serotonin reuptake inhibitors are approved for the use of major depressive disorder, generalized anxiety disorder, panic disorder, post-traumatic stress disorder, and obsessive-compulsive disorder. Their mechanism of action involves increasing the availability of serotonin in the synapse by decreasing reuptake and increasing serotonin release. Long-term effects of SSRIs include increased brain-derived neurotrophic factor (BDNF) leading to neurogenesis. Common side effects include GI upset, anorgasmia, and weight gain.

---

### What other diagnoses could be explored?

The patient has GERD, has been witnessed snoring, has recently gained weight, and has a family history of OSA. It would be appropriate to consider polysomnography testing to evaluate for OSA, either at home or through an attended sleep study, to exclude a breathing-related sleep

TABLE 29.2 ■ Nonpharmacologic Treatments for Insomnia

| Treatment | Explanation/Example |
| --- | --- |
| CBT-I | Repairs a faulty stimulus–response cycle by correcting maladaptive thoughts, feelings, and behaviors surrounding sleep. Implements stimulus control, behavioral interventions, sleep restriction, relaxation training, and cognitive therapy |
| Mindfulness-based Therapy for Insomnia | Meditation audiotapes, meditation classes, "brain dump" |
| Exercise | Aerobic and resistance training before 6 pm to regulate circadian rhythm |
| Sleep hygiene | Avoiding electronic devices (laptop, phone, television) and heavy meals 1–2 hours before bed time |
| Relaxation therapy | Progressive muscle relaxation |

condition, although this is not necessary to make a diagnosis of insomnia and is typically deferred in the absence of signs or symptoms of OSA.

---

Home sleep testing demonstrates mild snoring but no significant OSA. You proceed to treat her insomnia.

---

### What are first-line treatments for insomnia with the highest evidence rating?
Cognitive behavioral therapy for insomnia (CBT-I), exercise, relaxation therapy, mindfulness-based therapy, and sleep hygiene–lifestyle modifications are the preferred first line treatments with the highest evidence rating. Table 29.2 summarizes the nonpharmacologic first-line treatments for insomnia with explanations.

Your next six appointments consist of implementing a sleep diary, addressing sleep hygiene, using CBT-I techniques, and mindfulness audio recordings. Despite adherence to therapy, she continues to report taking up to 2 hours to fall asleep with an average of 5 hours of sleep per night.

### Which medications are to be avoided in this patient?
Benzodiazepines in this patient would be potentially detrimental, as she has a prior history of substance use disorder with alprazolam. They are also generally not recommended for insomnia even though they are often prescribed for sleep or sleep impairments secondary to disorders like generalized anxiety or depression.

---

**BASIC SCIENCE PEARL**  STEP 1/2/3

Benzodiazepines improve the efficiency of the brain chemical GABA on the GABAA receptor. GABA is the predominant inhibitory neurotransmitter in the central nervous system. Adverse effects of benzodiazepines can include respiratory suppression or hypoventilation, hypotension, bradycardia, and altered mental status, and they have a high potential for abuse. Withdrawal symptoms such as seizures may be life threatening. Benzodiazepine overdose is treated with flumazenil.

---

### Which medications can be considered for this patient?
Trazodone, hydroxyzine, mirtazapine, doxepin, and so-called Z drugs such as eszopiclone, zaleplon, and zolpidem should be considered. Ramelteon and suvorexant are newer medications

TABLE 29.3 ■ Common Sleep Medications and Their Mechanism of Action

| Medication | Description/Mechanism of Action |
|---|---|
| Zolpidem | GABA agonist at the GABAA receptor. Strong nonbenzodiazepine hypnotic with minimal anxiolytic properties. |
| Zaleplon | Similar to zolpidem with shorter half-life. |
| Eszopiclone | Similar to zolpidem with higher potency. |
| Melatonin | Naturally occurring neurohormone. Activates MT1 and MT2 receptors to shift circadian rhythm earlier. |
| Suvorexant | Antagonist at orexin receptors. Blocks the activity of wakefulness promoting neurotransmitters orexin A and B to orexin receptor type 1 and 2 suppressing wake drive. |
| Ramelteon | Melatonin receptor agonist with high affinity for MT1 and MT2. |
| Hydroxyzine | H1 receptor inverse agonist leading to antihistamine effects. Low potency for muscarinic acetylcholine receptors and thus has a low probability for anticholinergic side effects. Also used as anxiolytic. |
| Diphenhydramine | H1 receptor inverse agonist. Potent antagonist at muscarinic acetylcholine receptors and thus may cause anticholinergic side effects. |
| Trazodone | Atypical antidepressant. $5\text{-HT}_{2A}$ receptor antagonist and $\alpha_1$-adrenergic receptor antagonist. Sedation and orthostatic hypotension is thought to be due alpha-adrenergic blockade. Not anticholinergic. |
| Mirtazapine | Atypical antidepressant. Antihistamine via H1 inverse agonist, $\alpha_2$-adrenergic receptor antagonist, antagonist at 5HT2A, C, and 5HT3. Not anticholinergic. |
| Doxepin | Tricyclic antidepressant. Antihistamine, anticholinergic, antiserotonergic. |

with unique mechanisms of action. Melatonin may also be useful for individuals with delayed sleep phase disorder. Table 29.3 summarizes the medications used for sleep and their respective mechanism of action.

You prescribe zolpidem 5 mg nightly, as needed, and instruct the patient to continue her attention to sleep hygiene and other behavioral interventions. She begins taking it and reports excellent results after 1 week of use. One month later, you get another call from the patient. She reports she is out of the medication and has been taking two tablets, 10 mg, nightly. She also has noticed she has been waking up in locations with no recollection of how she got there and recently got into a fender bender while driving to an early morning job interview. You recommend that the patient reduce her dose back to 5mg and only use the medication on nights when she has at least 7 to 8 hours available for sleep and she agrees. She returns for follow up 6 weeks later and reports excellent control of her insomnia. She also reports starting a new job. Over subsequent weeks, she uses zolpidem less frequently and at her subsequent 3-month follow-up, she has completely discontinued zolpidem use and has resumed a normal sleep schedule. She continues to take sertraline and expresses a desire to continue seeing a psychologist at least monthly.

**CLINICAL SCIENCE PEARL**                                              **STEP 2/3**

The recommended dosing for immediate release zolpidem is 5 mg in women and 10 mg in men. For extended release zolpidem, the recommended dosing is 6.5 mg in women and 12.5 mg in men. This is because of concerns regarding decreased clearance in women and prolonged effects of next-day impairments in driving or other activities that require alertness.

**BEYOND THE PEARLS:**

- SSRIs are known to increase REM sleep latency. Decreased REM latency is seen in major depressive disorder.
- Alcohol and benzodiazepine in the short term provide sedation but have a harmful effect on sleep architecture in the long term (by reducing REM and N3 stage sleep). Abuse can lead to rebound insomnia and anxiety.
- Nonbenzodiazepine hypnotics do not suppress respiratory drive.
- MT1 and MT2 receptors are found in the suprachiasmatic nucleus.
- Benzodiazepines increase N2 phase sleep and suppress N3 phase sleep.
- Additional harmful effects of benzodiazepines may include cognitive dysfunction, memory impairment (anterograde amnesia), paradoxical disinhibition, delirium in elderly, and long-term worsening of psychiatric symptoms.
- The anticholinergic effects of diphenhydramine, such as urinary retention, constipation, mydriasis, increased heart rate, increased intraocular pressure, and dementia and confusion, are particularly of concern in geriatric patients at higher risk for delirium.
- Although trazodone is not anticholinergic it is still a problematic medication in geriatric patients because of orthostatic hypotension.

## References

American Academy of Sleep Medicine. (2014). *The international classification of sleep disorders, revised: diagnostic and coding manual.*, IL: Author.

American Psychiatric Association. (2013). *Diagnostic and statistical manual of mental disorders* (5th ed.). Washington, DC: Author.

Mai, E., & Buysee, D. (2008). Insomnia, prevalence, impact, pathogenesis, differential diagnosis and evaluation. *Sleep Medicine Clinics, 3,* 167–174.

Mendelson, W. (2011). Hypnotic medications: mechanisms of action and pharmacologic effects. In M. H. Kryger, T. Roth, & W. C. Dement (Eds.), *Principles and practices of sleep medicine* (5th ed.). St. Louis, MO: Saunders.

Nutt, D. J., & Stahl, S. M. (2010). Searching for perfect sleep: the continuing evolution of GABA-A receptor modulators as hypnotics. *Journal of Psychopharmacology, 24,* 1601–1612.

Schutte-Rodin, S., Broch, L., Buysee, D., Dorsey, C., & Sateia, M. (2008). Clinical guideline for the evaluation and management of chronic insomnia in adults. *Journal of Clinical Sleep Medicine, 4,* 487–504.

# CHAPTER 30

# Parasomnias

Lucas Cruz ■ Terese C. Hammond ■ Raj Dasgupta

---

A 25-year-old man presents to the sleep clinic with his wife, who reports that the patient has been having disturbing nightmares that wake him up from his sleep for the past 2 months. He does not recall these episodes and is only aware of them because his wife has been complaining about his abnormal behavior at night. He works in a marketing company and admits to an increased level of stress associated with an important deadline at work.

---

Parasomnias are defined as motor, verbal or experiential phenomena that occur in association with sleep. An evaluation for parasomnias is usually triggered by the observation of unusual or atypical behaviors at night, often by a roommate or spouse. Parasomnias are classified by the *International Classification of Sleep Disorders*, Third Edition (ICSD-3), in three groups depending on which phase of sleep they occur more frequently: non–rapid eye movement (NREM) related, rapid eye movement (REM) related, and other (Table 30.1). The complete evaluation for the condition starts with thorough history taking and physical examination, specifically a complete neurologic examination to assess for underlying neurologic disorders. Polysomnography (PSG) is an important component of the evaluation but is not required for every case. It is important to emphasize that the episodes of parasomnia may not occur every night and therefore multiple PSG evaluations may be required.

---

**CLINICAL PEARL**

Indications for evaluation of suspected parasomnias with polysomnography (PSG): (1) violent or injurious behavior; (2) behavior is extremely disruptive to household members; (3) excessive daytime sleepiness due to parasomnia; and (4) parasomnia associated with medical, psychiatric, or neurologic symptoms or findings.

---

The patient reports that he usually goes to bed around 11 p.m. and believes he falls asleep soon after. He sometimes wakes up at night to use the restroom but falls back asleep immediately after returning to bed. He wakes up around 7 a.m. and feels refreshed overall by his sleep time. He denies significant daytime sleepiness. He acknowledges that in the past, bed partners have complained of snoring, but denies any observed apnea episodes. His wife is present during the visit and relates that approximately 3 to 4 times per week, usually not long after falling asleep, he sits up in bed and appears confused, with his eyes open but staring blankly. Sometimes he also screams loudly, breathing heavily and sweating profusely. Attempts to interact with him during that time result in a blank stare, then he typically falls back to sleep almost immediately. The patient has no recollection of the events and does not remember dreams or nightmares associated with it.

### TABLE 30.1 ■ Parasomnia Classification

**NREM-related parasomnias**
Confusional arousals
Sleepwalking
Sleep terrors
Sleep-related eating disorder

**REM-related parasomnias**
REM sleep behavior disorder
Recurrent isolated sleep paralysis
Nightmare disorder

**Other parasomnias**
Exploding head syndrome
Sleep-related hallucinations
Sleep enuresis
Parasomnia due to a medical disorder
Parasomnia due to a medication or substance
Parasomnia, unspecified

Modified from American Academy of Sleep Medicine. (2014). *The International Classification of Sleep Disorders* (3rd ed.) Darien, IL: American Academy of Sleep Medicine.

During the initial evaluation of suspected parasomnias the history obtained by talking to the patient and other members of the household is essential and guides the differential. Features that are particularly important include age of onset, duration of the episodes, level of consciousness during the episodes, degree of recollection of the events, time of the night in which the events occur, and a detailed description of the behavior observed. It is important to note as well that different parasomnias can be observed in the same patient and even in the same night, especially in the case of the NREM parasomnias such as confusional arousal, sleepwalking, and sleep terrors.

---

**CLINICAL PEARL**

The abnormal behavior observed in parasomnias can be as simple as muscle jerks or as complex as walking, eating, and engaging in sexual behavior. A detailed description of the behavior provides important clues to specific clinical disorders.

---

The patient reports that when he was a child he used to have episodes that were like the ones described but has not had further events since he started middle school.

---

*What is your differential diagnosis for this patient's abnormal behavior at night?*
This patient's abnormal behavior complex behavior at night can be a manifestation of different conditions, including NREM parasomnias, REM parasomnias, nocturnal seizures, as well as other sleep-related disorders that can mimic parasomnias when not treated, such as obstructive sleep apnea (OSA). Important clues are provided in the history and physical examination. The fact that this patient has a previous history of similar events in childhood and now has recurrence in a time of stress is suggestive of an NREM parasomnia. Other features that support this conclusion are the lack of consciousness of the event and the amnesia following the episode.

Furthermore, his wife's description of these events has characteristics of both confusional arousal and sleep terrors. Confusional arousals represent brief episodes of incomplete arousal without sympathetic features such as tachycardia, tachypnea, and diaphoresis. In contrast, sleep terrors (also called *night terrors*) are characterized by sudden arousal with a loud screaming or crying and significant sympathetic response. They are frequently very distressing to those witnessing the episodes, but the patient typically falls asleep soon after and has no recollection of the events. The combination of two or more NREM parasomnias as seen in this patient is not uncommon, and the combination of behaviors can often be seen during the course of a single night.

---

**CLINICAL PEARL**

Non–rapid eye movement (NREM) parasomnias are more frequent in childhood and tend to disappear before adolescence. They can however reappear in adulthood and may be triggered by factors such as stress, sleep deprivation, sleep fragmentation, and medication use. Up to two-thirds of adults with NREM parasomnias have a history of similar events as a child.

---

REM sleep behavior disorder (RBD) is a REM parasomnia that should be in the differential for adult patients with abnormal nocturnal behaviors. RBD is extremely rare in childhood and, when seen, has associations with conditions such as pontine tumor, seizure disorders, and even as a harbinger of childhood narcolepsy.

This REM parasomnia is characterized by dream-enacting behavior, also called *oneirism*, that can be violent. One important feature of this condition is that the movements may be associated with the dream content, although the individual may not have full recollection of it. During the episodes, a close inspection of the patient's eyes would likely reveal that they are closed, and rapid eye movements are observed, as is typical of the REM stage. In contrast, episodes of NREM parasomnias are frequently characterized by open eyes, staring blankly or "glassy." Again, RBD is much more common in older adults, with an average age of onset about 50 years old, and this is not compatible with our patient's history (Table 30.2).

---

**TABLE 30.2 ■ Comparison Between NREM Parasomnias, RBD, and Nocturnal Seizures**

|  | NREM Sleep-Related Parasomnias | | | RBD | Nocturnal Seizures |
|---|---|---|---|---|---|
|  | Confusional Arousal | Sleepwalking | Sleep Terrors |  |  |
| Typical behavior | Sudden arousal followed by confusion | Sudden arousal and leaving the bed, variable complex behavior | Sudden arousal with screaming, crying, and sympathetic response | Dream enactment, frequently violent, fighting, punching, kicking | Stereotypical movements, possible vocalizations |
| Family history | Usually positive | | | Negative | May be positive |
| Age of onset | Usually before 10 years old, may recur in adulthood | | | Usually after 40 years old | Mean age 14 years old |
| Recollection of event | Partial or complete amnesia | | | Recall with details | Variable degree of amnesia |

---

**CLINICAL PEARL**

There is an important association between REM sleep behavior disorder (RBD) and neurodegenerative disease, including Lewy body dementia and Parkinson disease. Parkinson disease is one of the identifiable causes of RBD, along with multiple sclerosis (MS), dementia, cerebrovascular disease, and brain tumors. Of patients who have idiopathic RBD, up to 81% will subsequently develop Parkinson disease later in their lives. The development of the condition can be delayed by many years or decades.

---

Nocturnal seizure activity can appear similar to parasomnias, and it can be difficult to differentiate them from NREM parasomnia based on clinical features alone. They tend to occur during the day as well and typically present with more repetitive movements. Complete electroencephalography (EEG) during sleep is typically needed to evaluate for the condition in suspected cases.

Finally, untreated OSA can cause dream-enacting behavior in a condition called *pseudo-RBD*. The behaviors typically resolve with continuous positive airway pressure (CPAP) treatment.

---

**BEYOND THE PEARLS:**

- NREM parasomnias typically occur in children during N3 stage of sleep in the first half of the night. In adults it can also occur in stages N1 and N2, at any point during the night.
- NREM parasomnias have not been found to have a consistent association with any specific psychopathology.
- NREM parasomnias can be precipitated in children by fevers.
- RBD can be associated with severe neurologic disorders. In a woman with new onset RBD and other neurologic findings, multiple sclerosis should be considered as a potential cause.
- REM sleep without atonia (RSWA) is characteristic of RBD; however, it can be seen isolated in patients taking medications such as SSRIs.
- Parasomnia overlap disorder represents a combination of NREM parasomnia and RBD in the same patient. It has been associated with conditions such as narcolepsy, multiple sclerosis, brain tumors, and psychiatric disorders.
- RBD does not always require pharmacologic treatment, and environmental precautions may be sufficient.
- The most established treatment for RBD is clonazepam, given 30 minutes before bedtime.

---

The patient reports that he is generally healthy and denies neurologic complaints, including headaches, weakness, numbness, tingling, and tremors. The patient also denies recent weight changes, alcohol consumption, smoking, or illicit drug use. He denies any recent illnesses and does not take any medications. He recalls that his grandmother used to tell him that the patient's father had similar episodes when he was a child, but they resolved spontaneously. On physical examination, the patient's blood pressure is 110/64 mm Hg, pulse rate is 68/min, respiration rate is 13/min, temperature is 98.6 °F, and oxygen saturation is 98% on room air. Complete neurologic examination reveals no abnormalities in cognition, cranial nerves, motor, sensory, and cerebellar evaluation.

---

*What additional diagnostic testing would you order to further evaluate this patient's complaint and to distinguish between different possible causes?*

After a thorough history and physical examination, the next step to consider would be a PSG. In this case a PSG would be even more relevant as the patient does report a history of snoring, and it would be important to evaluate him for OSA, which could cause some of the symptoms described. In the evaluation of parasomnias, it is recommended to include both continuous video and audio monitoring throughout the test in order to better observe and characterize any abnormal behavior. In situations in which other neurologic disease is suspected based on history or examination, further diagnostic testing such as magnetic resonance imaging (MRI) and/or EEG may be appropriate.

### What are the main findings in PSG in cases of NREM parasomnias?

PSG with continuous video and audio monitoring performed for NREM parasomnia often captures the behavior in question. During these episodes or arousal, EEG typically reveals persistent slow wave (N3) activity, and there is increased muscle activity noted on electromyography (EMG). Signs of autonomic hyperactivity (e.g. tachycardia) can also be seen during the episode in sleep terror.

In contrast, PSG in patients with RBD usually reveals episodes of REM sleep without atonia (RSWA). Muscle tone as measured during polysomnography by EMG in the chin, arms, and legs is uncharacteristically elevated during REM sleep in patients with RBD.

---

**CLINICAL PEARL**

RBD is frequently associated with abnormalities in areas of the brain that are typically associated with muscle atonia during REM sleep, mostly the brainstem inhibitory centers.

---

**CLINICAL PEARL**

Zolpidem is a benzodiazepine receptor agonist and has been associated with significant increase in the risk of sleepwalking and other complex behaviors during sleep.

---

A complete PSG with video and audio monitoring is ordered. During the test, the patient has one episode in which he sits up in bed screaming and is noted to be tachycardic and tachypneic. His eyes are noted to be open, and he lies back down in bed after about 1 minute. EEG reveals slow waves, and no seizure activity is noted at any point during the night. The patient is noted to be snoring when lying supine, his apnea hypopnea index is measured at 2 events/hour. The lowest oxygen saturation recorded is 88% on room air.

---

### After performing the PSG, what is the most likely explanation of the patient's complaints?

The test confirms the previous suspicion of NREM parasomnia. More importantly it helps rule out conditions that may present similarly and may mimic this presentation, specifically OSA and nocturnal seizures.

---

The patient is reassured about his condition but reports that his wife is distressed with his atypical behavior. After a review of precipitating factors for the condition and environmental precautions, the patient is started on clonazepam at bedtime.

---

The treatment approach to NREM parasomnias involves mostly environmental precautions to avoid risk of injury to self and others (especially in cases of sleepwalking) as well as a review of possible precipitating factors that may be exacerbating the position. Common culprits are stress, sleep deprivation, and sleep fragmentation. This patient's approaching deadline at work appears to be causing significant levels of stress and may be the reason for the reappearance of these behaviors. Most patients do not require pharmacologic therapy for the condition. Experience with different agents is limited mostly to observational studies but some of the most commonly used drugs include clonazepam, tricyclic antidepressants, and selective serotonin reuptake inhibitors (SSRIs).

## BEYOND THE PEARLS:

- Treatment with continuous positive airway pressure (CPAP) has been shown to improve symptoms not only in patients with pseudo-RBD but also those with true RBD.
- Treatment with clonazepam is typically limited by its side effects: early morning sedation, memory dysfunction, and increased fall risk.
- Melatonin can also be used either alone or in combination with clonazepam in the treatment of RBD and may allow lower doses of benzodiazepines to be used.
- Melatonin is the only treatment for RBD that has been shown to decrease the number of REM sleep without atonia (RSWA) episodes.
- Sleep-related eating disorder (SRED) is a type of NREM parasomnia in which individuals consume peculiar and possibly dangerous foods during sleep, usually without recollection of the event afterward.
- SRED is much more common in females, and typical age of onset is 20–30 years-old.
- Benzodiazepine receptor agonists, especially zolpidem, tend to exacerbate SRED.
- The most used treatment for SRED is topiramate, although other agents, such as clonazepam, sertraline and pramipexole, have been used successfully.

Complaint/history: A 25-year-old man reports bizarre behavior during sleep.

Findings: No abnormal physical examination findings.

Labs/tests: Overnight PSG demonstrates evidence of NREM parasomnia, rules out OSA and seizure disorder.

Diagnosis: NREM parasomnia, sleep terror, and confusional arousal.

Treatment: Avoidance of precipitants, environmental precautions, clonazepam.

## References

American Academy of Sleep Medicine. (2014). *The international classification of sleep disorders, revised: Diagnostic and coding manual.* Darien, IL: Author.

Avidan, A. Y., & Kaplish, N. (2010). The parasomnias: Epidemiology, clinical features, and diagnostic approach. *Clinics in Chest Medicine, 31,* 353–370.

Boursoulian, L. J., Schenck, C. H., Mahowald, M. W., & Lagrange, A. H. (2012). Differentiating parasomnias from nocturnal seizures. *Journal of Clinical Sleep Medicine, 8,* 108–112.

Ohayon, M. M., Mahowald, M. W., & Leger, D. (2014). Are confusional arousals pathological? *Neurology, 83,* 834–841.

Pressman, M. R., Meyer, T. J., Kendrick-Mohamed J., Figueroa, W. G., Greenspon, L. W., & Peterson, D. D. (1995). Night terrors in adults precipitated by sleep apnea. *Sleep, 18,* 773–775.

Sheldon, S., H., & Loghmanee, D. A. (2014). REM behavior disorder. In S. H. Sheldon, R. Ferber, M. H. Kryger, & D. Gozal (Eds.), *Principles and practice of pediatric sleep medicine e-book* (p. 321). London: Saunders.

Tassinari, C. A., Rubboli, G., Gardella, E., Cantalupo, G., Calandra-Buonaura, G., Vedovello, M., ... Meletti, S. (2005). Central pattern generators for a common semiology in fronto-limbic seizures and in parasomnias. A neuroethologic approach. *Neurological Sciences, 26,* s225–s232.

Tinuper, P., Bisulli, F., & Provini, F. (2012). The parasomnias: Mechanisms and treatment. *Epilepsia, 53,* 12–19.

# CHAPTER 31

# Obstructive Sleep Apnea

Lucas Cruz ■ Kelly Fan ■ Edwin Valladares ■ Terese C. Hammond ■ Raj Dasgupta

A 63-year-old male is referred to you for excessive daytime sleepiness (EDS). His symptoms have been worsening for the past 3 years. He goes to sleep nightly around 9 PM and wakes up at 5 AM for his construction job. He falls asleep quickly and wakes up only once to use the restroom, falling back asleep within 5 minutes. He occasionally wakes up with a mild headache and feels fatigued throughout the day. He has been noted by his coworkers to "doze off" while reading the newspaper during his lunch break. His wife mentions loud snoring at night and has witnessed episodes in which he appears to stop breathing. His medical history is significant for difficult-to-control hypertension, gastroesophageal reflux disease, and worsening obesity, with a current body mass index (BMI) of 36 kg/m². Physical examination revealed a crowded oropharynx, with only hard and soft palates being visualized. His cardiopulmonary examination revealed no abnormal findings.

*What is the most likely diagnosis? What clues in the patient's history reinforce this diagnosis?*

Our patient presents with a chief complaint of excessive daytime sleepiness (EDS). Excessive daytime sleepiness is defined as the inability to maintain wakefulness or alertness during the major waking part of the day. Excessive daytime sleepiness can be a symptom of insufficient sleep, sleep disorders that interrupt sleep continuity, and medical or psychiatric disorders. Any evaluation for EDS should consider sleep-disordered breathing in the differential, specifically obstructive sleep apnea (OSA) because of its high prevalence and associated morbidity. The most important risk factors for OSA are outlined in Table 31.1. Our patient has, in fact, many such risk factors.

Although the clinical presentation of OSA can vary, the most common symptoms are daytime sleepiness and snoring. However, the single most useful symptom to identify patients with OSA is nocturnal choking or gasping during sleep. Many questionnaires have been created and validated to assist in screening for patients at risk for OSA. Among these, the STOP-Bang questionnaire (Table 31.2) was shown to be the most sensitive. A score of 3 or higher in this questionnaire has a high sensitivity for the diagnosis of OSA and warrants further diagnostic testing. Our patient's score is 8, indicating a high risk of OSA and making it the most likely diagnosis in this case.

Patients who develop OSA are at increased risk for a wide range of complications that can impact quality of life and other outcomes. Obstructive sleep apnea has been associated with hypertension, atrial fibrillation (AF), coronary heart disease, stroke, pulmonary hypertension, and heart failure, among others. Diurnal and nocturnal blood pressure have been shown to decrease with effective OSA treatment. However, the effect of OSA treatment with continuous positive airway pressure (CPAP) is variable on decreasing the risk and burden of these cardiovascular conditions and is still the subject of continued research.

TABLE 31.1 ■ Risk Factors for OSA

| | |
|---|---|
| Increased age | Family history of OSA |
| Male (sex) | Congestive heart failure |
| Obesity | End-stage renal disease |
| Craniofacial and upper airway abnormalities | Smoking |
| Nasal congestion | Hypothyroidism |

TABLE 31.2 ■ STOP-Bang Questionnaire

Snoring: Do you snore loudly?
Tired: Do you feel tired, fatigued, or sleepy during the daytime?
Observed: Has anyone observed you stop breathing or choking/gasping during your sleep?
Pressure: Do you have or are being treated for high blood pressure?
Body mass index more than 35 kg/m2?
Age older than 50 years old?
Neck circumference >17 inches in males or >16 inches in females?
Gender (male)
**Yes to three or more questions indicates an elevated risk for OSA and justifies further diagnostic testing.**

### CLINICAL PEARL

There is a strong association between obstructive sleep apnea (OSA) and atrial fibrillation (AF), independent of other confounding factors, such as obesity. Different mechanisms help explain this relationship, including autonomic dysfunction, hypoxia, hypercapnia, and increased negative intrathoracic pressures. Interestingly, OSA is a risk factor for recurrence of AF in patients who undergo ablation and treatment of OSA reduces the risk of recurrent AF.

*What are the changes in sleep respiratory physiology that predispose a patient to OSA?*
The hallmark of OSA is recurrent obstruction of the upper airway during sleep. Upper airway mechanics are significantly affected by sleep in different ways, including decreased activity in the pharyngeal musculature and increased upper airway resistance due to decreased airway caliber. In patients who have anatomic susceptibility, these factors increase the chance and severity of airway obstruction.

Different structural factors confer anatomic susceptibility to obstruction. These include craniofacial structure and the increased soft tissue surrounding the airway, such as increased tongue volume or increased adipose tissue deposition secondary to obesity. The Mallampati score (Fig. 31.1), initially devised to predict difficult laryngoscopies, is commonly used for assessment of airway patency. Higher scores are associated with more crowded and less patent airways.

### BASIC SCIENCE PEARL

The upper airway is surrounded by a skeletal structure that consists of the maxilla, mandible, skull base, and cervical spine. Anatomic changes such as retrognathia, the condition where the lower jaw is set further back than the upper jaw, can decrease the airway lumen and predispose to OSA. Studies have shown that increased mandibular length is associated with decreased risk of OSA in men.

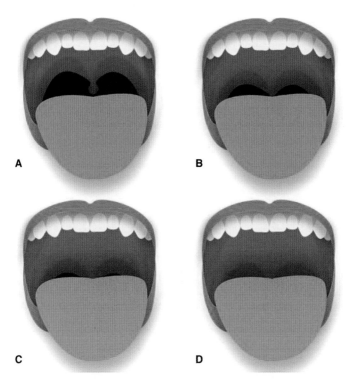

**Fig. 31.1** Mallampati score. (A) Class I: visibility of all of the soft palate, fauces, uvula, and pillars. (B) Class II: visibility of the soft palate, fauces, and only the base of the uvula. (C) Class III: visibility of the soft palate. (D) Class IV: visibility of the hard palate only. (Soydan, S.S. (2015). Changes in difficult airway predictors following mandibular setback surgery. *International Journal of Oral & Maxillofacial Surgery, 44*(11), 1351–1354. Copyright © 2015 International Association of Oral and Maxillofacial Surgeons.)

**CLINICAL PEARL**

Mandibular-advancement oral appliances can be used in the treatment of OSA in individuals with appropriate upper airway anatomy. These devices increase airway diameter by protruding the mandible and displacing soft tissues.

*What additional diagnostic tests would you need to complete to confirm a diagnosis of OSA?*
Our patient's clinical presentation and risk factors are highly suspicious for OSA. The American College of Physicians (ACP) recommends performing diagnostic testing for OSA in any patient with otherwise unexplained excessive daytime sleepiness. Other indications for performing additional testing in patients without excessive daytime sleepiness would include hard-to-treat hypertension or pulmonary hypertension.

The gold standard diagnostic test for OSA is in-laboratory polysomnography (PSG). Polysomnography provides breathing and other physiologic measures across sleep stage. Other physiologic measures include electroencephalogram (EEG) for establishing sleep stage, electrooculogram (EOG) and submental electromyogram (EMG) for identifying rapid eye movement (REM) sleep, one lead electrocardiogram (ECG) for arrhythmia identification, and anterior tibialis EMG for identification of leg movements during sleep. These measures assist in discriminating between

**TABLE 31.3 ■ Diagnostic Criteria for OSA**

One of two conditions must be present for the diagnosis:
Five or more obstructive sleep apnea or hypopnea respiratory events per hour of sleep.
AND
Symptoms or complications of OSA, including: sleepiness, gasping, choking, habitual snoring,
    hypertension, mood disorder, coronary artery disease, stroke, AF, or type 2 diabetes mellitus.
OR
Fifteen or more obstructive sleep apnea or hypopnea respiratory events per hour of sleep.

**TABLE 31.4 ■ Predominantly Obstructive Respiratory Events During a Sleep Study**

| Respiratory Event | Definition |
| --- | --- |
| Apnea | 90% or greater decrease in airflow for a minimum of 10 seconds with continued respiratory effort throughout event. |
| Hypopnea | At least 30% decrease in airflow for a minimum of 10 seconds associated with either a 3% or 4% oxygen desaturation from baseline, depending on accepted sleep laboratory criteria. |
| RERAs | Arousals associated with change in airflow that does not meet criteria for apnea or hypopnea. The events last at least 10 seconds and are associated with increased respiratory effort and terminate in an arousal seen on EEG. These are not included in the Apnea-Hypopnea Index (AHI). |

**TABLE 31.5 ■ Severity of Sleep-Disordered Breathing by Apnea-Hypopnea Index**

| AHI | Severity |
| --- | --- |
| Between 5 and 15 events per hour | Mild |
| Between 15 and 30 events per hour | Moderate |
| Greater than 30 events per hour | Severe |

conditions that can mimic features of OSA or occur concurrently with OSA. The American Academy of Sleep Medicine (AASM) recommends basing the diagnosis of sleep apnea on symptoms and the frequency of respiratory events per hour of sleep in a sleep study, which is called the *apnea-hypopnea index* (Table 31.3). Respiratory events identified during a sleep study include: apneas, hypopneas, and respiratory effort-related arousals (RERAs) (Table 31.4).

The most common measurement used to quantify respiratory events and classify the severity of sleep apnea is the apnea-hypopnea index (AHI). It is obtained by adding together the number of apnea and hypopnea episodes and dividing by the sum of the total sleep time in hours. Sleep-disordered breathing can be classified as mild, moderate, or severe (Table 31.5). An AHI of 5 or greater with symptoms of OSA, or 15 or greater without symptoms of OSA, is enough to diagnose it. These respiratory events can be either obstructive or central depending on the presence or absence of respiratory effort during the event.

**CLINICAL PEARL**

Another respiratory event metric in polysomnography reports is the respiratory disturbance index (RDI). The RDI is obtained by adding apneas, hypopneas, and RERAs and dividing the sum by the total sleep time in hours. The RDI can be greater than the AHI and may be more sensitive in diagnosing OSA.

In-laboratory PSG is the gold standard for the diagnosis of OSA; however, home sleep apnea testing (HSAT) is increasingly used to diagnose OSA given its convenience and lower costs. Home sleep apnea testing has been validated as an adequate tool for the diagnosis of OSA in otherwise uncomplicated patients. Home sleep apnea testing is also called *limited channel testing*, because it records breathing pressure for determination of breathing and snoring, breathing effort, pulse, oxygen saturation and body position. The obvious limitation is that sleep is inferred, because objective sleep is not measured using EEG signals. This can lead to misinterpretation and inaccurate results in less severe OSA patients. Home sleep apnea testing devices tend to underestimate the AHI and can lead to false negative results, especially in patients with mild OSA. A negative HSAT result should not rule out OSA when there is a high clinical suspicion and an in-laboratory PSG should be performed. The AASM also recommends the use of PSG rather than HSAT for diagnosis of OSA in patients with significant cardiorespiratory disease, neuromuscular disorder, awake hypoventilation, chronic opioid use, history of stroke, or severe insomnia.

---

You order a home sleep study which confirms an AHI of 45 per hour (Fig. 31.2). What would you do next for this patient?

---

Based on guidelines from the AASM, an AHI of 45/hr is diagnostic for severe OSA. An HSAT was able to capture the severity of this patient's OSA. In-laboratory polysomnography could have been excessive given his severity. See Fig. 31.3 for a sample of an in-laboratory PSG. The treatment goal is to reduce symptoms and AHI. Treating OSA can be multidisciplinary, as evidenced by the recommended clinical practice guidelines outlined by the American Academy of Sleep Medicine (AASM), American College of Physicians (ACP), the American Thoracic Society (ATS), and the International Geriatric Sleep Medicine Force (Fig. 31.3).

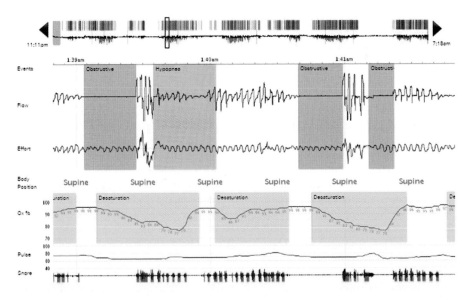

**Fig. 31.2** Three-minute home sleep apnea test snapshot. This is a snapshot outlining the entire night oxygen saturation at the top, with desaturation in blue and colored tick marks representing respiratory events. The black box represents the snap shot of the channels at 1:39 AM, with corresponding channels below it. Channels include: flow, effort, body position, saturation, pulse, and snoring.

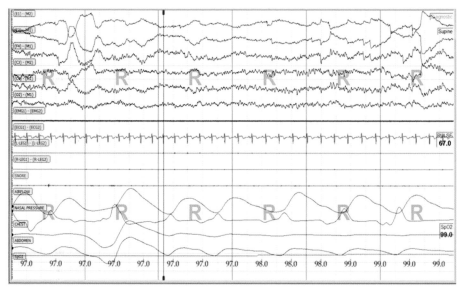

**Fig. 31.3** Sample of a 30-second polysomnography epoch during rapid eye movement (REM) sleep. This 30-second epoch demonstrates electrooculogram (EOG), electroencephalogram (EEG), submental electromyogram (EMG), electrocardiogram (ECG), anterior tibialis EMG, snore microphone, airflow, nasal pressure, chest and abdominal effort, and saturation, from top to bottom respectively. Pulse can be found on the side, and body position was entered manually by the sleep technologist as verified by continuous camera visualization.

---

**CLINICAL PEARL**

Benefits for treating OSA include a decrease in daytime sleepiness and health care costs, and an increase in quality of life and in select patient improvement in cardiac morbidity and mortality.

---

For all patients diagnosed with OSA, behavior modification is always recommended. Weight loss and exercise are encouraged for overweight and obese patients. In some cases, avoidance of supine sleep can ameliorate OSA severity by sleeping laterally or prone. Alcohol, cannabis use, and medications such as benzodiazepines, antihistamines, barbiturates, opiates, and antiepileptics should be avoided, if possible, because they exacerbate OSA by suppressing breathing.

Moreover, positive airway pressure (PAP) therapy is considered the standard treatment modality for OSA. Continuous positive airway pressure (CPAP) allows the maintenance of a constant positive pharyngeal transmural pressure and intraluminal pressure, while also increasing the end-expiratory lung volume. CPAP therapy benefits include reduction in AHI and clinical improvement in daytime sleepiness, sleep quality, cognitive function, depression, and blood pressure. Other reported benefits include improvement in gastroesophageal reflux, heart failure, and arrhythmias (Fig. 31.4).

For patients with mild to moderate OSA, who are unable to tolerate PAP therapy, the option to use an oral appliance is an alternative. These include mandibular advancement devices and tongue-retaining devices. Both devices are designed to maintain upper airway patency by holding the soft tissues of the oropharynx away from the posterior pharyngeal wall. For patients with severe OSA due to anatomic obstruction, upper airway surgery can be an option. Patients with tonsillar hypertrophy, adenoid hypertrophy, or craniofacial abnormalities who have surgically correctable anatomy benefit the most from this intervention. Finally, for selected patients with moderate to severe OSA who cannot tolerate CPAP therapy and do not have complete concentric collapse of the palate during simulated apneas, hypoglossal nerve stimulation via an implantable neurostimulator device is a viable option.

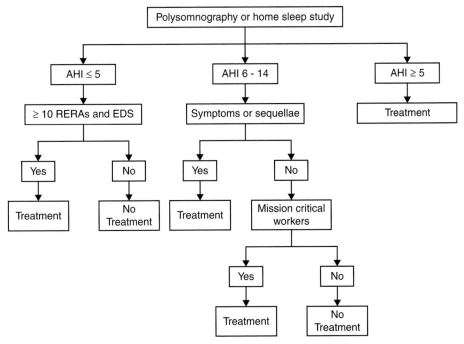

**Fig. 31.4** Obstructive sleep apnea (OSA) management algorithm. AHI, Apnea-hypopnea index (per hour); RERA, respiratory effort related arousals (per hour); EDS, excessive daytime sleepiness; mission critical workers (i.e., pilot, bus or truck drivers, air traffic controller).

For our patient with severe OSA, behavior modification and a trial of CPAP therapy would be the most appropriate.

You initiate auto-CPAP therapy and follow up with the patient in 4 weeks. You confirm excellent compliance but now note emergence of central sleep apneas.

### *What are some common causes of central sleep apnea?*

Our patient is exhibiting treatment emergence CSA. Central sleep apnea (CSA) occurs when both airflow and ventilatory efforts are absent during sleep. Causes of central sleep apnea can be divided into primary versus secondary. Primary CSA is due to idiopathic causes. In contrast, secondary CSA can be due to various causes such as heart failure, spinal cord injury, stroke, myasthenia gravis, and Cheyne-Stokes breathing. Substance abuse and medications that have an effect of suppressing the respiratory drive can lead to secondary CSA. Finally, treatment-emergent secondary CSA can be seen with the use of CPAP in a small group of OSA patients (1%–5%). For treatment-emergent CSA, the optimal treatment is unknown. However, this condition often resolves spontaneously within 3 months. For patients whose CSA persists, CPAP therapy may be decreased to a suboptimal level or different PAP therapy modes, such as adaptive servo-ventilation (ASV) or bilevel PAP (BPAP), may be trialed.

**CLINICAL PEARL**

Cheyne-Stokes breathing is an abnormal breathing pattern with recurrent apneas. It is a cyclic breathing pattern where respiratory frequency and tidal volume are initially increased but gradually decrease, which is then followed by a period of apnea. It is often found in patients with heart failure or stroke and is considered a type of central sleep apnea syndrome.

You continue CPAP therapy for the patient and continue to note excellent compliance. At 3-month follow-up, residual AHI is now down to two and his CSA has completely resolved. Overall the patient feels better but still notes excessive daytime sleepiness after eating lunch. What are additional treatment options that can help with this patient's symptoms?

It is important to distinguish EDS from complaints or symptoms of fatigue, which is a subjective lack of physical or mental energy. Major causes of EDS include insufficient sleep, other sleep disorders, medical and psychiatric conditions, and medications. Therefore it is important to obtain a detailed medical and sleep history. For patients already diagnosed with sleep-disordered breathing, it is important to confirm CPAP compliance, sufficient nightly sleep, and medication review.

Besides OSA, other sleep disorders that lead to EDS include idiopathic hypersomnia and narcolepsy. Although behavior modifications are important, pharmacologic agents can be considered for symptomatic treatment. Stimulants, such as modafinil, armodafinil, and methylphenidate, and amphetamines, can be prescribed. In particular, modafinil is often used, because it is better tolerated with less side effects.

## BEYOND THE PEARLS:

Treatment improvements for OSA.

**Technology in sleep apnea therapy:** Technology advances incorporated into CPAP therapy have empowered patients, thereby increasing compliance. Physicians have access to daily reports via cloud-based systems and can remotely make changes to CPAP settings from any computer via these cloud interfaces. Patients can receive daily feedback via smartphone applications and email messages, encouraging them on usage and compliance.

**CPAP mark fitting:** Optimal CPAP compliance is not only rooted in a patient's initial CPAP experience and AHI severity but also in using the most comfortable mask. Different patients find each mask type comfortable for different reasons. The nasal pillows mask is light and has minimal headgear; the nasal mask has minimal headgear and spreads pressure delivery around the nose as opposed to inside the nostril; and the full-face mask is comfortable because of the uniform pressure delivery between the nose and mouth although it is large in size.

**Travel CPAP devices:** These are CPAP devices the size of a smartphone that make travel with a CPAP more convenient. Continuous PAP therapy should be used whenever a person sleeps.

**The Pillars procedure:** This is a surgical procedure used to treat mild-to-moderate sleep apnea by placing small polyester rods in the soft palate. Once these rods have been implanted, the tissue around it heals, stiffening the soft palate and therefore reducing relaxation and vibration of the tissue and ameliorating the mild-to-moderate obstruction.

**Somnoplasty:** This is a surgical procedure used to treat snoring and mild-to-moderate OSA by using low-frequency heat to create burn areas in the mucosa of the soft palate. These areas eventually cause shrinking and stiffening of the tissue and resorption of the surrounding tissue, thereby leading to decreased snoring and OSA.

**Phrenic nerve stimulation:** This is a surgically implantable therapy for treating central sleep apnea by rhythmically and indirectly stimulating the phrenic nerve, which results in diaphragmatic pacing.

## References

American Academy of Sleep Medicine. (2014). *The international classification of sleep disorders, revised: Diagnostic and coding manual.* Darien, IL: Author.

Basyuni, S., Barabas, M., & Quinnell, T. (2018). An update on mandibular advancement devices for the treatment of obstructive sleep apnoea hypopnoea syndrome. *Journal of Thoracic Disease, 10*(Suppl 1), S48–S56.

Chung, F., Yegneswaran, B., Liao, P., Chung, S. A., Vairavanathan, S., Islam, S. ...Shapiro, C. M. (2018). STOP questionnaire: A tool to screen patients for obstructive sleep apnea. *Anesthesiology, 108*(5), 812–821.

Miller, J. N., Kupzyk, K. A., Zimmerman, L., Pozehl, B., Schulz, P., Romberger, D., & Berger, A. M. (2018). Comparisons of measures used to screen for obstructive sleep apnea in patients referred to a sleep clinic. *Sleep Medicine, 51*, 15–21.

Myers, K. A., Mrkobrada, M., & Simel, D. L. (2013). Does this patient have obstructive sleep apnea? The rational clinical examination systematic review. *Journal of the American Medical Association, 310*(7), 731–741.

Valladares, E. M., & Hammond, T. C. (2018). Novel therapies for sleep apnea—the implants have arrived! *Neurodiagnostic Journal, 58*(2), 116–125.

# CHAPTER 32

# Gender Dysphoria

Peter Ureste ■ Tammy Duong

---

A 68-year-old female presents with her husband after being referred to your clinic by her endocrinologist for concerns of worsening anxiety. She tells you that her anxiety started 1 year ago after she began transitioning from male-to-female and started hormone therapy. Her anxiety often occurs in social events such as dining out, due to fear of being scrutinized by others. For example, she talks about a lunch she had last week with her son and daughter-in-law, and sensed a marked fear of rejection. She states, "I felt like everyone was staring at me, I was afraid they'd judge me." As a result of the worsening fears of anxiety, she now rarely leaves her home. Before she began her transition, she was a runner, she enjoyed going to the movies, and she loved visiting new restaurants.

---

### What is gender identity?

The terms "sex," "gender," "gender identity," and "gender expression" are often confused but all have different meanings. *Sex* is a biological term for male or female assigned at birth by a healthcare provider based on the external genitals they are born with. Sex is what goes on a newborn's birth certificate. *Gender* is a social term for male or female set by societal expectations about one's behaviors, appearances, and views. Instead of referring to intimate body parts, gender is defined as the expected societal behavior based on sex. *Gender identity* is an early feeling of how a person feels internally about their gender. For most people, gender identity matches their assigned sex at birth, but for some, it feels different. It is important to know that gender identity is also more diverse than a binary framework allows (i.e., male or female, transfemale or transmale) and is on a spectrum. Some patients may also identify using nonbinary terms such as genderqueer, gender nonconforming, gender nonbinary, or they may use other terms. Always allow the patient to describe their own gender. *Gender expression* describes the way a person expresses their gender identity through personal appearance and behavior.

---

You learn that the patient identifies as a transwoman, and that her sexual orientation is heterosexual.

---

### How is gender identity different from sexual orientation?

Gender identity describes one's internal sense of their own gender (i.e., male, female, a blend of both, or neither). Sexual orientation describes whom the person is attracted to, falls in love with, or with whom they have sexual relationships. It is important to let the patient identify their sexual orientation. Similar to gender identity, sexual orientation is more diverse than a binary framework such as heterosexual or homosexual. Some may identify as bisexual (attracted to both male and female), asexual (lack of sexual attraction to others, or low-to-absent interest in or desire for sexual activity), pansexual (attraction toward people regardless of their sex or gender identity), or they may use some other term.

### *What cultural considerations should health care providers keep in mind when working with transgender patients?*

The initial encounter with a transgender patient (as with all patients) should focus on building rapport and establishing their name and pronouns. It is discouraged to use the phrase "preferred name" or "preferred pronoun," because to prefer something is providing an opinion. Sometimes a patient's current name may be different from their birth name, and their current pronoun may be different from their assigned sex at birth. Some patients may not identify themselves as male nor female, and may use other pronouns such as "they," "them," "theirs," or other terms. Allow patients to identify their own pronouns.

### *What is the differential diagnosis?*

This is a 68-year-old female who presents with worsening anxiety, reporting that she was assigned male sex at birth and now wears female clothing and identifies as a woman, resulting in rarely leaving her house. The following should be ruled out: gender dysphoria, transvestic disorder, body dysmorphic disorder, unspecified schizophrenia spectrum, and other psychotic disorder.

---

You learn that 1 year prior to her full transition, she intermittently wore women's clothing and used women's public restrooms.

---

### *Does this patient have transvestic disorder?*

Transvestic disorder is a paraphilic disorder that primarily occurs in heterosexual males with cross-dressing behaviors for sexual arousal and causes distress and/or functional impairment. Individuals with transvestic disorder do not cross-dress because they identify as transgender.

Some individuals such as drag queens or drag kings cross-dress for entertainment purposes. In regards to this patient, she does not cross-dress for sexual arousal or entertainment; rather, she cross-dresses to maintain conformity with her internal sense of being a female. Therefore, she does not have transvestic disorder.

---

**BASIC SCIENCE PEARL**                **STEP 1**

Paraphilias are intense and persistent sexual interests outside of "normophilic" behaviors. A paraphilic disorder requires a paraphilia for at least 6 months, may involve potentially nonadult or nonconsenting partners, and, when acted upon, lead to clinically significant distress, dysfunction, and/or criminal consequences.

---

**CLINICAL PEARL**                **STEP 2/3**

It is normal behavior for preschool boys and girls to dress up in clothes of the other sex as a way of trying out what it is like to be a man or a woman.

---

The patient expresses dissatisfaction with her chest, "I'd feel better about my breasts if I had implants." Her husband tells you that she is fixated on mastoplasty.

---

### *Does this patient have body dysmorphic disorder?*

In body dysmorphic disorder, the patient has one or more perceived defects or flaws in their physical appearance that results in significant distress and functional impairment. This perceived

**TABLE 32.1 ■ Diagnostic Criteria for Body Dysmorphic Disorder**

| | |
|---|---|
| A | Preoccupation with one or more perceived defects or flaws in physical appearance that are not observed or appear slight to others |
| B | The individual has performed repetitive behaviors or mental acts in response to the appearance concerns |
| C | Preoccupation causes clinically significant distress or impairment in daily functioning |
| D | Not better explained by concerns with body fat or weight in an individual whose symptoms meet criteria for an eating disorder |

defect or flaw with one's body is often not observable by others. Table 32.1 summarizes the diagnostic criteria for body dysmorphic disorder. Individuals with this disorder find a part of their body (possibly their genitalia or breasts) to be abnormal and want them removed, but they do not consider themselves a different gender. Furthermore, concerns in body appearance are not related to incongruence with one's expressed or experienced gender, as is observed in this patient. Hence, she does not have body dysmorphic disorder.

Even though the patient reports having an intense fear of rejection, no persecutory delusions are elicited, and she denies having auditory or visual hallucinations.

### Does she have a psychotic disorder?
A psychotic patient may report identifying with a gender different from the sex assigned at birth, as related to a delusion telling them they are a different gender; however, this is a rare clinical presentation, and the disorder is unlikely if there are no other psychotic symptoms. As for this patient, she denies having psychotic symptoms.

### What is gender dysphoria (GD)?
According to the *Diagnostic and Statistical Manual of Mental Disorders*, Fifth Edition (DSM-5), GD is a condition with marked incongruence between one's gender identity and their assigned gender at birth. For adolescents and adults, there must be at least two symptoms occurring for 6 months or greater, resulting in clinically significant distress or impairment in their social or occupational functioning. Table 32.2 summarizes the six symptoms of GD in adults. There are also two specifiers for the condition. First is whether the patient has a disorder of sex development

**TABLE 32.2 ■ Symptoms of Gender Dysphoria in Adults**

- Marked incongruence between one's experienced/expressed gender and primary and/or secondary sex characteristics.
- A strong desire to be rid of one's primary and/or secondary sex characteristics because of marked incongruence with one's experienced/expressed gender.
- A strong desire for the primary and/or secondary sex characteristics of some gender.
- A strong desire to be of the other or some alternative gender.
- Strong desire to be treated as the other or some alternative gender.
- A strong conviction that one has the typical feelings and reactions of the other or some alternative gender.
- *AND*, the previous symptoms are associated with significant distress or impairment in social or occupational functioning.

(intersex), which is a person born with a combination of male and female biological characteristics, such as chromosomes or genitalia. This may be due to congenital adrenal hyperplasia or androgen insensitivity syndrome. The second specifier is whether the patient is posttransition, or living full-time as the desired gender and has undergone (or is preparing to have) at least one cross-sex medical procedure or treatment regimen, such as hormone therapy or gender reassignment surgery confirming the desired gender.

| BASIC SCIENCE PEARL | STEP 1 |
|---|---|

Congenital adrenal hyperplasia is a group of inherited genetic disorders that affect the adrenal glands. The majority of cases is due to a deficiency in the 21-hydroxylase enzyme (autosomal recessive), which results in excess production of androgens and possible genital ambiguity in newborns with XX chromosomes.

| CLINICAL PEARL | STEP 2/3 |
|---|---|

Congenital adrenal hyperplasia is diagnosed by cortisol deficiency, high levels of cortisol precursors, and high androgen found in blood and urine.

| BASIC SCIENCE PEARL | STEP 1 |
|---|---|

Androgen insensitivity syndrome is a condition caused by mutations that result in severe impairment of the androgen receptor function. As a result, individuals with 46,XY chromosomes do not virilize normally, despite the presence of bilateral testes and serum testosterone concentration within or above the normal male range.

It is important to know that not all transgender individuals have clinically significant distress or impairment associated with their gender incongruence. Hence, not all trans people have GD. This diagnosis is also a controversial one and the subject of ongoing debate. Similar to the removal of homosexuality from the DSM due to changes in societal views, some argue that transgender is also a normal variant of gender identity and therefore should be removed as well. However, others argue that keeping the diagnosis in the DSM gives access to health care and insurance coverage for surgical and hormonal treatments, especially for those with lesser economic means.

You learn that the patient was assigned male at birth. The patient grew up in a strict religious household and was the youngest of five boys. The patient always had a sense of being a female but lived most of her life as a male despite secretly identifying as a female, even marrying a woman and having two children. Eventually the patient divorced and later met a man whom she married. At the age of 65 years old, the patient developed the courage to "come out of the closet" as a transwoman. She now sees an endocrinologist who prescribes her hormone therapy to feminize her secondary sex characteristics.

| BASIC SCIENCE PEARL | STEP 1 |
|---|---|

Primary sex characteristics refer to sexual organs themselves (uterus, vagina, penis, and testes) that appear at birth, whereas secondary sex characteristics refer to visible changes (breast development, fat deposition, development of the genitalia, changes in the larynx, and body hair growth) that begin at puberty and mark adult maturation.

> **BASIC SCIENCE PEARL**          **STEP 1**
>
> The sexual maturity rating, also known as the *Tanner stages,* is a five-stage systematized description of the development of the secondary sexual characteristics. Stage one represents prepuberty and stage five represents adult development. Each stage consists of changes in breast development in females, genital changes in males, and pubic hair changes in both males and females.

> **BASIC SCIENCE PEARL**          **STEP 1**
>
> Testosterone, the hormone that stimulates spermatogenesis, is responsible for the secondary sexual characteristics that develop in males during adolescence, and includes a deepening of the voice; the growth of facial, axillary, and pubic hair; and increased sex drive. Estrogen, the reproductive hormone that assists in endometrial regrowth, ovulation, and calcium absorption, is responsible for the secondary sexual characteristics of females, which include breast development, menarche, and widening of the hips.

---

The patient tells you that when she looks back at her childhood, she always knew that she was a girl since the age of 4 years old. "It was my very first conviction, the first thing I grew certain of as a young person, that I was a girl," she says. But given that the world told her that she was male, assigned her male sex at birth, and expected her to be masculine, it was easier to live her life as a male. As a result, she had a strong desire to be rid of her masculine secondary sex characteristics. She wanted to live and be treated as a woman and not as a man. Living her life as a man for many years (marrying a woman and portraying herself as a male) resulting in marital conflict, ultimately in divorce, and rejection by her religious siblings and daughter.

---

### Does this patient have GD?

For a diagnosis of GD, a person must have a marked incongruence between one's experienced and/or expressed gender and assigned gender. In this case the patient has many of the six symptoms: marked incongruence between her expressed gender and secondary sex characteristics, a strong desire to get rid of her secondary sex characteristics, and a conviction to be female, and be treated as such, although having been assigned male gender at birth. Because she is receiving cross-sex hormone treatment, posttransition may also be used as a specifier. These symptoms have resulted in strain in some of her relationships (divorce and no longer speaking with her siblings and daughter due to their rejection) and daily functioning (leaves her home less frequently). Hence, she does meet criteria for GD.

### What is the treatment for GD?

Treatment for GD is gender-affirming care, which includes a combination of psychotherapy, hormones, and surgery. Psychotherapy can help individuals feel more comfortable in their own bodies. Hormone therapy has demonstrated stress reduction without significant adverse psychological or physical effects. Plastic surgeons can conduct gender-confirming surgeries like top surgery (mastectomy or breast augmentation) and bottom surgery (vaginoplasty or phalloplasty). The Standards of Care for the Health of Transsexual, Transgender, and Gender Nonconforming People, published by the World Professional Association for Transgender Health (WPATH), recommends against physical interventions before the age of 16 years old. Additionally, they recommend that surgery only be performed after the age of 18, and after the individual has lived in their desired-gender role for at least 2 years. It is important to know that not all transgender individuals wish to take hormones or undergo surgery.

The role of a psychiatrist within gender care is to facilitate the diagnosis of gender dysphoria, assess for psychiatric comorbidity, explore the readiness for gender-affirming medical interventions (hormone therapy, gender reassignment surgery), and emotionally support the trans individual. Treatment of GD is best made by a multidisciplinary team consisting of a psychiatrist, endocrinologist, social worker, and possibly a lawyer for assisting with legal issues related to changing one's gender identity.

---

The patient shares that for the last 6 months, she has been worrying about negative evaluations and rejection by others for being a transwoman. You explore this further and learn that her anxiety is related only to social situations in which she may be judged for being transgender. She denies having periods of being tremulous, short of breath, chest pain, fear of dying, or other panic symptoms. She also denies having generalized worries in other areas of her life, such as finances, relationship with her husband, or friends who are accepting of her transgender. She abstains from alcohol (her last drink was 20 years ago) and denies past or present use of illicit drugs.

---

### How common is comorbid mental illness in transgender patients?
Like other minority groups, sexual minorities, including transgender individuals, may present with co-occurring psychiatric illnesses. It is argued that this is due to the stress of being a member of a stigmatized minority group, also known as *minority stress*. Cross sectional studies suggest that the transgender population has a higher prevalence of depression, suicide, anxiety, personality disorders, and substance use compared with their cis-gender counterparts. Additionally, gender-affirming care is associated with improvement in mental health for those with GD. Risk factors associated with co-occurring mental disorders among the trans population include victimization (i.e. social stigma, discrimination, transphobia), reduced social support (i.e. family rejection, societal rejection), and difficulties accessing health care and social services (i.e. no health insurance, lack of awareness by health care providers).

### What is your differential diagnosis for this patent's anxiety?
This patient likely does not have panic disorder because she is not having panic symptoms. She also does not have generalized worries so likely does not have generalized anxiety disorder. Given that she does not use alcohol, and her symptoms do not occur in the context of using substances, she likely does not have alcohol/substance-induced anxiety disorder. Because her anxiety occurs only in the context of social situations then social anxiety disorder is high on the differential.

### What is social anxiety disorder?
Social anxiety disorder is a condition with marked fear or anxiety about one or more social situations in which the individual is exposed to possible scrutiny by others. This can occur while being observed eating or drinking in social settings. The individual often fears of acting in such a way that will be negatively evaluated by others and lead to rejection. Social situations almost always provoke fear or anxiety that results in either avoidance or intense fear. These symptoms occur for at least 6 months and result in impairment in daily functioning. As for this patient, she meets criteria for social anxiety disorder.

---

**CLINICAL PEARL**                                                                 **STEP 2/3**

The treatment for social anxiety disorder can include cognitive behavioral therapy, selective serotonin reuptake inhibitor, low-dose benzodiazepines, or beta-blockers (for performance anxiety).

The patient is started on sertraline for social anxiety disorder, which is uptitrated to a therapeutic dose. She also undergoes cognitive behavioral therapy with the goal to be more comfortable with her own body. She continues to receive hormone therapy from her endocrinologist and receives breast augmentation. The patient is happier in her own body, has returned to regularly jogging outdoors, and is now going to restaurants to meet friends and her son.

## BEYOND THE PEARLS:

- GD is best treated from a multidisciplinary team consisting of an endocrinologist, psychiatrist, surgeon, social worker, and lawyer, among others
- It is discouraged to use the phrase "preferred name" or "preferred pronoun" because to prefer something is providing an opinion. It is not a preferred opinion on how someone wants to be addressed.
- It is important when working with patients to establish their current name and pronoun. Always let the patient identify their own gender and pronoun, as some do not identify with terms that fall into a binary model.
- Not all transgender individuals have GD, but only those with clinically significant distress or impairment associated with a perceived incongruence between their experienced gender and their assigned gender at birth.
- Do not assume that all trans people want to undergo hormone therapy and/or gender reassignment surgery.
- Compared with cis people, transgender people have a higher prevalence of comorbid psychiatric illness, which longitudinal studies suggest improve after gender-affirming treatment.
- The role of a psychiatrist in gender care is to facilitate the diagnosis of gender dysphoria, assess for psychiatric comorbidity, explore the readiness for gender-affirming medical interventions, and emotionally support the trans individual.
- A transmale who still has a cervix and breast tissue should be screened for cervical and breast cancer. A transfemale who still has a prostate should be screened for prostate cancer.

## References

American Psychiatric Association. (2013). *Diagnostic and statistical manual of mental disorders* (5th ed.). Washington, DC: Author.

Berlin, F. S. (2016). A conceptual overview and commentary on gender dysphoria. *Journal of the American Academy of Psychiatry and the Law, 44,* 246–252.

Byne, W., Karasic, D. H., Coleman, E., Eyler, A. E., Kidd, J. D., Meyer-Bahlburg, H. F. L., ... Pula, J. (2018). Gender dysphoria in adults: An overview and primer for psychiatrists. *Transgender Health, 3*(1), 57–73.

Dhejne, C., Van Vlerken, R., Heyelens, G., & Arcelus, J. (2016). Mental health and gender dysphoria: A review of the literature. *International Review of Psychiatry, 28*(1), 44–57.

Gonzales, G., & Henning-Smith, C. (2017). Barriers to care among transgender and gender nonconforming adults. *Milbank Quarterly, 95*(4), 726–748.

# CHAPTER 33

# Paraphilias

Reza Safavi

---

A 19-year-old Caucasian male college student presents to the local mental health clinic with 3 months of depressed mood, sleep disturbance, and poor performance at school. He reports that he is unable to sleep at night and feels tired all day. He also reports he is unable to focus on schoolwork and feels hopeless. He denies any loss of interest in hobbies or activities he used to enjoy. He sarcastically says his family forced him to see a psychiatrist after becoming aware of his "weird interests," quoting his family. He denies any feelings of worthlessness, excessive guilt, or thoughts of hurting himself or others. He reveals that 3 months ago, his mother discovered "toys" in his bedroom and kicked him out. Since then, he frequently hears his mother's voice, calling him a "pervert." He reports that he feels on edge and becomes irritated when thinking about his family. Tearfully, the patient explains that his family has discovered he is a "pup."

---

### What are possible causes for these symptoms?

Most of these symptoms seem to be depressive in nature: depressed mood, insomnia, hopelessness, diminished ability to concentrate, significant decline in school performance, and relationship issues with his family. The differential diagnosis is summarized in Table 33.1. Even though depressive mood disorders are at the top of the differential diagnosis list, other psychiatric conditions cannot be ruled out. He reports irritability and speaks about his "weird interests," which sound related to the ongoing issues around being considered perverted by his family. He says he hears his mother's voice (possible auditory hallucination) and addresses himself as a "pup" (possible delusion). Given his age, a first psychotic episode in schizophrenia is a considerable possibility. Substance use with substance-induced mood or psychotic disorders should also be considered. In addition to the standard mental status examination, a detailed medical and psychiatric assessment is essential in evaluating a patient with these symptoms. To rule out psychiatric disorders caused by other medical conditions or substances, routine laboratory testing and urine drug screening are also indicated.

---

He remains guarded during the first half of the interview. When asked about the events that led to his visit, he says "you are probably going to think I am a freak like everybody else." The patient is assured that the goal of the interview is to better understand his situation. He becomes less guarded and explains that he joined the local "pup community" about 1 year ago, where he has been enjoying his time meeting other like-minded "kinky" men. He clarifies that he does not believe he is an actual dog. He feels he belongs to this community and that he has found his "pack." He attends "puppy play" events where he gets to wear his "puppy gear." Puppy play is erotic to him, but more importantly, he feels he can be as free as he wants when he spends time with other "puppies." It provides him a chance to take a break from his schoolwork and daily stress. He denies any past episodes of depression or other psychiatric symptoms. His mother's discovery of his puppy tail, muzzle, and puppy mitts led to a major argument with his parents, who asked him to leave the house. He has been staying with a friend's family and is thankful for them helping him out, but he cannot forget his mother constantly calling him a pervert and his father shouting, "I did not raise a sick son." When asked about auditory hallucinations, he denies any and reports he was referring to flashbacks from the heated arguments.

Table 33.2 outlines the patient's mental status examination. The remainder of the psychiatric assessment, including past medical and psychiatric history, is negative with no manic or psychotic symptoms. He does not take any medications and denies any psychiatric illnesses in his family. He denies any traumatic childhood events, including sexual abuse. He reports that he grew up with his parents and had a good childhood. He is currently enrolled at the local community college and hopes to transfer to the local university soon and pursue a degree in psychology. He denies any substance use and tries to cope with stress by going to the gym and hanging out with his friends. The initial intake time is up. He agrees to return to the clinic the following week to discuss his ongoing issues and provide a detailed sexual history. He is informed about the routine medical laboratory testing and urine drug screening, and samples are collected before he leaves the clinic.

### TABLE 33.1 ■ Differential Diagnosis for Depressive Symptoms

**Depressive disorders**
- Major depressive disorder
- Substance/medication-induced depressive disorder
- Depressive disorder due to another medical condition

**Trauma- and stressor-related disorders**
- Adjustment disorders
- Posttraumatic stress disorder

**Bipolar and related disorders**
- Bipolar I disorder
- Bipolar II disorder
- Substance/medication-induced bipolar disorder
- Bipolar disorder due to another medical condition

**Schizophrenia spectrum and other psychotic disorders**
- Delusional disorder
- Brief psychotic disorder
- Schizophrenia
- Substance/medication-induced psychotic disorder
- Psychotic disorder due to another medical condition

### TABLE 33.2 ■ Mental Status Examination

**Appearance:** 19-year-old male, dressed in regular street clothes, good hygiene, wearing a chain around his neck with a silver bone-shaped dog tag reading "JAX"

**Sensorium:** Alert and oriented to person, place, time, and condition

**Behavior:** Guarded initially, becomes cooperative through the interview, tearful intermittently when discussing family issues

**Motor activity:** No psychomotor agitation or retardation

**Speech:** Normal tone, prosody, latency, and volume

**Mood:** "Depressed"

**Affect:** Congruent with normal range

**Thought process:** Linear

**Thought contents:** Denies any suicidal or homicidal ideations. Denies any auditory or visual hallucinations. No delusions appreciated on the examination.

**Cognition:** Normal

**Insight:** Fair

**Judgment:** Fair

**TABLE 33.3 ■ Clinical Evaluation for Sexual History**

- Puberty onset and age when first aware of his/her sexuality, including fantasies
- Personal belief about sex
- Safe sex awareness, current methods of prevention and compliance
- Development of sexual relationships (e.g., when they experienced their first crush, how the person first learned about sex, the nature of his or her first sexual contact)
- Gender and age range of sexual contacts and fantasies
- The nature of his or her sexual contacts (e.g., kissing, touching, oral sexual contact, anal sexual contact, intercourse) and sexual position (e.g., top, bottom, versatile)
- Number of sexual contacts in the past and current partners
- Exposure to sexually stimulating materials (e.g., magazines, Internet, sexual text messaging, sexual telephone calls, adult bookstores, strip clubs)
- Use of substances during sex (e.g., alcohol, methamphetamines, inhalants)
- Personal feelings about his or her body, sexual organs, and any sexual dysfunctions
- Specific focus on nonliving objects (e.g., shoes) or nongenital body parts (e.g., feet) and ability to perform sexually without those objects
- Sexual fantasies and any possible legal or social consequences in the past due to sexual behaviors
- History of gender identity concerns or disorders

He returns to the clinic the following week. At first, he is concerned about the questions he must answer during his sexual history interview, but he is assured he could answer questions up to his comfort level and skip questions if he felt uncomfortable. Table 33.3 summarizes components of a detailed sexual history interview.

He reports that he reached puberty around age 14. He knew he was attracted to men since childhood, but he kept this information from his family until now. He used the Internet to find answers to his questions about sexuality, as he felt uncomfortable talking to his family, who always assumed he was interested in women. His current boyfriend is 2 years younger than him and is the only sexual partner he has had. They met a year ago at a local coffee shop. They are sexually active; he reports that he is a "submissive top." He usually assumes the "top" sexual position, but also enjoys it when his boyfriend takes control and orders him around. He enjoys sex and feels positive about it. He has a healthy sexual relationship with his partner. They are both on preexposure prophylaxis (PrEP) and get tested for human immunodeficiency virus and other sexually transmitted infections every 3 months. He reports that their foreplay sometimes involves his puppy gear. He refers to his boyfriend as his "handler" during foreplay. He feels excited when his handler puts a leash on his neck and gives him "treats." He points to the chain around his neck with the bone-shaped dog tag and explains that he was "collared" by his boyfriend a few months ago. He feels strongly about his collar as it symbolizes the dynamics of his relationship with his partner. Despite numerous requests from his family to remove it, he never takes it off.

He reports that he became familiar with the puppy community when he started searching the Internet. He has met other members in the community who are good friends. They help him cope with his recent stressors and educate him about the puppy community. The patient was at first shy about sharing his interests with his partner, but now they both enjoy his interests equally. He reports being a puppy is "more than just sex"—on an emotional level, it helps him connect with his partner and his new community. He denies experiencing any sexual difficulties without his gear. He smiles and exclaims, "Vanilla sex is fun, but puppy play makes it more special! Arf!"

The laboratory results are back, and all within normal range. Urine drug screening is negative for controlled substances.

## What is a paraphilia?

Paraphilias are intense and persistent sexual interests outside of "normophilic" behaviors (phenotypically considered common or "normal" foreplay and genital stimulations). Some paraphilias may involve use of nonliving objects (e.g., shoes) or a nongenital body part (e.g., feet). Some other paraphilias are defined by interests in participating in specific activities (e.g., urination), and are defined by the role of the individual during the paraphilic activity such as watching others versus being watched by others when naked or during sexual intercourse. If these paraphilic fantasies, urges, or behavior are greater than or equal to an individual's normophilic sexual interests, then the individual is considered to have a specific paraphilia. However, if these urges are not intense or persistent, not suppressing normophilic sexual interests, and mostly are used as an occasional part of an individual's sexual practice, then the individual is not considered to have a paraphilia. These nonintensive, nonnormophilic sexual tendencies are usually described as fetishes or kinks in the general community.

Most fetishes fall under the broader nonclinical umbrella of BDSM (BD = bondage and discipline, Ds = dominance and submission, and SM = sadism and masochism). For most individuals involved with BDSM, mutual agreement and consent are essential. These practices may include physical restraints, control, pain, body fluids, and/or humiliation, and individuals participating are consenting adults. In general, the two key components defining BDSM activities are (1) mutual sexual gratification by all participants and (2) no long-lasting severe distress or impairment from these activities.

The gap between normo- and paraphilic behaviors is highly influenced by the society and changes with time. The boundaries of paraphilic behaviors are changing rapidly. With homosexuality once considered a paraphilia, both the professional and general communities are becoming more accepting of atypical sexual fantasies as normal variations of human sexuality.

---

**CLINICAL PEARL**                                                                 **STEP 2/3**

**Normophilia:** a clinical term defining sexual behaviors considered phenotypically common, or "normal" sexual behaviors, including foreplay and genital stimulations.
**Fetish:** a nonclinical term defining sexual behaviors socially considered "unconventional."
**Paraphilia:** a clinical term including intense and persistent nonnormophilic sexual urges or fantasies that suppress normophilic sexual interests.
**Paraphilic disorder:** a clinical term defining the presence of paraphilia that leads to severe social, occupational, or functional impairment.

---

## What is a paraphilic disorder?

A paraphilic disorder requires presence of a paraphilia for at least 6 months that, when acted upon, leads to clinically significant distress, dysfunction, and/or criminal consequences; and may involve potentially nonadult or nonconsenting partners. A paraphilic disorder is diagnosed when paraphilic fantasies and urges are acted upon, and those actions create severe social, occupational, and/or functional impairments. Despite a vast number of fetishes, kinks and paraphilias, the *Diagnostic and Statistical Manual of Mental Disorders*, Fifth Edition (DSM-5), defines eight paraphilic disorders with specific related paraphilias. These disorders are outlined in Table 33.4.

All paraphilic disorders require at least 6 months of recurrent and intense sexual arousal from the related paraphilia as manifested by fantasies, urges, or behaviors, which may cause clinically significant distress or impairment in social, occupational, or other important areas of functioning, or involve a nonconsenting partner.

Some of these conditions become a clinical condition when the associated paraphilia might be benign in nature, but the intensity of those urges cause significant social, occupational, or functional impairment. For example, if an individual has strong and intense sexual fantasies around use of a nonliving object, but these urges are not opposed by that person's spouse, then it remains within the definition of a paraphilia. However, if that person's spouse is strongly oppositional in

TABLE 33.4 ■ **Paraphilic Disorders**

| Paraphilic Disorder | Related Paraphilia |
|---|---|
| Voyeuristic disorder | Observing an unsuspecting person who is naked, in the process of disrobing, or engaging in sexual activity |
| Exhibitionistic disorder | Exposure of one's genitals to an unsuspecting person |
| Frotteuristic disorder | Touching or rubbing against a nonconsenting person |
| Sexual masochism disorder | Being humiliated, beaten, bound, or otherwise made to suffer |
| Sexual sadism disorder | Causing the physical or psychological suffering of another person |
| Pedophilic disorder | Involving sexual activity with a prepubescent child or children<br>*** Individual must be at least 16 years old and at least 5 years older than the child or children |
| Fetishistic disorder | Use of nonliving objects or highly specific focus on nongenital body part<br>***Nonliving objects are not limited to clothing used in cross-dressing or devices designed for the purpose of tactile genital stimulation (e.g., dildo or vibrator) |
| Transvestic disorder | Cross-dressing |

that regard, up to the point it leads to marital issues, then the condition is considered a paraphilic disorder (fetishistic disorder).

In contrast, some paraphilic disorders by definition include nonconsenting and/or nonadult victims and are inevitably a disorder once those urges are acted upon (e.g., pedophilic disorder). The associated paraphilias with these disorders are generally considered criminal activities if acted upon, as they violate or endanger others.

---

He consents to his mental health provider contacting his mother for collateral information. He reports feeling less stressed after today's visit and feels he was able to discuss his interests in a nonjudgmental environment. He agrees to return to the clinic the following week. His mother is contacted and reports that she would love to do anything she could do to "cure" her son. She reports that he had a normal childhood and was a wonderful son with no issues at school or within the family. However, things changed 3 months ago. She becomes tearful over the phone and reports that she found his "things" in his bedroom. She became suspicious and checked his phone, where she found pictures and videos of him "in a puppy costume, rubbing himself against others, and acting freakish at those sick parties he goes to." She explains that she went online to research "what was happening to the family" and that she "came across some weird stuff like voyeuristic, exhibitionistic, or frotteuristic." She says she knew that her son was gay, even before he told the family—she had heard from his friends that he was dating another man. She elaborates that she was happy for him, but did not realize his boyfriend was underage: "Tell me doctor, is my son a pedophile?"

---

### *Does he have a paraphilia?*
He provides a detailed sexual history, which is very essential in assessing his condition. He describes his puppy play as erotic, but he also associates those behaviors with community-related social activities. He reports that he retains sexual function with his partner regardless of the presence of puppy gear. His interests in puppy play do not exceed his normophilic sexual behaviors. He does not meet the criteria for paraphilia. However, his behavior may fall within the broader spectrum of BDSM, which is not a psychiatric condition.

### *Does he have a paraphilic disorder?*
The diagnosis of a paraphilic disorder requires the presence of a paraphilia for at least 6 months in addition to social, occupational, and/or functional impairment secondary to the paraphilia. As

**TABLE 33.5 ■ Differential Diagnosis for Paraphilic Disorders**

**Nonpathologic use of sexual fantasies, behaviors, or objects**
- Does not cause clinically significant stress
- Does not involve nonconsenting or nonadult partners

**Sexual behavior with impaired judgment or impulse control due to another mental disorder**
- Not individual's typical behavior
- Occurs during the course of another mental disorder
- Accompanied by other symptoms of another mental disorder
- Examples include manic episode, neurocognitive disorders, or schizophrenia

**Sexual behavior in conduct disorder or antisocial personality disorder**
- Accompanied by other norm-breaking and antisocial behaviors
- Accompanied by other nonsexual or nonparaphilic behaviors toward victims
- Lack of empathy or respect for the rights of other individuals

**Substance induced**
- In presence of substance intoxication or medication (e.g., dopamine agonist medications)
- Not typical of patient's behavior when not under the influence of substance/medication

**Obsessive-compulsive disorder**
- Ego-dystonic thoughts or worries about the presence of paraphilias with absence of any paraphilic urges or behaviors

discussed previously, his detailed history does not indicate the presence of a paraphilia. His current condition with mood symptoms and conflict with his parents is not a direct consequence of his sexual tendencies, but rather, brought about by his family's lack of understanding. If he were not able to perform sexually without his puppy gear, or puppy play were more arousing to him than normophilic sexual behaviors, and these sexual fantasies had directly created significant impairment in his relationship with his partner, then those behaviors would be diagnostic for paraphilic disorder.

Another example of a paraphilic disorder would be if the patient were unable to perform in school due to overinvolvement with his sexual fantasies. For example, missing classes or performing poorly in his academic tasks secondary to excessive time spent on his sexual fantasies, then it would be considered functional impairment as a direct consequence of his paraphilia. However, in this case, his poor performance at school is caused by social stressors, such as family conflict and loss of housing. Table 33.5 outlines a detailed differential diagnosis for other conditions that may present similarly to this case and how they differ from this patient.

**CLINICAL PEARL**        STEP 2/3

For all paraphilic disorders:
- The intense sexual arousal must be present for at least 6 months.
- Related to a paraphilia, manifested by fantasies, urges, or behaviors.
- Must cause clinically significant social, occupational, or functional impairment.

**BASIC SCIENCE/CLINICAL PEARL**        STEP 1/2/3

- **Cisgender:** a person whose gender identity corresponds with their birth sex.
- **Transgender:** a person whose gender identity does not correspond with their birth sex.
- **Transsexual:** old medical term describing a person seeking medical assistance to transition from one sex to another. The medical community has replaced this term with *gender dysphoric* or *gender incongruent*.
- **Transvestite:** an individual who derives pleasure from wearing clothes of the opposite sex.

*His mother is concerned about voyeurism, exhibitionism, or frotteurism. Does his history indicate any of these behaviors?*

His mother is very concerned after seeing pictures and videos of the events her son attends. According to her, these pictures show him in his puppy gear, exposing himself, and rubbing himself on others. It is important to keep in mind that these events are social events in which all participants are consenting adults and are aware of the sexual activities involved. Voyeurism, exhibitionism, and frotteurism, on the other hand, involve unsuspecting and/or nonconsenting partners. Consent and awareness of the person being watched, exposed to, or touched is the key factor defining these behaviors—therefore his behaviors are not considered frotteuristic, exhibitionistic, or voyeuristic.

*Does he have sexual masochism disorder?*

He makes some comments about desires to be controlled by his partner whom he calls his handler. However, he does not report any desires to be in pain nor does his partner enjoy inducing pain. Sexual sadism and masochism are common practices in the BDSM community; however, these are not considered paraphilic disorders as all individuals participating are consenting participants, and no long lasting or permanent injuries or suffering are caused. In contrast, sexual sadism disorder and sexual masochism disorder include physical or psychological pain involving a nonconsenting partner and/or cause severe impairment or long-lasting injuries. Consent is, once again, a key component of the definition of these disorders.

*He is 19 years old and his boyfriend is under 18 years old. Does he have pedophilic disorder?*

Different countries and states have different definitions of consenting age for sexual activities. Clinically, an individual to be considered suffering from pedophilic disorder is at least 16 years old and sexually aroused by a younger child (or children) at least 5 years younger. He is 19 years old and his partner is 2 years younger than him. Additionally, during the interview, he does not indicate being sexually aroused by younger children specifically.

Even though he does not meet the clinical criteria for pedophilic disorder, there might be some legal restrictions about his sexual activities with his partner in his state of residence. These legal regulations are outside the scope of this case report. However, you may find additional legal information regarding this topic for your state by visiting the *Child Welfare Information Gateway* website at www.childwelfare.gov.

---

**CLINICAL PEARL**                                                        **STEP 2/3**

Most states require mandatory reporting by clinicians to the local child protective services or federal agencies regarding individuals with sexual activities involving minors or access to child pornography. For more details regarding your state's regulations, please visit the **Child Welfare Information Gateway** website at www.childwelfare.gov or contact the local child protective agency.

---

*What is the diagnosis?*

The diagnosis is adjustment disorder with depressed mood.

This patient presents with 3 months of depressive symptoms and significant impairment in school performance, amid the setting of increased family issues, after his family discovered his involvement with the BDSM community and nonnormophilic sexual behaviors. He does not demonstrate any manic or psychotic symptoms, and his sexual behaviors did not occur or change during an episode of a mental health disorder. Therefore bipolar disorder or schizophrenia spectrum disorders can be ruled out. He does not have any medical issues, nor does he use any medications or recreational substances—therefore, mood or psychotic disorders secondary to another medical condition or substance use are not accurate diagnoses.

Adjustment disorder is defined as development of emotional or behavioral symptoms in response to an identifiable stressor occurring within 3 months of the onset of the stressor. The disorder could be specified further based on primary symptoms as with depressed mood, with anxiety, with disturbance of the conduct, or a combination of these symptoms. These symptoms are expected to resolve within 6 months after the stressor or its consequences have terminated.

In regard to his sexual history, his nonnormophilic fantasies do not suppress his normophilic sexual behavior and are not pathologic. Even though his distress is indirectly related to his fetish, the primary stressor leading to his symptoms is his family's lack of understanding, and possibly different values. In his case, it is crucial to differentiate between adjustment disorder versus pathologic paraphilic disorders, as treatment options for these disorders are not the same. The goal of treatment for his condition (adjustment disorder) is to provide emotional support and to help him learn effective coping skills and stress management. A short trial of medications may also be indicated to manage his depressive symptoms while he copes with the stressful events. In contrast, the goal of treatment in paraphilic disorders is to control and to prevent relapse of sexual interests and/or behaviors that have caused harm to the patient or others.

---

The patient returns to the clinic the following week to discuss his diagnosis and treatment options. He prefers not to start a medication and reports feeling less stressed since he started coming to the clinic and is interested in enrolling in weekly therapy to manage his stress and cope with his ongoing situation.

---

### What are the available treatments for paraphilic disorders?

When considering the appropriate treatment, it is important to remember paraphilias per se do not cause distress or harm. However, paraphilic disorders are diagnosed when a paraphilia causes distress and/or harm to the patient or others. The purpose of treatment is to prevent recurrence of those behaviors that can be harmful to the individual or those surrounding them. Treatment can range from less invasive interventions, including psychotherapy (see Table 33.6) and pharmacologic approaches (see Table 33.7), to more restricted living environments to limit opportunities for the sexual behavior. The DSM-5 includes a specifier "in a controlled environment" that primarily applies to those individuals who live in institutional or other settings where opportunities to act upon sexual urges are restricted.

The primary goal of treatment for paraphilic disorders is to assist the patient in gaining an understanding of how his/her paraphilias cause impairments and to prevent relapses of associated disturbing behaviors. It is important to differentiate between preventing these impairing behaviors specifically rather than becoming asexual. Therapy and medications may be used to help the patient gain normal daily functioning with minimal restrictions and have sexual gratification via normophilic or harmless paraphilic means.

---

TABLE 33.6 ■ Psychotherapy for Paraphilic Disorders

| Psychotherapy | Goal of Treatment |
|---|---|
| Cognitive behavioral therapy | • Increase control over problematic sexual interests<br>• Equip with skills to achieve goals in healthy ways |
| Relapse prevention | • Identify, anticipate, and cope with triggers that may lead to problematic behavior<br>• Modeled after psychotherapy for addictive behaviors |
| Good living model | • Focus on maximally fulfilling human potentials and strengths<br>• Achieve happiness and well-being without the problematic behaviors |

TABLE 33.7 ■ **Psychopharmacology for Paraphilic Disorders**

| Medication | Goal of Treatment |
| --- | --- |
| Selective serotonin reuptake inhibitors | • Mood improvement and impulse control<br>• Decrease obsessive urges<br>• Higher doses may cause anorgasmia, which may increase risk of relapse |
| Testosterone reducing agents | • Regulation of sexual desire, fantasy, aggression, and cognition<br>• Gold standard only when overall reduced sex drive is desired |

Selective serotonin reuptake inhibitors (SSRIs) are commonly used to manage any present mood symptoms and to improve impulse and obsession control. Most SSRIs share a common side effect of sexual dysfunction that is avoided when treating paraphilic disorders as these side effects may increase the risk of recurrence of those harmful paraphilic behaviors. If the medication causes sexual dysfunction while the patient is encouraged to gain sexual gratifications via normophilias or harmless paraphilias, he/she may conclude that treatment is not effective and return to the old harmful sexual behaviors.

Once called *chemical castration,* hormonal medications are considered only in extreme cases to decrease patient's overall sexuality when other treatments have failed.

A few months after completion of therapy, the patient sends a thank-you card to his psychiatrist. During therapy he was able to achieve better skills for managing his stress and focusing on school. He now lives in the dorms and works at the school library. His parents decide to attend peer support classes at the LGBT center, and their relationship with him has significantly improved. He remains active with his puppy community and plans to participate as a contestant in the upcoming local puppy contest. He is very thankful for the neutral and nonjudgmental therapy environment.

**BEYOND THE PEARLS:**

• There is a wide range of sexual interests and most are not harmful or pathologic.
• Normo- and paraphilias are defined by society and vary culture to culture. It is very important to consider and to be sensitive to patient's cultural background.
• Not every individual with paraphilic disorder is a criminal and vice versa.
• There are multiple treatment options for paraphilic disorders, and treatments are effective.
• There is no end to learning in medicine, and as medical providers, we are privileged to learn from our patients while we treat them. It is very important to respect our patients and remain nonjudgmental when helping them as they help us become better providers in the future.

## References

American Psychiatric Association. (2013). Paraphilic disorders. *Diagnostic and statistical manual of mental disorders* (5th ed.). Washington, DC: Author.

Barnhill, J. W. (2014). Paraphilic disorders. In *DSM-5 clinical cases.* Washington, DC: American Psychiatric Publishing.

Becker, J. V., et al. (2014). Chapter 26. Paraphilic Disorders. In *The American Psychiatric Publishing textbook of psychiatry* (6th ed.). Washington, DC: American Psychiatric Publishing. Retrieved from https://psychiatry-online.org/doi/10.1176/appi.books.9781585625031.rh26.

First, M. B. (2014). Differential diagnosis for paraphilic disorders. In *DSM-5 handbook of differential diagnosis.* Washington, DC: American Psychiatric Publishing.

Hembree, W. C., Cohen-Kettenis, P. T., Gooren, L., Hannema, S. E., Meyer, W. J., Murad, M. H., ... T'Sjoen, G. G. (2017). Endocrine treatment of gender-dysphoric/gender-incongruent persons: An Endocrine Society clinical practice guideline. *Journal of Clinical Endocrinology and Metabolism, 102*(11), 3869–3903.

Murphy, L., et al. (2014). Paraphilias and paraphilic disorders. In G. O. Gabbard (Ed.). *Gabbard's treatments of psychiatric disorders* (5th ed.). Washington, DC: American Psychiatric Publishing.

# CHAPTER 34

# Neuroleptic Malignant Syndrome

Jeffrey Michael Bonenfant ■ Aarti Chawla Mittal

A 24-year-old male presents to the emergency department with a 2-day history of progressive altered mental status. His family, always at his bedside, brought him for evaluation because he was being "stiff" and "delusional" since yesterday. Table 34.1 outlines his vital signs at presentation and repeated measures 15 minutes later.

TABLE 34.1 ■ **Vital Signs**

| At presentation | Repeated 15 minutes later |
| --- | --- |
| Blood pressure 134/80 mm/Hg | 170/100 mm/Hg |
| Respiration rate 20/min | 25/min |
| Oxygen saturation 95% on room air | 97% on room air |

On physical examination, you note a young, thin male with incoherent speech and nonpurposeful head movements. He appears to be visually hallucinating. He is diaphoretic and warm to the touch. You are unable to passively flex or extend the upper and lower extremities, which remain in midflexion. There is dark-colored urinary incontinence, and the patient is not following commands. Hospital records show he was recently hospitalized with a new diagnosis of bipolar disorder and discharged 7 days ago with risperidone 2 mg daily. Family confirms this has been his only medication. He received meningococcal vaccination 2 years ago and has not been in contact with anyone sick.

## What is your initial differential diagnosis?

A young male with bipolar disorder on risperidone is presenting with fevers and altered mental status. Infection, namely meningitis, should be at the top of the differential. Hypercalcemia, parathyroid, and thyroid dysfunction are also considerations. Other etiologies that may be difficult to distinguish in this presentation are drug toxicities, such as methamphetamine, cocaine, ketamine, or other synthetic drugs. Consideration for status epilepticus is appropriate. Malignant catatonia, a subtype of catatonia, may present in this fashion, although it is usually associated with schizophrenia, not bipolar disorder. Finally, do not forget that the patient is on risperidone and thus at risk for neuroleptic malignant syndrome (NMS). Although the patient does not have specific history to support them, conditions such as serotonin syndrome, malignant hyperthermia, heat stroke, and retarded-type catatonia should be considered.

## What is your initial approach with this patient? What labs would you like to order?

You should first put in two large bore needles and begin aggressive cooling measures for his elevated temperature. To evaluate for infection, you need blood cultures, urinalysis, urine culture,

### TABLE 34.2 ■ Results of Laboratory and Diagnostic Studies

| Serum Chemistry | Urinalysis and UDS | CSF Analysis | Diagnostic Studies |
|---|---|---|---|
| WBC count 12.8 K/μL (normal differential) | Clear, amber color | Color: clear | CT head: normal |
| Na 134 mEq/L | Large blood | WBC: <5/mm³ | EEG: Normal, no |
| K⁺ 4.8 mEq/L | Protein negative | RBC: 3 X 10⁶/L | epileptiform |
| Cl 108 mEq/L | Leukocyte esterase | Protein: 48 mg/dL | discharges |
| CO2 20 mEq/L | negative | Glucose: 84 mg/dL | |
| BUN 43 mg/dL | Nitrite negative | Gram stain: negative | |
| Cr 2.1 mg/dL | Trace ketones | | |
| Albumin 4 mg/dL | WBC 5/hpf | | |
| Ca 10.1 mg/dL | RBC 1/hpf | | |
| AST 25 U/L | Hyaline casts 35/hpf | | |
| ALT 22 U/L | pH 5.5 | | |
| Alk Phos 109 U/L | UDS: negative | | |
| Total bilirubin 0.9 mg/dL | | | |
| TSH 3.2 mIU/L | | | |
| Total CK 3,255 U/L | | | |

*Alk Phos,* Alkaline phosphatase; *ALT,* alanine aminotransferase; *AST,* aspartate aminotransferase; *CK,* creatine kinase; *CSF,* cerebral spinal fluid; *CT,* computed tomography; *EEG,* electroencephalogram; *RBC,* red blood cell; *TSH,* thyroid-stimulating hormone; *UDS,* urine drug screen; *WBC,* white blood cell.

serum lactate, and a complete blood count with differential. Given that the suspected infectious source is meningitis, this patient would need a lumbar puncture for further evaluation of his cerebrospinal fluid. For the toxicities, you could start with a urine drug screen panel, which generally checks for amphetamines, methamphetamines, benzodiazepines, barbiturates, marijuana, cocaine, phencyclidine, and opiates. It will not detect many of the synthetic drugs or ketamine. An electroencephalogram (EEG) is needed to evaluate for status epilepticus, and you should also check creatine kinase because of the presence of dark-colored urine. If the patient is in status epilepticus, the muscle breakdown from seizures could cause rhabdomyolysis. A complete metabolic panel would also be indicated to evaluate his electrolytes, calcium level, kidney function, and liver function. Given his altered mental status, a computed tomography (CT) scan of the head and thyroid-stimulating hormone (TSH) level would also be warranted. Results of laboratory and diagnostic studies for our patient are given in Table 34.2.

### Does this change your differential diagnosis?

First, the normal EEG results make status epilepticus unlikely. The patient has leukocytosis, and thus infection is still high on the differential. You can confidently say that a urinary tract infection and meningitis are not the source. Normal calcium level with normal albumin level (corrected calcium for albumin = measured calcium + [normal albumin of 4] − [measured albumin] × 0.8), altered mental status and psychiatric alterations of hypercalcemia or parathyroid dysfunction can be ruled out, as can thyroid dysfunction such as hyperthyroid storm. The urine drug screen is negative, so you can rule out methamphetamine and cocaine toxicities; however, this does not rule out ketamine or synthetic toxicities. We are still unable to rule out neuroleptic malignant syndrome and malignant catatonia, which are diagnoses of exclusion (meaning all other diagnoses must be ruled out).

Further analysis of the laboratory results shows an elevated blood urea nitrogen and creatinine indicating acute kidney injury. This may be caused by the elevated creatine kinase (CK) and an early sign of rhabdomyolysis. Fever lends to increased insensible losses and acute kidney injury may be due to intravascular fluid depletion. Although generally, a CK of 10,000 mg/dL or higher is the marker for rhabdomyolysis, we should continue to monitor his CK as it may continue to rise. Although he is not technically in rhabdomyolysis, there are signs of elevated CK as well as a urinalysis with large blood on macroscopy without elevated red blood cell count on microscopy. This latter finding is the machine erroneously sensing the myoglobin from muscle breakdown as hemoglobin.

Our current running assessment for this patient would be acute encephalopathy, pyrexia, and acute kidney injury. Our differential for the acute encephalopathy is still infection, neuroleptic malignant syndrome, malignant catatonia, and synthetic toxicities.

### Are there any medications or treatments you would like to start?
Given the increasing mortality with delay of antibiotic administration in sepsis, early and broad dosing of antibiotics would be very appropriate. Additionally, with the suspicion of neuroleptic malignant syndrome, administration of risperidone or other antipsychotic medications should be discontinued. You would also want to avoid antiemetic medications, as they could potentiate neuroleptic malignant syndrome.

A bedside ultrasound can evaluate this patient's inferior vena cava collapsibility to assess for intravascular volume depletion. If it is greater than 50% collapsible, the patient will tolerate some intravenous (IV) fluids and thus should be fluid resuscitated with crystalloid fluids, either normal saline or lactated ringers.

### Can you confirm a diagnosis of neuroleptic malignant syndrome on the indicated findings?
At this point, and with multiple other etiologies ruled out, it seems as though this patient does have neuroleptic malignant syndrome. You have not completely ruled out infection, as blood cultures take 5 days for final results, so continuation of empiric antibiotics is warranted. According to the workup completed so far, the patient's symptoms are congruent with a diagnosis of NMS—autonomic dysregulation, early rhabdomyolysis, altered mental status, and hyperthermia in the setting of risperidone use.

### What further management is warranted based on this workup?
Patients with suspected NMS require admission to an intensive care unit for close observation, including frequent vital sign measurement and neurologic examinations, regulation of hyperthermia, and control of autonomic dysfunction. Both nonpharmacologic and pharmacologic cooling measures should be employed, such as cooling blankets and acetaminophen, respectively. Toxicology and psychiatric consultations will provide appropriate support and should be obtained. Potential comorbidities include rhabdomyolysis, circulatory or respiratory failure, aspiration pneumonia, pulmonary embolism, disseminated intravascular coagulation, and long-term cognitive deficit caused by hypoxia and prolonged hyperthermia.

| BASIC SCIENCE PEARL | STEP 1 |
| --- | --- |

Muscle rigidity and eventual rhabdomyolysis is caused by calcium release from sarcoplasmic reticulum of skeletal myocytes.

### How common is NMS? What is the typical presentation, diagnostic criteria, and duration?
The incidence of NMS is 0.02%–3.23%. It is a rare and potentially fatal reaction to a neuroleptic agent, having a mortality rate as high as 20%. The cardinal clinical manifestations include **altered mental status, muscle rigidity, fever,** and **autonomic instability** in association with antipsychotic medication administration. The most commonly associated antipsychotics are first-generation, high-potency agents such as haloperidol and fluphenazine. Table 34.3 lists medications associated with NMS.

## TABLE 34.3 ■ Medications Most Commonly Associated with NMS

**Neuroleptics**
- First-generation, or typical, antipsychotic (highest association)
  - haloperidol (high potency)
  - fluphenazine (high potency)
  - chlorpromazine (low potency)
- Second-generation, or atypical, antipsychotic
  - risperidone
  - clozapine
  - olanzapine
  - aripiprazole

**Antiemetics**
- metoclopramide
- promethazine
- domperidone

---

**CLINICAL PEARL**                                                        **STEP 2/3**

Risk factors for developing NMS include being young, male, use of long-acting depot antipsy-chotics, or brain disease (lesions due to infection, traumatic brain injury, or epilepsy).

Mental status change and muscle rigidity are typically first in the presentation, followed by fever and autonomic dysfunction. Symptoms develop within 4 weeks of initiating an antipsychotic medication in 96% of cases. The majority, 66%, occur within the first week, whereas 16% occur within the first 24 hours. NMS is not a dose-dependent phenomenon, meaning that the strength of the medication dose does not correlate with the severity of disease. It is unclear if concomitant use of lithium or anticholinergic drugs increases risk. Typical laboratory findings are leukocytosis, elevated total creatinine kinase level, anion gap metabolic acidosis, elevated catecholamine levels, and electrolyte disturbances. Predisposing factors include prior episodes, dehydration, agitation, and the rate and route of neuroleptic administration. Symptoms last 7 to 10 days in uncompli-cated cases receiving oral neuroleptics.

To confirm the diagnosis, the following criteria must be met: exposure to a dopamine antago-nist or dopamine agonist withdrawal within the past 72 hours; mental status change; muscle rigid-ity; oral temperature of greater than 100.4 °F (or 38 °C) on at least two occasions; total creatinine kinase level equal to or greater than four times the upper limit of normal; sympathetic nervous system lability; and negative workup for infectious, toxic, metabolic, and neurologic etiologies. Sympathetic nervous system lability in NMS has been determined by expert panelists as having at least two conditions within the parameters of a systolic or diastolic blood pressure change of greater than 25% above baseline, systolic change of equal to or greater than 25 mm Hg or diastolic change of equal to or greater than 20 mm Hg within 24 hours; diaphoresis; urinary incontinence; or hypermetabolism defined as a heart rate increase of equal to or greater than 25% above base-line and a respiratory rate of equal to or greater than 50% above baseline. Table 34.4 presents the diagnostic criteria for NMS.

### What is the underlying pathophysiology?

The exact mechanism is not understood. A neuroleptic agent is defined as contributing to decreased stimulation of dopaminergic pathways within the nervous system. The clinical observation is that NMS can be triggered by any antipsychotic medication that functions as a dopamine antagonist, the with-drawal of a dopamine agonist such as in Parkinson disease, and other medications involving dopamine

TABLE 34.4 ■ Diagnostic Criteria for NMS

Exposure to dopamine antagonist <u>or</u> dopamine agonist withdrawal within the past 72 hours, in addition to:
- mental status change
- muscle rigidity
- oral temp >100.4 °F or 38 °C on at least two occasions
- CK level ≥ four times upper limit of normal
- sympathetic nervous system lability, defined as having ≥ two of the following:
  - SBP or DBP ≥25% above baseline
  - ≥25 mm Hg systolic *or* 20 mm Hg diastolic change within 24 hours
  - diaphoresis
  - urinary incontinence
  - hypermetabolism, defined as:
    - HR increase ≥25% above baseline and RR increase ≥50% above baseline

*CK*, creatine kinase; *DBP*, diastolic blood pressure; *HR*, heart rate; *mm Hg*, millimeters of mercury; *RR*, respiratory rate; *SBP*, systolic blood pressure.

manipulation such as antiemetics. In addition, NMS can be treated with dopamine agonists. Due to these observations, D2 receptor antagonism has been postulated as having a mechanistic influence.

Dopaminergic mechanisms regulate muscle tone, movement, and temperature. The three major dopaminergic pathways in the central nervous system associated with the clinical presentation of NMS are the nigrostriatal, mesocortical, and tuberoinfundibular. The nigrostriatal pathway encompasses neuronal projections from the substantia nigra to the dorsal striatum, which is the pathway affected in Parkinson disease. The mesocortical pathway projects from the ventral tegmentum to the prefrontal cortex. The tuberoinfundibular pathway projects from the arcuate nucleus of the hypothalamus to the pituitary.

Clinical implications of decreased dopamine stimulation to these pathways may manifest in rigidity from the nigrostriatal pathway, altered level of consciousness from the mesocortical pathway involving the reticular activating system, and temperature alterations from the tuberoinfundibular pathway involving the hypothalamus. Table 34.5 summarizes the major dopamineric pathways involved in NMS and their clinical implications. First-generation antipsychotic medications, such as haloperidol and fluphenazine, have greater affinity for D2 receptors than second-generation antipsychotics, which may provide insight into their greater association with NMS. Roles for norepinephrine, gamma-aminobutyric acid (GABA), and serotonin, in addition to adrenal-associated sympathetic activity, increase the ratio of noradrenaline-to-dopamine levels, and genetic predisposition have been postulated.

TABLE 34.5 ■ Distinguishing Factors of NMS from Serotonin Syndrome, Malignant Hyperthermia, and Heat Stroke

| NMS | Serotonin Syndrome | Malignant Hyperthermia | Heat Stroke |
|---|---|---|---|
| • onset in days<br>• fever<br>• rigidity<br>• diaphoresis<br>• associated with antipsychotic and antiemetic agents | • GI symptoms<br>• myoclonus<br>• hyperreflexia | • onset in minutes to hours<br>• associated with inhaled anesthetics and neuromuscular blockade agents | • fever<br>• hypotonia<br>• dry skin |

| BASIC SCIENCE PEARL | STEP 1 |

The mesolimbic pathway connects the ventral tegmental area of the midbrain to the ventral striatum of the basal ganglia. This pathway is implicated in schizophrenia and is the intended target for anitpsychotics.

*How can you distinguish NMS clinically from other etiologies with similar presentations?*
Multiple conditions have overlapping signs and symptoms in comparison to NMS.

| BASIC SCIENCE/CLINICAL PEARL | STEP 1/2/3 |

The dopamine pathways include the nigrostriatal, mesocortical, mesolimbic, and tuberoinfundibular pathways.
The nigrostriatal pathway is typically responsible for initiation of movement. Its inhibition in NMS leads to extrapyramidal symptoms such as rigidity. In turn, this causes increased muscle metabolism and rhabdomyolysis.
The mesocortical pathway is implicated in cognition. Disruption in this pathway causes altered mental status.
The tuberoinfindibular pathway normally controls the toninic inhibition of prolactin release. However, because it also innervates the hypothalamus, its disruption in NMS causes uncontrolled temperature regulation resulting in hyperthermia.

Serotonin syndrome, malignant hyperthermia, and heat stroke may all present in a similar fashion to NMS and therefore must be included in the differential diagnosis. There are factors in the clinical presentation that can help distinguish between these overlapping conditions (Table 34.5). Serotonin syndrome involves gastrointestinal symptoms, myoclonus, and hyperreflexia which are not typical of NMS. Malignant hyperthermia occurs typically in the surgical setting postanesthetic administration. Heat stroke presents with hypotonia and dry skin whereas NMS presents with rigidity and diaphoresis.

| CLINICAL PEARL | STEP 2/3 |

An episode of NMS does not confer an increased risk for developing malignant hyperthermia or vice versa. However, a prior episode of NMS is a risk factor for future episodes of NMS.

*What other management strategies have been suggested for severe cases? Can neuroleptic medications be administered after resolution of an episode of NMS?*
In severe, prolonged, or refractory cases, the use of dopamine agonists or dantrolene, individually or in combination, may be indicated. Examples of agents with dopamine agonist effects include bromocriptine and levodopa. Amantadine may also be considered. Bromocriptine is a dopamine agonist that is typically used in those with parkinsonism, a disease caused by inefficient dopamine effects. Levodopa is enzymatically converted to dopamine after crossing the blood-brain barrier. Similarly, in NMS, bromocriptine may reduce symptoms through the same mechanistic action of increased dopamine stimulation. Dantrolene works through blockade of a calcium channel in the sarcoplasmic reticulum of muscle cells, inhibiting release of calcium from the sarcoplasmic reticulum and thus inhibiting actin-induced muscle contraction. The exact mechanism of amantadine in extrapyramidal symptoms is not well understood; however, it is a *N*-methyl-D-aspartate (NMDA) receptor antagonist whose effects are elicited through blockade of NMDA-stimulated glutamate and muscarinic cholinergic receptors, which, in turn, stimulate dopamine release.

Nitroprusside for use in blood pressure control, may have the added benefit of cutaneous vasodilation to assist in reduction of hyperthermia. Clonidine is also effective, possibly due to its centrally acting antihypertensive mechanism via alpha-2 receptor antagonism.

After recovery from an NMS episode, neuroleptics may be reintroduced in the majority of patients. Risk of recurrence does exist and requires careful monitoring.

### BEYOND THE PEARLS:

- NMS is an adverse reaction to neuroleptic medication, most commonly a first-generation antipsychotic such as haloperidol.
- Symptoms typically begin within 3 to 7 days after initiation of a neuroleptic agent; however, may occur at any time during pharmacologic therapy.
- Patients with suspected NMS should be admitted to an intensive care unit.
- Duration lasts 7 to 10 days in uncomplicated cases receiving an oral neuroleptic.
- Major clinical symptoms include altered mental status, muscle rigidity, hyperthermia, and autonomic dysfunction.
- Clinical observation correlates with nigrostriatal, mesocortical, and tuberoinfundibular pathways of the central nervous system.
- Although the exact mechanism for NMS is unknown, a decrease in agonist effect on dopaminergic pathways in the central nervous system, primarily D2 receptors, has been implicated in disease pathogenesis.
- Treatment consists of airway and circulation support, immediate discontinuation of the offending medication, nonpharmacologic and pharmacologic cooling measures, electrolyte monitoring, and hydration.
- In severe, prolonged, or refractory cases the introduction of dopamine agonists, dantrolene, or amantadine may be indicated. Electroconvulsive therapy has also been used in refractory cases.
- Neuroleptic agents may be introduced after resolution of an NMS episode, but risk of recurrence exists and requires careful monitoring.

### References

American Psychiatric Association. (2013). *Diagnostic and statistical manual of mental disorders* (5th ed.). Washington, DC: Author.

Caroff, S. N., & Mann, S. C. (1993). Neuroleptic malignant syndrome. *Medical Clinics of North America, 77*(1), 185–202.

Gregorakos, L., Thomaides, T., Stratouli, S., & Sakayanni, E. (2000). The use of clonidine in the management of autonomic overactivity in neuroleptic malignant syndrome. *Clinical Autonomic Research, 10*(4), 193–196.

Gurrera, R. J. (1999). Sympathoadrenal hyperactivity and the etiology of neuroleptic malignant syndrome. *American Journal of Psychiatry, 156*(2), 169–180.

Gurrera, R. J., Caroff, S. N., Cohen, A., Carroll, B. T., Deroos, F., Francis, A., ..., & Wilkinson, J. R. (2011). An international consensus study of neuroleptic malignant syndrome diagnostic criteria using the Delphi method. *The Journal of Clinical Psychiatry, 72*(09), 1222–1228.

Gurrera, R. J., Mortillaro, G., Velamoor, V., & Caroff, S. N. (2017). A validation study of the international consensus diagnostic criteria for neuroleptic malignant syndrome. *Journal of Clinical Psychopharmacology, 37*(1), 67–71.

Kawanishi, C. (2003). Genetic predisposition to neuroleptic malignant syndrome. *American Journal of PharmacoGenomics, 3*(2), 89–95.

Mann, S. C., Caroff, S. N., Fricchione, G., & Campbell, E. C. (2000). Central dopamine hypoactivity and the pathogenesis of neuroleptic malignant syndrome. *Psychiatric Annals, 30*(5), 363–374.

Sibley, D. R., Hazelwood, L. A., & Amara, S. G. (2018). 5-Hydroxytryptamine (serotonin) and dopamine. In L. L. Brunton LL, R. Hilal-Dandan, B. C. Knollmann, (Eds.), *Goodman & Gilman's: The Pharmacological Basis of Therapeutics* (13th ed.). New York, NY: McGraw-Hill; 2018.

Simon, R. P., Aminoff, M. J., & Greenberg, D. A. (2018). Movement disorders. In *Clinical neurology* (10th ed.). New York, NY: McGraw-Hill.

Strawn, J. (2007). Neuroleptic malignant syndrome. *American Journal of Psychiatry, 164*(6), 870.

Velamoor, R. (2017). Neuroleptic malignant syndrome: A neuro-psychiatric emergency: Recognition, prevention, and management. *Asian Journal of Psychiatry, 29*, 106–109.

Velamoor, V. R. (1998). Neuroleptic malignant syndrome. *Drug Safety, 19*(1), 73–82.

Velamoor, V. R. (1994). Progression of symptoms in neuroleptic malignant syndrome. *Journal of Nervous and Mental Disease, 182*(3), 168–173.

Wilson, M. P., Vilke, G. M., Hayden, S. R., & Nordstrom, K. (2016). Psychiatric emergencies for clinicians: Emergency department management of serotonin syndrome. *Journal of Emergency Medicine, 51*(1), 66–69.

# CHAPTER 35

# Serotonin Syndrome

Earl Andrew B. De Guzman

An 85-year-old female presents with her husband to the emergency department after he found her at home to be confused, lethargic, and diaphoretic. Her husband informs you that earlier in the day she complained of shortness of breath, pleuritic chest pain, coughing, and yellow-green sputum. Her past psychiatric history is significant for major depressive disorder that has been in remission for several years as well as taking daily sertraline. On physical examination, her blood pressure is 92/57 mm Hg, pulse rate is 135/min, respiration rate is 22/min, oxygen saturation is 86% on room air, and temperature is 100.3 °F. There are diffuse expiratory rhonchi on lung examination. The remainder of the examination is normal. Urine toxicology was negative. She is started on vancomycin, levofloxacin, and piperacillin-tazobactam and admitted to the intensive care unit for suspected community acquired pneumonia (CAP).

### What are some causes of altered mental status?

There are various causes of an acute-onset, fluctuating state of consciousness, known as *delirium*, which may include vascular, infectious, neoplastic, degenerative, intoxication, and congenital etiologies. Other causes may include traumatic, vitamin/metabolic derangements, heavy metals, or anoxia. These various causes are summarized in Table 35.1.

Delirium can further be characterized as hypoactive (lethargic, apathetic, psychomotor slowing), hyperactive (combative, paranoid, mood lability), or mixed, with characteristics of the former two and which represents the most common presentation. Among the elderly, risk factors for developing delirium include frailty, chronicity of medical problems, depression, pain, and falls.

The results of her blood culture are positive for methicillin-resistant *Staphylococcus aureus* (MRSA), which is sensitive to vancomycin. Her rapid antigen testing is positive for *influenza A*. She is placed on oseltamivir, and vancomycin is switched to linezolid because of her worsening condition, which corresponds to computed tomography (CT) chest findings of multiple cavitary lesions. She is suspected to have CAP that is complicated by *influenza A*.

### In general, when should you consider toxidrome as a diagnosis?

A toxidrome represents a unique constellation of signs and symptoms that are associated with exposure to a class or subset of substances at toxic levels. A toxidrome should be considered in cases in which a combination of these toxic signs and symptoms are concomitant with an acute-onset confusional state and exposure to substances or medications. Some agents that can lead to a toxidrome include anticholingerics, sympathomimetics, narcotics, hyponotics, serotonergics, antipsychotics, and anesthetics. With this particular case, there are four similar differential diagnoses: serotonin syndrome, malignant hyperthermia, neuroleptic malignant syndrome, and malignant catatonia (Table 35.2).

### TABLE 35.1 ■ Causes of Delirium

| | |
|---|---|
| Vascular | Cerebral arteriosclerosis, circulatory collapse (shock), emboli from atrial fibrillation, patent foramen ovale, endocarditic valve, hypertensive encephalopathy, hyperviscosity syndrome, intracranial hemorrhage or thrombosis, polyarteritis nodosa, sarcoid, systemic lupus erythematosus, thrombotic thrombocytopenic purpura |
| Infectious | Bacterial/viral/fungal meningitis, encephalitis, Behcet's syndrome, brain/epidural/subdural abscess, general paresis, human immunodeficiency virus, Lyme disease, malaria, mumps, parasitic, typhoid fever, sepsis |
| Neoplastic | Carcinomatous meningitis, paraneoplastic syndromes, space-occupying lesions (gliomas, meningiomas, abscesses) |
| Degenerative | Senile and presenile dementias (Alzheimer's or Pick's dementia, Creutzfeldt-Jakob disease, Huntington's chorea, Wilson's disease) |
| Intoxication | Chronic intoxication or withdrawal effect of sedative-hypnotic drugs (anticholinergics, anticonvulsants, bromides), carbon monoxide from burn inhalation, dissociative anesthetics, opiates, tranquilizers |
| Congenital | Aneurysm, complex partial seizures, status epilepticus, postictal states |
| Traumatic | Contusion, fat emboli syndrome, heat stroke, laceration, postoperative trauma, subdural and epidural hematomas |
| Intraventricular | Normal pressure hydrocephalus |
| Vitamin deficiency | B12 (pernicious anemia), niacin (pellagra), thiamine (Wernicke-Korsakoff syndrome) |
| Endocrine-metabolic | Carcinoid, Cushing's/Addison's syndromes, diabetic coma/shock, hepatic/renal failure, hyperthyroidism, hypoglycemia, myxedema, paraneoplastic syndromes, parathyroid dysfunction, porphyria, sleep apnea, severe electrolyte or acid/base disturbance, uremia, Whipple's syndrome |
| Metals | Heavy metals (lead, manganese, mercury), other toxins |
| Anoxia | Hypoxia and anoxia due to pulmonary or cardiac failure, anemia, anesthesia |
| Depression-other | Depressive pseudodementia, catatonia, hysteria |

Cassem et al., 2004

---

| BASIC SCIENCE/CLINICAL PEARL | STEP 1/2 |
|---|---|

Toxidromes presenting with altered mental status are particularly challenging and require a detailed history and physical examination to distinguish one toxidrome from other variants. An acute change in vital signs and mental status in the context of a systemic illness is most likely a cause of an underlying medical derangement and not a primary psychiatric disorder.

---

*How do you distinguish the particular toxidrome as the etiology of this patient's presentation?*
As there are many conditions that may closely mimic toxidrome, a detailed history and physical examination can elucidate which conditions are treatable and even reversible, especially in the context of an acute mental status change and suspected drug-drug interactions. It is not uncommon for neuropsychiatric patients to have a concomitant toxidrome that clouds or even mimics primary psychotic, mood, and neurologic disorders. To complicate matters more, certain toxidromes may present similarly to other types of toxidrome despite exposure to a different class of substances.

---

Approximately 6 hours later, she appears more diaphoretic, has agitation, and is grasping in the air at visual hallucinations. On physical examination, she has dilated pupils, dry mucous membranes, muscle rigidity, and ankle clonus bilaterally.

TABLE 35.2 ▪ Differential Diagnoses

| Condition | Primary Neurotransmitter Involved | Time Course of Onset | Vitals | Signs | Labs |
|---|---|---|---|---|---|
| Serotonin syndrome | Agonism of 5HT, primarily 5HT-2A receptors | <24 hr | Hyperthermia (>41.1°C), hypertension, tachycardia, tachypnea | Delirium, clonus, hyperreflexia, shivering, muscle rigidity, hyperactive bowels, ataxia | Leukocytosis, elevated CPK, decreased sodium bicarbonate |
| Malignant hypertherma | Stimulation of end-plate ACh receptors (Succinylcholine); volatile anesthetics | <24 hr | Hypercarbia, tachycardia, hyperthermia (>39°C) | Muscle rigidity, hyporeflexia, mottled skin with flushing/cyanosis | Hyperkalemia, myoglobinuria, elevated CK, mixed metabolic/respiratory acidosis |
| Neuroleptic malignant syndrome | Antagonism of Dopamine, primarily D2 receptors | 1-3 days | Hypertension, tachycardia, tachypnea, hyperthermia (>38°C) | Delirium, lead-pipe rigidity, diaphoresis | Elevated CK, leukocytosis, elevated LFTs, hyperkalemia, hypocalcemia, hypomagnesemia, hypo-/hypernatremia, metabolic acidosis, low serum iron concentration, myoglobinuria |
| Malignant catatonia | Dysfunction of GABA-A receptors | 1-3 days | Hypertension, tachycardia, tachypnea, hyperthermia (>38°C) | Waxy flexibility, catalepsy, stupor, negativism, delirium, muscle rigidity. Also, can have preceding mania, depression, psychosis | Elevated CK, leukocytosis, low serum iron |

*What is your differential diagnosis?*

This is an 85-year-old female with a history of major depressive disorder who is treated with sertraline who presents with cough, fever, and sputum production, and is diagnosed with CAP from MRSA that is complicated by influenza A. She has worsening mental status and autonomic signs despite addition of linezolid and now has dilated pupils, dry mucous membranes, muscle rigidity and ankle clonus bilaterally.

Serotonin syndrome, especially in the context of this patient who is taking sertraline (a selective serotonin reuptake inhibitor, or SSRI) with addition of linezolid for MRSA, is highest on the differential at this time. Although this patient appeared to have autonomic signs and altered mental status associated with delirium from CAP, additional clinical signs after adding of linezolid 6 hours later is highly suspect for serotonin syndrome.

As with other toxidromes, serotonin syndrome is a clinical diagnosis and is exclusionary of other etiologies. It is a life-threatening illness that requires a high degree of suspicion and with prompt delivery of treatment. The onset, time course, and description of symptoms along with a history of home medications and recent changes or additions of new medications are important to consider, even in a patient who has a stable psychiatric illness well-managed by antidepressants.

**BASIC SCIENCE PEARL**                                                              **STEP 1**

Serotonin, also known as *5-hydroxytryptamine* or *5-HT,* is a monoamine neurotransmitter in the central nervous system. It is synthesized from the amino acid tryptophan using two enzymes. L-tryptophan is converted to 5-hydroxy-L-tryptophan (5-HTP) by the enzyme-tryptophan-5-monooxygenase tryptophan hydroxylase (TPH), which is then converted to serotonin by the enzyme 5-hydroxytryptophan decarboxylase. Serotonin is mostly synthesized in the ralphe nuclei of the brainstem but is also synthesized in the gastrointestinal tract and can be found stored in platelets.

Supplementary diagnostic tests can help clarify the diagnosis, especially if a toxidrome closely resembles other etiologies, such as sepsis, encephalitis, neuroleptic malignant syndrome, anticholinergic/cholinergic syndrome, malignant hyperthermia, or thyroid storm. However, obtaining drug levels of serotonin or other drugs should not delay prompt treatment and may not necessarily correlate with the severity of the toxidrome. A complete metabolic panel may detect underlying electrolyte disturbances with liver and renal metabolism and functioning. A urine toxicology test may detect potential drugs of abuse (such as stimulants), and a quantitative drug level test can be obtained if there is a suspicion of ingestion and with corresponding signs or symptoms suggestive of toxicity associated with a medication (valproic acid, lithium, tricyclic antidepressants). An electrocardiogram may also be helpful in determining associated arrhythmias. A CT scan of the head may be useful in acute mental status change to rule out acute neurologic disorders (stroke, mass shift), whereas a lumbar puncture may help determine an underlying encephalitis or autoimmune process, such as paraneoplastic encephalitides. A urinalysis may also be helpful in detecting an underlying urinary tract infection or myoglobinuria suggestive of rhabdomyolysis from other hyperthermic toxidromes, such as neuroleptic malignant syndrome. A venous blood gas analysis can identify underlying hypoxia and acidosis.

**BASIC SCIENCE/CLINICAL PEARL**                                                    **STEP 1/2**

Serotonin syndrome is life threatening and requires prompt treatment based on careful history and physical examination. Diagnostic testing may be helpful in clarifying the diagnosis but is highly based on clinical suspicion and should not delay treatment.

*What is Serotonin Syndrome?*

Serotonin syndrome is an acute toxidrome caused by excess levels of circulating serotonin in the central nervous system and the periphery. Serotonin toxicity can develop because of disturbances of uptake inhibition, decreased metabolism, increased synthesis, increased release, activation of relevant receptors, and cytochrome (CYP) P450 inhibition by SSRIs, such as CYP2D6 and CYP3A4.

TABLE 35.3 ■ Severity of Serotonin Syndrome

| Mild | Moderate | Severe |
|------|----------|--------|
| Tachycardia | Hypertension | Metabolic acidosis |
| Shivering | Hyperthermia | Hypotension |
| Diaphoresis | Hyperactive bowel sounds | Rhabdoymyolysis/Kidney failure |
| Mydriasis | Inducible/Ocular clonus | Seizures |
| Myoclonus | Agitated delirium | Disseminated intravascular |
| Hyperreflexia | Muscle rigidity | coagulation |
| | | Coma |

---

**CLINICAL PEARL**             **STEP 2/3**

Most cases of serotonin syndrome develop within 6 hours of initiation of serotonergic agents, overdose, or change in medication that increases levels of serotonin. Mild symptoms may have a subacute presentation whereas more severe symptoms may be progressively lethal.

---

### What are the clinical manifestations of serotonin syndrome?

Serotonin syndrome is characterized as a triad of acute mental status changes, autonomic hyperactivity, and neuromuscular abnormalities, ranging from mild to severe, as summarized in Table 35.3. Mild cases may be afebrile but with tachycardia, shivering, diaphoresis, mydriasis, tremor or myoclonus, and hyperreflexia. In moderate cases, patients may develop added hypertension, hyperthermia, hyperactive bowel sounds, diaphoresis, notable hyperreflexia and clonus along the lower extremities, horizontal ocular clonus, and worsening delirium. Lastly, severe cases may be characterized by shock, muscle rigidity and hypertonicity more along the lower extremities, life threatening core temperature more than 107 °F, metabolic acidosis, rhabdomyolysis, seizures, renal failure, elevated liver transaminases and creatinine, and disseminated intravascular coagulopathy.

As it is a clinical diagnosis, serotonin syndrome can be diagnosed effectively using Hunter's criteria, which is 84% sensitive and 97% specific. These criteria are summarized in Fig. 35.1.

---

**CLINICAL PEARL**             **STEP 2/3**

Clonus is the most sensitive and specific sign of serotonin syndrome. A high degree of suspicion should not delay treatment, especially in close temporal approximation to starting a serotonergic agent.

---

### How does linezolid cause serotonin syndrome?

Linezolid was originally developed as a psychotropic with antidepressant effects via its mechanism as a mild reversible nonselective monoamine oxidase inhibitor (MAOI), but was found to be an effective antibiotic for vancomycin-resistant enterococci (VRE) and MRSA. As an MAOI, linezolid increases synaptic concentrations of serotonin, dopamine, and norepinephrine. When combined with serotonergic agents such as SSRIs (in this case sertraline), serotonin levels can increase further to toxic levels (Table 35.4).

### What is the treatment for serotonin syndrome?

The primary treatment is immediate discontinuation of the offending agent. Thereafter, providing supportive therapy with attention to airway, breathing and circulation with placement on monitoring, intravenous fluids, and oxygen is the basic form of treatment to normalize vital signs.

For the agitated delirious patient, benzodiazepines and dexmedetomidine, an α-2 receptor agonist, are preferred in the agitated delirious patient as they are effective in blunting the hyperadrenergic state. Antipsychotics and anticholinergic agents may worsen hyperthermia and are not recommended. Patients who require restraints are placed at an increased risk for hyperthermia, lactic acidosis, and mortality.

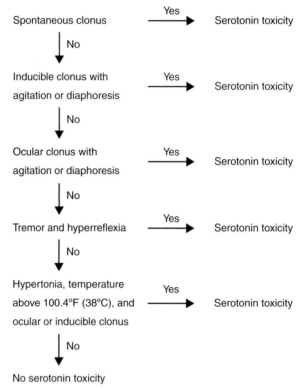

**Fig. 35.1** Hunter's criteria for serotonin syndrome (Dunkley et al., 2003).

### TABLE 35.4 ■ Medications That Interact with Linezolid to Cause Serotonin Syndrome

| | |
|---|---|
| Increased Synthesis | Increased Substrate (L-tryptophan) |
| Decreased metabolism | **Monoamine oxidase inhibitors (MAOIs):** phenelzine, tranylcypromine, moclobemide, selegiline, isocarboxazid, linezolid, methylene blue |
| Increased release | Amphetamines, cocaine, fenfluramine, sibutramine, ecstasy, phenanthrene, opioids (oxycodone, buprenorphine), tramadol |
| Serotonin (5-hydroxy-tryptamine) receptor agonism | Buspirone, lysergic acid diethylamide (LSD), dihydroergotamine (DHE), triptans, mirtazapine |
| Increased serotonin (5-hydroxy-tryptamine) receptor sensitivity | Lithium |
| Decreased reuptake | **Tricyclic antidepressants (TCAs):** amitriptyline, imipramine, clomipramine, desipramine, doxepin<br>**Selective serotonin reuptake inhibitors (SSRIs):** paroxetine, sertraline, fluoxetine, fluvoxamine, citalopram, escitalopram<br>**Serotonin noradrenaline reuptake inhibitors (SNRIs):** venlafaxine, duloxetine, milnacipran<br>**Other antidepressants:** trazodone, nefazodone<br>**Opioids:** fentanyl, meperidine, methadone, dextromethorphan, tramadol<br>**Miscellaneous:** ondansetron, granisetron, St. John's Wort |

Rastogi et al., 2011

In treating hyperthermia, cooling measures, not antipyretics, especially among patients with core temperatures greater than 107 °F should be considered. Acetaminophen and antipyretics should be avoided as serotonin syndrome is a disorder caused by increased muscle activity, not a change in central temperature set point. If necessary, intubation, sedation, and paralysis with a long-acting nondepolarizing agent such as cisatracurium can better manage core temperature.

In managing autonomic instability, esmolol and nitroprusside have been effective as short-acting agents for treating tachycardia and hypertension. Direct-acting vasoactive agents that include epinephrine, norepinephrine, and phenylephrine are effective in treating MAOI-associated hypotension. Longer-acting beta blockers such as propranolol may lead to circulatory shock.

The patient should be observed for any emergent signs of serotonin syndrome after withdrawal of the offending agent. Depressed patients being treated with MAOIs, and SSRIs with long half-lives such as fluoxetine may require up to a 5-week washout period.

The antihistamine cyproheptapine is a potent serotonin 2A antagonist that may be helpful as an antidote, but its efficacy remains unclear.

| CLINICAL PEARL | STEP 2/3 |
| --- | --- |

Bromocriptine and dantrolene, agents often used in the treatment of neuroleptic malignant syndrome, are to be avoided, as the former can precipitate serotonin syndrome, and the latter did not improve survival in animal models. The combination of both may cause further autonomic instability and mortality. Although with similar presentations, serotonin syndrome must be clinically differentiated from neuroleptic malignant syndrome in order to provide the best evidence-based treatment.

---

After a review of the most recent changes in the regimen, sertraline is discontinued because of high suspicion of its interaction with linezolid in developing serotonin syndrome. The patient's core temperature abruptly rises to 107 °F with ankle clonus and muscle rigidity, and she is intubated. She is administered further cold intravenous fluids and cooling blankets with ice packs to the groin and armpits. Her core temperature normalizes over 4 hours. For agitation, the patient receives intravenous lorazepam with adjuvant cyproheptadine. Her rigidity and agitation resolve, facilitating successful extubation. She improves after 4 days, at which time she continues her antibiotic treatment, with improvement of her vital signs, and is transferred to the inpatient medical unit.

---

### BEYOND THE PEARLS:

- Serotonin syndrome is a rare but potentially fatal toxidrome that requires a high degree of suspicion (especially in the setting of proserotonergic agents) and prompt delivery of treatment.
- Acute mental status changes, autonomic hyperactivity, and neuromuscular abnormalities are the triad presentation of serotonin syndrome.
- Hunter's criteria is a standardized method of diagnosis that is 84% sensitive and 97% specific. Clonus is the single most sensitive and specific sign of serotonin syndrome.
- Serotonin syndrome is primarily a clinical diagnosis and one exclusive of other similar toxidromes, though diagnostic tests may be considered as adjuvant methods for confirmation of the diagnosis or progression of overall disease.
- Linezolid, an antibiotic used in the treatment of VRE and MRSA, is also an MAOI that may interact with other proserotonergic agents, such as opioids and antidepressants to potentiate toxic serotonin blood levels.
- Prompt withdrawal of the offending agent with careful attention to immediate normalization of vital signs, airway, breathing, circulation, and neuromuscular tone are the hallmarks of supportive treatment.
- Bromocriptine and dantrolene are contraindicated as they increase the risk for autonomic instability and mortality.

- The antihistamine cyproheptadine is a potent serotonin-2A antagonist that may be helpful as an antidote, but its efficacy remains unclear.
- Depressed patients being treated with MAOIs and SSRIs with long half-lives, such as fluoxetine, may require up to a 5-week washout period.

## References

Bienvenu, O. J., Neufeld, K. J., & Needham, D. M. (2012). Treatment of four psychiatric emergencies in the intensive care unit. *Critical Care Medicine, 40*(9), 2662–2670.

Bijl, D. (2004). The serotonin syndrome. *Netherlands Journal of Medicine, 62,* 309–313.

Boyer, E. W., & Shannon, M. (2005). The serotonin syndrome. *New England Journal of Medicine, 352*(11), 1112–1120.

Cassem, N. H., Murray, G. B., Lafayette, J. M., et al. (2004). Delirious patients. In T. A. Stern, G. L. Fricchione, N. H. Cassem et al., (Eds.), *Massachusetts General Hospital Handbook of general hospital psychiatry* (5th ed., pp. 119–134). Philadelphia, PA: Mosby/Elsevier.

Dunkley, E. J. C., Isbister, G. K., Sibbritt, D., Dawson, A. H., & Whyte, I. M. (2003). The hunter serotonin toxicity criteria: Simple and accurate diagnostic decision rules for serotonin toxicity. *QJM : Monthly Journal of the Association of Physicians, 96*(9), 635–642.

Quinn, D. K., & Stern, T. A. (2009). Linezolid and serotonin syndrome. *Primary Care Companion to the Journal of Clinical Psychiatry, 11*(6), 353–356.

Rastogi, R., Swarm, R. A., & Patel, T. A. (2011). Case scenario: Opioid association with serotonin syndrome: Implications to the practitioners. *Anesthesiology, 115*(6), 1291–1298.

Volpie-Abadie, J., Kaye, A. M., & Kaye, A. D. (2013). Serotonin syndrome. *Ochsner Journal, 13*(4), 533–540.

# CHAPTER 36

# Lithium Toxicity

Courtney Eaves ■ Jessica Reis

---

A 34-year-old female with bipolar disorder is brought to the emergency department by family after they noticed she seemed confused and less alert than usual. She is noted to be drowsy, have slurred speech, and have an unsteady gait. Shortly after arrival, she has a seizure. The family provides history that the patient has recently been depressed, but they believe she has been compliant with her lithium. The family member also tells you that the patient slipped and fell 1 week ago and has been taking over-the-counter medication for knee pain.

---

### *What other information do you want to know?*

You would want to obtain more information about the patient's recent psychiatric symptoms, injuries sustained during the fall, and current medication list, including over-the-counter medications. Given the patient's history of bipolar disorder treated with lithium, as well as the clinical presentation, lithium toxicity should be high on your differential diagnosis list. A thorough review of the medication list to check for drug-drug interactions is very important in this case because many medications can affect lithium absorption and elimination by the kidneys. If medication bottles are present, it is important to count remaining medication to assess for intentional or unintentional overdose. Other diagnoses to consider would be an acute change in psychiatric illness, intracranial hemorrhage sustained during the fall, and medication or drug ingestion, possibly as a suicide attempt.

### *If you suspect lithium toxicity, what laboratory or other diagnostic testing should be ordered?*

Serum lithium level: The serum lithium level should be checked; this can give information about the severity of the overdose and help guide treatment decisions.

0.7–1.2 mEq/L = therapeutic range

> 1.5 mEq/L = toxic

> 2.0 mEq/L = lethal

Electrocardiogram (ECG): Cardiovascular manifestations of lithium toxicity include cardiac arrhythmias, conduction delays, and nonspecific ST-segment and T wave abnormalities.

Basic metabolic panel: Blood urea nitrogen (BUN) and creatinine (Cr) should be checked because lithium toxicity can cause acute renal failure. Electrolytes and BUN/Cr ratio should be used to assess fluid status and guide fluid replacement.

Complete blood count: It is always important to check for signs of an infectious process in a case of altered mental status. In addition, hemoglobin and hematocrit can give clues to the fluid status of the patient.

Toxicology: Toxicology screening is recommended to rule out coingestion of medications and/or illicit substances.

TABLE 36.1 ■ Types of Lithium Toxicity

| Type of Toxicity | Cause | Clinical Findings | Diagnosis |
|---|---|---|---|
| Acute | Acute ingestion of a supratherapeutic dose in a patient not already on lithium | **GASTROINTESTINAL FINDINGS MOST PROMINENT** Early—nausea, vomiting, diarrhea Later—sluggishness, ataxia, confusion, tremor, seizures | • History and examination findings • Serum lithium concentration (*may not correlate well with degree of toxicity*) |
| Acute on Chronic | Acute ingestion of supratherapeutic dose in a patient already taking lithium | Similar to acute | Similar to acute |
| Chronic | Increased absorption or decreased elimination of lithium in a patient on lithium therapy | **NEUROLOGIC FINDINGS MOST PROMINENT** Gradual emergence of sluggishness, ataxia, confusion, tremors, seizures | • History and examination findings • Serum lithium concentration (*more likely to correlate well with degree of toxicity*) |

---

**CLINICAL PEARL**                                                            **STEP 2/3**

Multiple randomized clinical trials have shown that treatment with lithium can reduce the risk of suicide in patients with both unipolar depression and bipolar disorder. Although the exact mechanism is unknown, lithium can prevent recurrence of mood episodes and may also help reduce impulsivity and aggression.

---

*What are the most important signs and symptoms of lithium toxicity?*
Three patterns of lithium toxicity are commonly recognized and have different presentations and implications for treatment (see Table 36.1). Acute lithium toxicity occurs when a supratherapeutic dose of lithium is ingested by a patient who is not currently maintained on lithium, such as an intentional overdose. Acute on chronic toxicity results when a patient who is maintained on lithium ingests a supratherapeutic dose, such as in the case of a dosage escalation or overdose. In contrast, chronic intoxication results from increased absorption or decreased elimination of lithium in a patient maintained on lithium therapy.

---

The family member presents the medication bottles that they found in the patient's purse. She is currently prescribed lithium 600 mg twice a day, ibuprofen 200 mg three times a day as needed for pain, and oral contraceptive pills. There is an appropriate amount of medication remaining based on the prescription dates. Initial laboratory values reveal a white blood cell count of 15,000 k/μL, normal hemoglobin and platelets, sodium 142 mg/dL, potassium 4.3 mEq/L, chloride 105 mEq/L, carbon dioxide 23 mEq/L, blood urea nitrogen 17 mg/dL, creatinine 2.1 mg/dL, and an initial lithium level of 3.4 mEq/L. Her initial ECG appeared normal, and toxicology screening is negative.

The patient remains very drowsy and confused. Vital signs are within normal limits. Based on these findings, you suspect chronic lithium toxicity as a result of a drug interaction between the lithium and newly prescribed ibuprofen. You decide to start intravenous (IV) hydration with isotonic saline and recommend emergent hemodialysis based on the clinical picture and lithium level.

**TABLE 36.2 ■ Determining When Dialysis Is Needed**

| Need for Dialysis Based on Lithium Level | |
| --- | --- |
| Lithium level (in mEq/L) | Should patient receive hemodialysis? |
| <2.5 | Usually not required, only if decreased consciousness, seizures, or life-threatening complications present |
| 2.5–4 | Presence of decreased consciousness, seizures, or life-threatening complications |
| 4–5 | If any complications or any renal impairment present |
| >5 | ALWAYS |

### What are the most important aspects of lithium toxicity treatment?

The first step in treatment of lithium toxicity is to assess the "ABCs," or airway, breathing, and circulation. Once stabilized, IV hydration with isotonic saline should be started to restore sodium and water balance and maximize lithium clearance. Activated charcoal binds poorly to lithium, making it ineffective in preventing lithium absorption. The use of activated charcoal should be reserved for cases where you suspect ingestion of other substances. Whole bowel irrigation is indicated in acute ingestions of lithium such as after an overdose. Gastric lavage may be used if time from ingestion to treatment is very short (less than 1 hour). Hemodialysis is an effective method for removing lithium, and its indication is dependent on the clinical picture and serum lithium levels (see Table 36.2).

### Why do lithium levels sometimes increase again even after they have started to decrease with one session of hemodialysis?

It takes time for lithium to distribute itself evenly between extracellular and intracellular fluids. As lithium is removed from the extracellular space via hemodialysis, blood levels will initially decrease. As intracellular lithium equilibrates into the extracellular space, the lithium level may actually increase initially. Serum lithium concentration should be measured 6 hours after dialysis to ensure levels are decreasing.

### How is lithium absorbed, metabolized, and excreted?

Lithium is absorbed in the gastrointestinal (GI) tract and is unaffected by food ingested. Lithium is not metabolized. Levels of immediate release lithium peak after 1 to 2 hours, whereas the extended release lithium levels peak after 4 to 5 hours. It is primarily excreted through the kidneys. The half-life of immediate release lithium in healthy adults is about 24 hours; however, as renal function declines the half-life will increase.

| CLINICAL PEARL | STEP 1/2/3 |
| --- | --- |
| Decreased volume of distribution (e.g., intravascular hypovolemia, elderly population), impaired renal function, and the use of certain medications, including thiazide diuretics, angiotensin-converting enzyme (ACE) inhibitors, and nonsteroidal antiinflammatory drugs (NSAIDs), will all increase lithium levels. | |

Increased volume of distribution (increased total body water, such as during pregnancy) and increased dietary sodium, caffeine, acetazolamide, and theophylline will reduce lithium levels.

### What are some long-term side effects of lithium use?

In addition to monitoring for short-term side effects of both acute and chronic toxicity, it is important to consider long-term side effects of lithium use. These side effects can occur with prolonged therapeutic use or with chronic toxicity. Renal injury can occur in the form of either nephrogenic diabetes insipidus or chronic tubulointerstitial nephropathy leading to renal insufficiency. Progression to end-stage renal disease is rare.

Lithium can also lead to hypothyroidism or, less frequently, hyperthyroidism. It can also cause hyperparathyroidism and increased calcium levels. Lithium is considered teratogenic because of an increased risk of Ebstein's anomaly in neonates, which is an abnormality of the tricuspid valve. The absolute risk of a neonate developing this cardiac malformation remains small even with lithium therapy, thus lithium can still be used in some cases of pregnancy when the benefit of the medication outweighs the risk.

---

**CLINICAL PEARL**                                                              **STEP 2/3**

Advise patients that if they are losing a lot of water from their bodies (e.g., diarrhea, vomiting, excessive sweating), they should increase their intake of water or reduce the amount of lithium they are taking to avoid lithium toxicity.

---

After several sessions of hemodialysis, the patient's serum lithium level drops within therapeutic range and her mental status improves. She is evaluated by the psychiatry service to assess suicidality and make treatment recommendations. The patient does have a history of suicide attempts but denies over-taking her medication; this is supported by the number of pills remaining in her pill bottles. The psychiatrist recommends continued lithium treatment, as it is an effective treatment for her bipolar disorder and may reduce suicidality in the future.

---

**BEYOND THE PEARLS:**

- It is well-known that lithium has many effects on biological systems, affecting both signal transduction pathways and various neurotransmitters. However, lithium's specific mechanism of therapeutic effect remains elusive, and it is still not known whether it is the same mechanism by which lithium exerts its toxic effects.
- Except for the widely known hypothesis that lithium reduces inositol by inhibiting inositol monophosphatase and inositol polyphosphate-1-phosphatase, other reported molecular targets for lithium were glycogen synthase kinase-3β and akt/β-arrestin-2. Neurotransmitter hypotheses include possible lithium effects on cholinergic, glutamatergic, and serotonergic systems.
- Lithium may increase gray matter volume and improve integrity of white matter. It also may have neuroprotective factors.
- Lithium should not be used when severe renal impairment, hyponatremia, dehydration, or severe cardiovascular disease are present. It should also be used with caution in patients with psoriasis as it can exacerbate this condition.
- Long-term neurologic sequelae of lithium toxicity can occur even after lithium is removed with hemodialysis. This is known as *the syndrome of irreversible lithium effectuated neurotoxicity* (SILENT) and involves a wide range of neurologic and psychiatric symptoms.

### References

Adityanjee Munshi, K. R., & Thampy, A. (2005). The syndrome of irreversible lithium-effectuated neurotoxicity. *Clinical Neuropharmacology*, *28*, 38–49.

Chen, K. P., Shen, W. W., & Lu, M. L. (2004). Implication of serum concentration monitoring in patients with lithium intoxication. *Psychiatry and Clinical Neurosciences*, *58*, 25–29.

Decker, B. S., Goldfarb, D. S., & Dargan, P. I. (2015). Extracorporeal treatment for lithium poisoning: systematic review and recommendations from the EXTRIP workgroup. *Clinical Journal of the American Society of Nephrology*, *10*, 875–887 2015.

Geddes, J. R., Burgess, S., Hawton, K., Jamison, K., & Goodwin, G. M. (2004). Long-term lithium therapy for bipolar disorder: Systematic review and meta-analysis of randomized controlled trials. *American Journal of Psychiatry*, *161*, 217–222.

Greller, H. A. (2015). Lithium. In R. S. Hoffman, M. A. Howland, N. A. Lewin, L. S. Nelson, & L. R. Goldfrank (Eds.), *Goldfrank's toxicologic emergencies* (10th ed.). New York, NY: McGraw-Hill Education.

Haussmann, R., Bauer, M., von Bonin, S., Grof, P., & Lewitzka, U. (2015). Treatment of lithium intoxication: Facing the need for evidence. *International Journal of Bipolar Disorders*, *3*, 23.

Paul, R., Minay, J., Cardwell, C., Fogarty, D., & Kelly, C. (2010). Review: Meta-analysis of the effects of lithium usage on serum creatinine levels. *Journal of Psychopharmacology*, *24*, 1425–1431.

Sadock, B. J., Sadock, V. A., & Ruiz, P. (2015). *Kaplan & Sadock's synopsis of psychiatry: Behavioral sciences/ clinical psychiatry* (11th ed.). Philadelphia, PA: Wolters Kluwer.

Ward, M. E., Musa, M. N., & Bailey, L. (1994). Clinical pharmacokinetics of lithium. *Journal of Clinical Pharmacology*, *34*, 280.

# CHAPTER 37

# Suicide Risk Assessment

Susie Morris

---

A 67-year-old white male with a history of recurrent major depressive disorder and alcohol use disorder (in full sustained remission) presents for an annual physical examination. He has a past medical history significant for type 2 diabetes, obstructive sleep apnea, and obesity.

---

### What is the definition of suicide?

The Centers of Disease Control and Prevention define suicide as "death caused by self-directed injurious behavior with an intent to die as a result of the behavior." Conversely, a suicide attempt is a nonfatal, self-directed, injurious behavior made with an intent to inflict death. Suicidal ideation is "thinking about, considering, or planning suicide." These distinct definitions are necessary for both clinical and research purposes.

### What is a suicide risk assessment?

Suicide risk assessment is a formalized evaluation of an individual patient's risk for completed suicide. It is a clinical assessment that should be documented in the medical record in an organized fashion. The suicide risk assessment can be documented in a narrative format or completed using any number of accepted, clinical scales developed for that purpose. Just like an abnormal laboratory value or concerning physical finding, a suicide risk assessment that indicates cause for alarm warrants an appropriate clinical response from the provider.

### Who can perform a suicide risk assessment?

Any clinician can perform a suicide risk assessment, and every member of the treating team must evaluate for suicide risk. In the outpatient setting, sometimes nurses and nursing assistants will do the first suicide risk assessment by administering a formalized questionnaire to each patient. It is the responsibility of the physician to follow up with the patient regarding the content of that questionnaire and complete an additional screening with each patient. Remember that a patient's comfort in disclose may vary by provider, which is why risk assessment is paramount at each step of the clinical interaction.

---

Intake staff document a suicide risk screening, which is negative for current thoughts of suicide.

---

### Which patients require a suicide risk assessment?

All patients require a suicide risk assessment. This assessment of risk should be documented in the patient's medical record. Multiple screening tools are in use and available to aid in assessing and documenting suicide risk. Asking about suicidal ideations and behaviors does not increase the risk of completed suicide. In fact, asking about risky symptoms and behaviors is protective in that it facilitates access to appropriate health care services to ensure patient safety.

---

**CLINICAL PEARL**                                                            **STEP 2/3**

Some commonly used suicide risk screening tools include the Columbia-Suicide Severity Rating Scale (C-SSRS), the Suicide Assessment Five-Step Evaluation and Triage (SAFE-T), and the Patient Health Questionnaire (PHQ).

---

Mental status examination: Overweight white male in casual attire, intact eye contact, no psychomotor disturbances, appears stated age, no observed response to internal stimuli. Calm, cooperative, and polite. Linear thought process with normal speech rate, rhythm, volume, and latency. Thought content negative for suicidal or homicidal ideations; no delusions elicited. Mood is "fine" with full range of affect. Insight/ judgment intact.

---

***What are some common static risk factors for completed suicide?***

Risks for completed suicide can be divided into static and dynamic risks factors, meaning mutable and immutable factors that impact a person's overall risk category. Risk factors for completed suicide have been identified in epidemiologic research and differ by culture and country. The most serious risk factor for completed suicide is a history of suicide attempts. That being said, the majority of victims of suicide do not have a history of suicide attempts. Another important risk factor for suicide is advanced age. Data indicate that the risk for suicide increases with each decade of life, with a particular rise in risk in the sixth decade. Persons aged 75 years and older are at three times higher risk for completed suicide than young persons aged 15 to 24.

Risk of completed suicide in Caucasians is approximately twice the rate reported in other races; although the risk of suicide in African Americans has increased in recent years. Suicide rates are generally higher among men than women, and this is true among all age groups; although, women more commonly experience suicidal ideation compared with men, and adolescents report suicidal ideation more often than do elderly people.

---

**CLINICAL PEARL**                                                            **STEP 2/3**

Sexual minorities are at greater risk for suicide than their heterosexual peers, especially in adolescence and early adulthood. Transgender individuals are also at increased risk for suicide.

---

A history of mental illness is certainly a risk factor for suicide; however, data indicate that over half of the victims of suicide in the United States were not diagnosed with any psychiatric condition before death. Diagnoses of major depression, bipolar affective disorder, schizophrenia, anxiety disorder, or personality disorder confer a greater risk for suicide compared with the general population. Depression is thought to be a factor in 65% to 90% of completed suicides and is the most commonly diagnosed psychiatric disorder in those who commit suicide. Borderline personality disorder is the psychiatric diagnosis associated with the greatest number of lifetime suicide attempts. Specific symptoms of hopelessness, helplessness, and impulsivity are also associated with increased risk. Substance use disorders also play an important role in suicidality. In the United States at least one-fourth of suicide victims have an alcohol use disorder; though other substance use disorders are also risk factors for completed suicide.

Family history of completed suicide is a powerful risk factor as well. Research indicates that there is likely a genetic risk factor that is confounded by certain environmental phenomena. Twin studies demonstrate that monozygotic twins have a higher concordance rate for suicide and suicide attempts than do dizygotic twins. Adoption studies corroborate the hypothesis that a genetic factor exists, showing that persons who are adopted who have a biological history of completed suicide have a higher personal risk for suicide. Neurobiological theories have been posited as possible explanations for these observed risks.

---

**BASIC SCIENCE PEARL**                                                      **STEP 1**

Studies show that victims of suicide have lower posthumous levels of cerebrospinal fluid serotonin metabolites compared with persons who did not die of suicide.

---

On interview, the patient reveals a trauma history significant for childhood sexual abuse.

---

### What are some common dynamic risk factors for completed suicide?

Environmental risk factors play a significant role in overall suicide risk assessment for any individual. Childhood abuse has a profound impact upon suicide risk, and childhood sexual abuse, in particular, portends a sizable increase in a person's risk for completed suicide.

Although marital status is thought to be a protective factor against suicide in the United States, divorce, separation, and loss of a spouse are risk factors for suicidality. Socially isolative behaviors can be predictive of suicidality and coincide with increased risk. Persons who complete suicide are often retrospectively described to have become more isolative just before the death. Although the data are variable, higher rates of suicide have been observed in rural areas and are thought to be attributable to limited access to health care, social isolation, and lower levels of education. Suicidal behavior is more common among unemployed individuals compared with employed persons, and the risk is highest if the job loss is sudden. Indeed, higher rates of suicide are observed in times of economic recession. Poor physical health is also a prominent risk factor (Table 37.1 and Fig. 37.1).

---

He enjoys spending time with his two adult daughters and reading. He attends church with his wife on a weekly basis. Regarding his health, his diabetes is under tight control, and he has an active gym membership.

---

### Are there any protective factors against suicide?

Marital status is thought to be a protective factor against suicide. A current pregnancy and/or having the responsibility of raising children have also been observed to be protective. Religious faith can also be a deterrent against completed suicide. Employment is also protective.

---

TABLE 37.1 ■ **Risk Factors for Completed Suicide**

| Risk Factors |
| --- |
| Caucasian race |
| Male gender |
| Sexual minority |
| Mental illness |
| Previous suicide attempts |
| Older age |
| Military service |
| Poor physical health |
| Family history |
| Childhood abuse |
| Substance use disorder |
| Unemployment |
| Permissive view |
| Access to firearms |

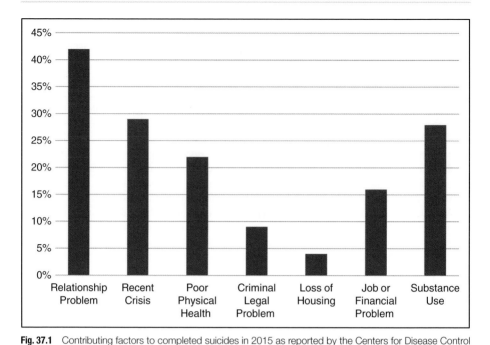

**Fig. 37.1** Contributing factors to completed suicides in 2015 as reported by the Centers for Disease Control and Prevention (CDC).

| CLINICAL PEARL | STEP 2/3 |
|---|---|

Being a skilled worker is generally thought to be a protective factor against suicide; however, of all skilled workers, physicians are at the greatest risk for suicide. Moreover, medical students are also at incongruous risk for suicide, and resident physicians are at greater risk of developing depression compared with their nonresident peers.

The patient reveals that he is an avid hunter, and one of his hobbies is tactical pistol-shooting.

### What is the link between firearms access and suicidality?

Data from the Centers for Disease Control and Prevention indicate that, in 2016, about 45,000 deaths resulted from suicide in the United States. Half of those suicides were committed using firearms. Data also demonstrate that having a gun in the home is associated with an increased risk of firearm-related suicide and homicide. In fact, a gun kept in the home is 11 times more likely to be used in the commission or attempt of a suicide rather than used in an act of self-defense. This underscores the clinical importance of asking patients about access to firearms as part of a thorough suicide risk assessment (Fig. 37.2).

| CLINICAL PEARL | STEP 3 |
|---|---|

Involuntary commitment for psychiatric treatment can result in restrictions on firearms ownership.

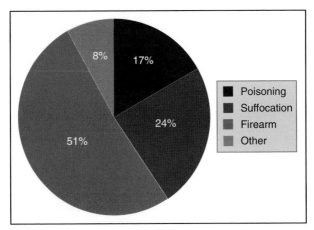

**Fig. 37.2** Means of suicide in the United States, 1999 to 2016 (CDC, Centers for Disease Control and Prevention).

---

The patient is currently being treated for his depression with escitalopram 20 mg daily. He sees a therapist on a weekly basis. He reports that his last drink was 20 years ago, and he attends monthly Alcoholics Anonymous meetings.

---

### What is this patient's suicide risk?

This patient's current risk for suicide is low. Though he does have a number of static risk factors, his dynamic risk factors are less concerning and suggest against suicidal intent at the present evaluation.

### If this patient's risk for acute suicide was elevated, what are some evidence-based interventions that decrease suicide risk?

Access to appropriate mental health treatment is an evidence-based therapeutic intervention that can be protective against completed suicide. Specifically, psychopharmacotherapy can have a therapeutic impact on patients. Some studies show a decrease in suicidal behavior in patients with depression who are treated with selective serotonin reuptake inhibitors. Research demonstrates that treatment with clozapine or lithium, specifically, is associated with decreased incidence of suicide.

Psychotherapeutic strategies are also helpful in combating suicidality. Research shows that dialectical behavioral therapy conducted in patients with borderline personality disorder reduces the number of suicide attempts by those patients. A number of outreach programs, both in communities and schools, increase accessibility of crisis intervention and mental health care, which, in turn, decrease completed suicides.

Restricting access to lethal means is a controversial intervention that does have some evidentiary support. For instance, measures in Australia that reduced access to barbiturates appeared to cause a relative decrease in suicide rates. As previously noted, there is some link between suicidality and firearms access. It has been suggested that limiting access to firearms and increasing availability of firearms safety education may reduce injuries related to firearms (both in the context of homicide and suicide).

Another controversial topic is media reporting of suicides. Suicide contagions have been a noted cultural phenomenon wherein one suicide results in a number of "copycat" suicides.

Adolescents are particularly susceptible to suicide attempts and completed suicides in the wake of contagions. Data suggest that the manner in which such suicides are reported by the media can impact subsequent behaviors. It is recommended that media sources exercise caution in reporting the material, taking careful steps to avoid either normalizing or romanticizing suicidality.

---

Although this patient has a number of risk factors for suicidality, he does not presently exhibit an elevated risk for completed suicide. You document that his overall suicide risk assessment is low.

---

### What can be done if you suspect a patient to have elevated risk for acute suicide?

Acute suicidality is a psychiatric emergency and warrants inpatient psychiatric admission to ensure the patient's safety. Involuntary commitment laws for psychiatric treatment vary between states; however, each state allows for involuntary detainment for treatment in the event that a patient is an acute harm to her/himself. Although it is important to protect a patient's confidentiality in the context of medical treatment, if a patient reports suicidal intent, you are obligated to facilitate treatment for that patient, which may require you to contact emergency medical services.

### BEYOND THE PEARLS:

- Borderline personality disorder is the psychiatric diagnosis associated with the greatest number of lifetime suicide attempts. Major depressive disorder is associated with the greatest number of completed suicides.
- Psychopharmacotherapy can have a therapeutic impact on patients. Research demonstrates that treatment with clozapine or lithium, specifically, is associated with decreased incidence of suicide in patients with schizophrenia or bipolar disorder, respectively.
- Adolescents are particularly susceptible to suicide contagions wherein one suicide results in a number of "copycat" suicides.
- Childhood sexual abuse portends a sizable increase in a person's risk for completed suicide.
- Adoption studies corroborate the hypothesis that a genetic factor exists, showing that persons who are adopted and have a biological history of completed suicide have a higher personal risk for suicide. It is important to ask patients whether they have a family history of completed suicide.
- A 2010 prospective cohort study of interns across 13 U.S. hospitals found that the incidence of physician interns' thoughts of death increased by 370% in the first 3 months of their intern year. The Accreditation Council for Graduate Medical Education established the Symposium on Physician Well-Being. One of the aims of this symposium is to increase awareness of the crisis of burnout, depression, and suicide by physicians.

### References

Centers for Disease Control and Prevention. (n.d.). Suicide, 2016. Retrieved from www.cdc.gov/violenceprevention/suicide

Goldman, M. L., Shah, R. N., & Bernstein, C. A. (2015). Depression and suicide among physician trainees: Recommendations for a national response. *JAMA Psychiatry*, 72(5), 411–412.

Kessler, R., Borges, G., & Walters, E. E. (1999). Prevalence of and risk factors for lifetime suicide attempts in the national comorbidity study. *Archives of General Psychiatry*, 56(7), 617–626.

Melamed, Y., Bauer, A., Kalian, M., Rosca, P., & Mester, R. (2011). Assessing the risk of violent behavior before issuing a license to carry a handgun. *Journal of the American Academy of Psychiatry and the Law, 39*(4), 543–548.

Posner, K., Brown, G. K., Stanley, B., Brent, D. A., Yershova, K. V., Oquendo, M. A., ... Mann, J. J. (2011). The Columbia-Suicide Severity Rating Scale: Initial validity and internal consistency findings from three multisite studies with adolescents and adults. *American Journal of Psychiatry, 168*, 1266–1277.

World Health Organization. (2002). Self-directed violence. *World Report on Violence and Health.* Geneva: Author.

# CHAPTER 38

# Medication-Induced Movement Disorders

Tammy Duong ■ Peter Ureste

A 22-year-old male with a history of schizophrenia is admitted to the inpatient psychiatric unit for psychosis. He has been nonadherent with his outpatient medication regimen and has developed auditory hallucinations of voices telling about "demons stalking him" and delusions that helicopters are following him. He smashed all the televisions in the house because he believes that the local news anchorwoman was broadcasting his location to the authorities. His mother, with whom he lives, called the police.

He has no past medical history other than schizophrenia. Basic metabolic panel, complete blood cell count, thyroid function tests, and urine analysis are normal. Urine toxicology is negative. When he arrives on the unit, he is started on risperidone 4 mg daily.

Within the next 24 hours, nursing calls to request an urgent evaluation of the patient. He is circling the nursing station, appears anxious, and is having trouble speaking. Through clenched teeth he calls out, "My jaw is stuck!" His lower mandible is clenched, locked into position, and resists passive movement. His neck is slightly extended, and his eyes appear to be forcefully rolled in the direction of the upper right quadrant. He lacks rigidity in his upper or lower extremities.

## What are medication-induced movement disorders?

Antipsychotics and other dopamine blocking agents such as metoclopramide can cause dramatic involuntary movements in patients. Although exact mechanisms are unclear, it is hypothesized that dopamine blockade at the D2 receptor alters the balance between dopaminergic and cholinergic transmission within the nigrostriatal tract, which is responsible for movement initiation. Symptoms can be varied. It can affect a focal group of muscles or be generalized. Medication-induced movement disorders are broadly categorized into those that occur acutely or chronically (tardive). Table 38.1 lists medication-induced movement disorders.

Vital signs are taken for this patient. His temperature is 98 °F, blood pressure is 125/82 mm Hg, pulse rate 88/min, respiratory rate is 18/min, and oxygen saturation is 98% on room air. Although it is difficult for him to speak, he is awake, alert, and oriented to person, place, time, and current situation. He is not diaphoretic.

## What is the differential diagnosis for this patient?

Acute onset of involuntary muscle contraction soon after initiation or dose of change of an antipsychotic medication should raise high suspicion for an acute medication-induced movement disorder. These include acute dystonia, occulyogyic crisis which is a specific type of acute dystonia, akathisia, parkinsonism, and neuroleptic malignant syndrome (NMS). NMS is potentially lethal and should be ruled out first. It presents with a constellation of symptoms, including confusion, hyperthermia,

TABLE 38.1 ■ **Medication-Induced Movement Disorders**

| Acute | Chronic (Tardive) |
|---|---|
| • Dystonia:<br>   • Oculogyric crisis<br>   • Torticollis<br> • Akathisia<br> • Neuroleptic malignant syndrome<br> • Parkinsonism | • Dystonia<br> • Akathisia<br> • Dyskinesia<br> • Tremors<br> • Tics |

diaphoresis, generalized "lead pipe" rigidity, autonomic instability, respiratory distress, and creatinine kinase greater than four times the upper limit of normal. This diagnosis is unlikely in this patient, as his vital signs are normal and he is fully alert, oriented, and displaying only focal rigidity.

Parkinsonism is a constellation of symptoms that consist of: (1) resting tremor, (2) muscle rigidity, and (3) bradykinesia. Other symptoms can develop, including masked facies, stooped posture, shuffling or festinating gait, micrographia, and hypophonia. Other than muscle rigidity, none of these symptoms are present in our patient. As such, parkinsonism is unlikely.

Acute dystonia consists of sudden and sustained contraction of a specific muscle group. These usually occur in the trunk, neck, facial muscles, or less often in the limbs. Acute dystonias occur in isolation or in combination with each other. It can be potentially lethal if occurring in laryngeal muscles that aid in respiration. The muscle contractions force the patient to assume odd positions or postures. Torticollis occurs when cervical muscles spasm, forcing the neck to turn to one side or the other. Oculogyric crisis is an acute dystonia affecting the extraocular muscles and forces the eyes to deviate in the direction of the dystonia.

Acute dystonias can occur after the first dose of an antipsychotic but can also occur at any time point during treatment. Approximately half of cases occur within 48 hours of treatment initiation. In 90% of cases, acute dystonia occurs within the 5 days of treatment.

This patient is experiencing mandibular and ocular muscle spasms shortly after the initiation of a high-potency antipsychotic. This is most consistent with acute dystonia and oculogyric crisis.

| CLINICAL PEARL | STEP 2/3 |
|---|---|

Acute dystonia may occur in combinations. Cervical or mandibular dystonia commonly occur in combination with oculogyric crisis.

| CLINICAL PEARL | STEP 2/3 |
|---|---|

Risk factors for acute dystonia include: male gender, young age, history of ECT, history of substance use (especially cocaine), and brain damage.

| BASIC SCIENCE/CLINICAL PEARL | STEP 1/2/3 |
|---|---|

All antipsychotics have the potential to cause medication-induced movement disorders. However, first-generation antipsychotics have a higher risk of inducing acute dystonia than second-generation antipsychotics. Also, high-potency antipsychotics such as haloperidol and risperidone are more likely to lead to these side effects compared with their low-potency counterparts.

### What is the treatment for acute dystonia?

In untreated cases, acute dystonia can spontaneously resolve in 12 to 48 hours. However, as this side effect can cause surprise and acute distress in patients, it should be treated urgently.

Parental treatment of anticholinergics is the treatment of choice for acute dystonia. Intramuscular diphenhydramine 50 mg or benztropine 1 to 2 mg are commonly used. Treatment can resolve symptoms within a few minutes. In all cases of medication-induced movement disorders, consider alternative treatments and discontinuing the offending agent if appropriate. On occasion, anticholinergic medications are given prophylactically in younger patients taking high-potency antipsychotics. This practice is not recommended for older adults.

---

Diphenhydramine 50 mg is given intramuscularly to the patient. Within 20 minutes the patient regains voluntary movement of his extraocular muscles and mandible. "Doctor, you are my hero!" he exclaims down the hallway.

Two days later, the patient is seen pacing the hallways. When brought into the interview room, he sits down momentarily and then quickly stands back up. He marches in place for the duration of the interview. He comments, "I'm so uncomfortable. I can't stay still."

---

### What is akathisia?

This patient's feeling of restlessness and inability to sit still after the introduction of an antipsychotic is consistent with akathisia. Akathisia is a medication-induced movement disorder characterized by hyperkinetic motor movements. It most often affects the legs, but arms and trunk can also be involved. Patients characterize the sensation as internal restlessness and the irresistible urge to move. This can present as stereotypic movements such as marching in place, shifting weight from one foot to the other, rocking back and forth, or motions to sit then stand. Akathisia is often mistaken for psychosis, untreated anxiety, agitated depression, restless leg syndrome, tics, or excessive levodopa dosing. Despite having the urge to move, movement does not alleviate the sensation. Many patients also report feeling anxious. Akathisia is a psychiatrically urgent condition, as some patients cannot tolerate the side effect, and is considered a risk factor for suicide.

### What are treatments for akathisia?

As with all medication-induced movement disorders, reduction or discontinuation of the offending agent should occur. Otherwise, beta-blockers such as propranolol are used as a first-line treatment for akathisia and can be helpful to alleviate the restless sensation. Use of anticholinergic medications are less effective in akathisia than treating other medication-induced movement disorders. Benzodiazepines have also been traditionally used but have lacked statistical significance in some studies. Other agents such as α-agonist clonidine and 5HT2A antagonists, such as mirtazapine, trazodone, and mianserin may also have a positive effect on reducing akathisia severity.

---

Patient is started on propranolol 10 mg twice a day, and his feelings of restlessness improve throughout the next day. While administering medications to the patient, the nursing staff notices the front side of the patient's shirt is wet and has stains over the chest. The patient is examined, and there is a milky white discharge bilaterally from both nipples.

---

### What is galactorrhea and why is the patient experiencing this?

Galactorrhea is the expression of milk from the breast outside of childbirth or breast feeding. It can be associated with hyperprolactinemia. However, it is important to note that many cases of prolactinoma can be asymptomatic.

---

**BASIC SCIENCE PEARL**                                                                 **STEP 1**

Lactotroph cells reside in the anterior pituitary and secrete prolactin. Prolactin can influence milk production.

---

Lactotroph cells in the anterior pituitary secrete prolactin, which is responsible for milk production. Prolactin secretion is under tonic inhibitory control by dopamine on lactotroph D2 receptors via the tuberoinfundibular pathway. This means that dopamine secreted from the hypothalamus inhibits prolactin secretion and thus inhibits milk production.

Although galactorrhea is not a medication-induced movement disorder, it is still a potential side effect of antipsychotics. These medications antagonize D2 receptors; this prevents dopamine from inhibiting prolactin secretion and results in hyperprolactinemia.

---

**BASIC SCIENCE PEARL**                                                                 **STEP 1**

Several dopaminergic pathways exist. Four pathways that are affected by antipsychotics are:
- mesolimbic pathway
- mesocortical pathway
- nigrostriatal pathway
- tuberoinfundibular pathway

---

Other associated symptoms with hyperprolactinemia include gynecomastia, amenorrhea, sexual dysfunction, or infertility. Aside from amenorrhea, these symptoms occur in both men and women. Approximately 18% of men and 47% of women treated with antipsychotics have an elevated prolactin level. In clinical practice, prolactin levels are not drawn in asymptomatic patients taking antipsychotics, as there is a fair likelihood of the levels being elevated without providing additional useful diagnostic information.

---

As a result of the side effects, the patient is cross-titrated from risperidone to aripiprazole. Over the next week, his auditory hallucinations begin to resolve, and his feelings of paranoia are less bothersome. Because of his history of medication nonadherence, a long-acting injectable antipsychotic is considered. It is ultimately deferred given the number of side effects he has had during this hospitalization. Patient is discharged home with his mother on aripiprazole 20 mg every morning.

---

**What are the risks and benefits of long-acting injectable antipsychotic medications?**

Medication nonadherence is a major issue for many patients with a schizophrenia diagnosis. The medication discontinuation rate can be as high as 50% to 75% within 6 months of initiation. There are several antipsychotics available in depot formulation that can be administered intramuscularly on a monthly basis in lieu of oral medications. This can enhance adherence, delay time to rehospitalization, and lower the overall number of psychiatric hospitalizations.

Concerns with use of long-acting injectable antipsychotics include redness, swelling, and pain at the injection site. Many clinicians are concerned about loading a patient with a large dose of antipsychotic medication and being unable to discontinue the medication quickly should an adverse event arise. Long-acting injectable antipsychotics are associated with more akinesia, change in low-density lipoproteins, and anxiety compared with oral antipsychotic medication. However, there is no statistical difference between long-acting injectable and oral antipsychotics in regard to extrapyramidal side effects, weight change, or discontinuation rate due to side effects.

The patient returns to the outpatient clinic the next week for his postdischarge follow-up with his mother. His grooming and hygiene have improved. He reports he still feels as though he is being watched sometimes but can ignore the feeling. He is adherent with his medications. Abnormal involuntary movement scale (AIMS) is performed and he scores 0/40. He asks what the examination is testing.

### What is tardive dyskinesia (TD)?

TD is the stereotyped, sustained, and twisting involuntary movement seen in a patient taking antidopaminergic medication on a long-term basis. Oral-buccal-lingual variety of TD appears as involuntary muscle contractions in the face, jaw, and tongue. It can appear as chewing motions, tongue darting, or lip puckering. TD can also affect the trunk and extremities, which appears as twisting or thrusting movements. In milder cases, the patient may not be aware of these involuntary movements.

Like many other medication-induced movement disorders, first-generation antipsychotics carry a higher risk than second generation antipsychotics. A popular explanation is that first generation antipsychotics have a higher binding affinity for D2 receptors, which is a major risk factor for TD. Second-generation antipsychotics also work on other receptors such as 5HT2A receptors and adhere more transiently to the D2 receptor.

---

**CLINICAL PEARL**          **STEP 2/3**

Primary risk factors for tardive dyskinesia include use of a medication with strong D2 receptor affinity, duration of treatment, total medication dose, age greater than 60 years, and female gender. Other risk factors are presence of a major neurocognitive disorder, other extrapyramidal side effects, and antipsychotic treatment for an affective disorder instead of a psychotic disorder.

---

### Dopamine is needed in the substantia nigra to initiate movement. Why would long-term dopamine blockade lead to hyperkinetic movements seen in TD?

The dopamine receptor hypersensitivity theory posits that long-term blockade of D2 receptors will lead to their hypersensitization. This means that a relatively lower level of dopamine is needed to cause movement, and these receptors can be overstimulated. The movements in TD can resemble those in Parkinson disease patients with excessive levodopa treatment. In clinical practice, immediately stopping an antipsychotic may temporarily worsen TD because the dopamine blockade will cease, but the D2 receptor will still be hypersensitized. Increasing the dose of antipsychotic will temporarily improve the hyperkinetic movements before worsening them.

### What is a scale that can be helpful in monitoring for signs of TD?

The abnormal involuntary movement scale (AIMS) is a standardized scale to quantify the severity, location, and progression of TD. It is recommended to conduct an AIMS assessment on patients before initiating an antipsychotic and then yearly afterward.

This patient scores a 0/40 on the AIMS and does not exhibit signs of tardive dyskinesia.

### What are treatments for tardive dyskinesia?

The use of antipsychotics should be limited, if possible, especially in patients who are elderly or who have a major neurocognitive disorder. Caution should be used not to discontinue antipsychotic medication too quickly in order to prevent a withdrawal and temporarily worsen TD. If the patient requires antipsychotic treatment, then consider a second generation antipsychotic if not already on one or clozapine in refractory cases.

The medication class vesicular monoamine transporter (VMAT)-2 may be helpful for treating TD. VMAT is a protein that packages monoamine neurotransmitters (dopamine, norepinephrine,

TABLE 38.2 ■ VMAT2 Inhibitors for Treatment of Tardive Dyskinesia

|  | Tetrabenazine | Deutetrabenazine | Valbenazine |
|---|---|---|---|
| Dosing | Three times daily | Twice daily | Daily |
| Half-life | 5–7 hours | 9–10 hours | 15–22 hours |
| Adverse effects | Sedation, parkinsonism, akathisia, depression, suicidality | Same | Same |

VMAT2, Vesicular monoamine transporter-2.

serotonin, and histamine) into presynaptic vesicles for release into the synaptic cleft. The transporter is found in two forms: VMAT1 is expressed in the peripheral nervous system, whereas VMAT2 is expressed in the central nervous system. Studies suggest that blocking transporter-2 has resulted in some improvement in TD. There are three VMAT2 inhibitors, one of which is used off-label whereas the other two are approved by the Food and Drug Administration (FDA).

Tetrabenazine, which is FDA approved for treating chorea associated with Huntington disease, is used off-label for treating TD. Deutetrabenazine, the deuterated form of tetrabenazine, was the first medication approved for TD, followed by valbenazine in 2017. Studies showing their long-term efficacy and safety are still pending, and there are no studies comparing these agents head to head with other VMAT2 medications. These medications have common adverse side effects, which include somnolence, parkinsonism, akathisia, depression, and suicidality. Table 38.2 summarizes the three VMAT-2 inhibitors for treating TD, including dosing, half-life, and adverse effects.

Unfortunately, even with these interventions, TD can persist longitudinally or irreversibly.

---

After 2 months of treatment on aripiprazole, the patient is experiencing no side effects and psychosis continues to be reasonably controlled. He decides to start treatment with depot formulation aripiprazole. After 6 months of stable treatment on the long-acting injectable, the patient decides to return to school part time. He enrolls in classes at the local community college and works for the local radio station sorting mail.

---

## BEYOND THE PEARLS:

- Chronic anticholinergic medication use in older adults to prevent acute dystonia is not recommended because of the negative effects on cognition.
- Advanced age and female gender are risk factors for developing medication-induced parkinsonism.
- Unlike acute dystonia, gender and age are not risk factors for akathisia.
- Akathisia is a psychiatric urgency, as it is a risk factor for suicide.
- First generation antipsychotics and risperidone have a higher risk of inducing prolactinemia. Relative prolactin-sparing antipsychotics include clozapine, olanzapine, and aripiprazole.
- TD may be treated with VMAT2 inhibitors. Because their side effects include akathisia and suicidality, then patients treated with these medications should be closely monitored.
- An AIMS assessment should be performed before initiating an antipsychotic and then yearly afterward.

## References

Besnard, I., Auclair, V., Callery, G., Gabriel-Bordenave, C., & Roberge, C. (2014). Antipsychotic-drug-induced hyperprolactinemia: Physiopathology, clinical features and guidance. *L'Enchephale*, *40*(1), 86–94.

Kaufman, D. M., & Milstein, M. J. (2013). *Kaufmans clinical neurology for psychiatrists*. Bronx, NY: Elsevier.

Khan, A. Y., Salaria, S., Ovais, M., & Ide, G. D. (2016). Depot antipsychotics: Where do we stand?" *Annals of Clinical Psychiatry*, *28*(4), 289–298.

Laoutidis, Z. G., & Luckhaus, C. (2014). 5-HT2A receptor antagonists for the treatment of neuroleptic-induced akathisia: A systematic review and meta-analysis. *International Journal of Neuropsychopharmacology*, *17*(5), 823–832.

Solmi, M., Pigato, G., Kane, J. M., & Correll, C. U. (2018). Treatment of tardive dyskinesia with VMAT-2 inhibitors: a systematic review and meta-analysis of randomized controlled trials. *Drug Design, Development and Therapy*, *12*, 1215–1238.

# CHAPTER 39

# Alcohol Withdrawal

Aarti Chawla Mittal ■ Destry Washburn

A 56-year-old male is admitted to the medical/surgical ward for right middle lobe pneumonia. He is unable to provide a detailed history, and you have not been able to contact any family to find out about his medical history. His physical examination reveals palmar erythema, gynecomastia, and spider angiomata on his upper chest and nose, as well as a mildly distended but soft abdomen.

He is placed on antibiotics for a community acquired pneumonia. His labs are outlined in Table 39.1.

*What significant medical history are you suspicious for given his physical examination and laboratory findings?*

The findings of palmar erythema, gynecomastia, spider angiomata, and distended abdomen are suspicious for liver pathology. This is further confirmed with his laboratory findings of pancytopenia (leukopenia, anemia, and thrombocytopenia). An elevated INR is further proof of compromised synthetic liver function. The patient also has an elevated AST and ALT in a 2:1 ratio. Highest on our differential diagnosis for his liver disease is alcohol cirrhosis, followed by hepatitis C, hepatitis B, hepatocellular carcinoma, and portal vein thrombosis.

| CLINICAL PEARL | STEP 2/3 |
|---|---|
| Greater serum AST than ALT is 90% sensitive for liver disease. A ratio of AST:ALT in a 2:1 ratio is often seen in alcohol liver disease. | |

TABLE 39.1 ■ Patient Lab Values

| Laboratory Test | Result |
|---|---|
| WBC | 2.7 K/μL |
| Hg | 11.2 g/dL |
| MCV | 104.3 × 10$^{15}$L |
| Platelets | 92 K/μL |
| INR | 1.7 |
| AST | 183 U/L |
| ALT | 91 U/L |
| T. Bili | 1.4 mg/dL |

*ALT*, Alanine transaminase; *AST*, aspartate aminotransferase; *Hg*, hemoglobin; *INR*, international normalized ratio; *MCV*, mean corpuscular volume; *T. Bili*, total bilirubin; *WBC*, white blood cells.

**BASIC SCIENCE PEARL**                                              **STEP 1**

Aspartate Aminotransferase (AST) is located in mitochondria. Alcohol is a toxin that causes the release of AST.

**CLINICAL PEARL**                                                  **STEP 2/3**

Increased serum Υ-glutamyltransferase is also indicative of alcohol use.

On hospital day 3, the patient starts to become tachycardic to 157/min, hypertensive to 169/92 mm/Hg, diaphoretic, and restless. He has a resting hand tremor. He is having visual hallucinations, as he is preoccupied with making sure the medical team feeds the cat that is living in his hospital room.

*What do you think has caused this acute change in mental status?*
Although you do not have more definitive history, your physical examination and laboratory findings point to this patient having alcoholic cirrhosis. Given that he has now gone up to 3 days without drinking alcohol, he may be going into alcohol withdrawal. Remember that patients are at risk of alcohol withdrawal within hours to 4 days after cessation of alcohol. The symptoms of alcohol withdrawal are anxiety, tremors, headache, nausea, vomiting, and diaphoresis.

The patient has many of the previously mentioned symptoms, and given his visual hallucinations and hyperadrenergic state, his condition should be classified as severe alcohol withdrawal.

*What other diagnoses should be considered?*
As discussed previously, alcohol withdrawal is a clinical diagnosis. Other possible etiologies must be considered and ruled out. Altered mental status has a broad differential and causes include infection, such as meningitis, encephalitis, sepsis due to infection from any source; structural as in stroke (hemorrhagic or ischemic or trauma); or metabolic derangements. Many of these etiologies can present very similarly to alcohol withdrawal and a premature diagnosis may lead to a delay in discovering the accurate diagnosis and the treatment.

*What causes alcohol withdrawal symptoms?*
In the normal state, the brain maintains a balance between its inhibitory system and excitatory systems. Gamma-amino butyric acid (GABA) neurotransmitters act on GABA receptors causing neuronal inhibition. The neurotransmitter glutamate acts on N-methyl-D-aspartate (NMDA) receptors causing neuronal excitement.

With chronic alcohol use, alcohol enhances the effect GABA and favors the inhibitory state. To compensate, the body will down regulate GABA-A receptors. In addition, alcohol inhibits NMDA receptors. In a similar compensatory measure, NMDA receptors are upregulated.

When alcohol is suddenly removed, there are now fewer GABA-A receptors compared to NMDA receptors. The central nervous system (CNS) is now favoring a hyperexcitable state. This can lead to tachycardia and hypertension. CNS hyperexcitability can also cause tremor, anxiety, insomnia, and irritability. Table 39.2 outlines the criteria for alcohol withdrawal.

*Once the diagnosis of alcohol withdrawal is established, what is your priority in treating this patient?*
The initial approach should be directed toward controlling the patient's symptoms and providing supportive care. Special attention should then be made in correcting any metabolic derangements. Psychomotor agitation is treated with benzodiazepines, and dose adjustments are made

**TABLE 39.2 ■ Diagnostic Criteria for Alcohol Withdrawal**

1. Sudden cessation or relative reduction of prolonged and heavy alcohol use.
2. At least two of the following symptoms:
   a. diaphoresis or tachycardia
   b. tremor
   c. insomnia
   d. nausea or vomitting
   e. hallucinations
   f. psychomotor agitaion
   g. anxiety
   h. generalized tonic-clonic seizures

based on severity. Close monitoring of vital signs and frequent reassessment of the patient's clinical status is very important. Nutritional support and intravenous (IV) fluids should be provided as necessary. Clinical evaluation of volume status should be performed, and any volume deficits should be replaced until the patient is determined to be euvolemic.

Prevention and treatment of Wernicke's encephalopathy requires administration of glucose and thiamine. Other vitamins should be provided intravenously, as alcohol withdrawal patients often are deficient in folate, magnesium, potassium, and phosphate. The term *banana bag* refers to an IV infusion containing 100 mg thiamine, 1 mg folic acid, 3 gm magnesium sulfate, and 1 ampule of multivitamins, usually mixed in 5% dextrose solution. Higher doses of thiamine may be warranted (500 mg IV 2–3 times daily).

---

**CLINICAL PEARL**                                                                    **STEP 2/3**

Wernike's encephalopathy consists of confusion, ataxia, nystagmus, and opthalmoplegia.

---

**BASIC SCIENCE PEARL**                                                                 **STEP 1**

Thiamine (vitamin B1) deficiency is often implicated in Wernike's encephalopathy. It is a cofactor needed to produce adenosine triphosphate (ATP). It is important to replenish thiamine at the same time or before giving glucose-containing fluids to prevent precipitation of Wernicke's encephalopathy.

---

Because of altered mental status, the patient should initially be kept nil per os (NPO) to prevent aspiration. Malnutrition, however, is often present in alcohol withdrawal patients and therefore should be addressed as soon as possible. Glucose-containing fluids are usually sufficient in the first 2 days. If the patient continues to be at high risk of aspiration after 1 to 2 days then a nasogastric tube may need to be inserted for parenteral nutrition.

*What should you anticipate as you continue to manage this patient?*
In severe forms of withdrawal, one can see auditory and visual hallucinations (delirium tremens), seizures, and a hyperadrenergic state, which can be life threatening. Physical restraints may be required for the safety of both the patient and the care providers. These should be removed as soon as it is determined that it is safe to do so. Fighting against restraints places the patient at risk of increased temperature and rhabdomyolysis.

Risk factors for delirium tremens (DT) include:
- A history of sustained drinking
- A history of previous DT

- Age greater than 30 years
- The presence of a concurrent illness
- The presence of significant alcohol withdrawal in the presence of an elevated ethanol level
- A longer period (more than 2 days) between the last drink and the onset of withdrawal

Delirium caused by alcohol withdrawal should be managed the same as other forms of delirium. Nonpharmacologic measures such as frequent reorientation of the patient to date, place, and time; providing adequate lighting and reassurance; and, if possible, mimicking day/night cycles as closely as possible.

### What is the mainstay of medical treatment for alcohol withdrawal?

Benzodiazepines are the most commonly used treatment. Ideally, symptom-driven use of short-acting benzodiazepines is preferred. Although there can be cross-tolerance with alcohol, remember to use benzodiazepines with caution, as an adverse effect of the drug is respiratory suppression.

Benzodiazepines stimulate GABA receptors and are first-line in treating alcohol withdrawal symptoms. There are several of these classes of medications to choose from, each with different properties.

Longer acting medications (diazepam or chlordiazepoxide) are often chosen as they sometimes provide a smoother treatment course with less risk of recurrent withdrawals and possible seizures. Shorter acting medications, including lorazepam or oxazepam have also been used and are preferred in patients with cirrhosis or acute alcoholic hepatitis in order to prevent oversedation. Not all benzodiazepines are available in IV form, and therefore this must be considered when selecting the medication. IV is preferred initially because of risk of aspiration as stated previously.

---

The patient is started on intravenous thiamine, potassium, magnesium, phosphate, and glucose. You decide to start a benzodiazepine to address his withdrawal symptoms.

---

| CLINICAL PEARL | STEP 2/3 |
|---|---|

Lorazepam, oxazepam, and temazepam are benzodiazepines metabolized extrahepatically. They are preferred in patients with significant liver disease.

### How do we know how much benzodiazepine to give?

There is good evidence to support the use of titration of medications based on risk factors and severity of symptoms. Younger, healthier patients may require less sedation, with the goal of insuring safety and comfort while enabling an accurate neurologic examination. Older patients with cardiopulmonary compromise for any reason may need heavier sedation in order to decrease systemic stress. Again, close monitoring is essential in order to anticipate and intervene in case of deterioration of clinical status or oversedation.

The Clinical Institute Withdrawal Assessment for Alcohol Scale (CIWA-Ar) is a validated scoring tool that can guide the clinician to when medication is necessary to treat alcohol withdrawal. Fig. 39.1 outlines the CIWA-Ar.

When using such a system, medication is only given if symptoms are seen and then dose adjustments are made according to severity. Frequent evaluations are made before administering treatment. Initial evaluations should be made every 10 to 15 minutes and then hourly once symptoms have stabilized. This approach has been found to achieve adequate symptom control and therapy while requiring less sedative medications and even decreasing hospital length of stay compared with fixed-dose regimens. It should be noted that very high doses of benzodiazepines may be required to control symptoms.

---

According to the CIWA-Ar scale, the patient is requiring high doses of benzodiazepines every hour.

---

## Clinical Institute Withdrawal Assessment Scale for Alcohol, Revised (CIWA-Ar)

### Nausea and Vomiting
0 – No nausea or vomiting
1
2
3
4 – Intermittent nausea with dry heaves
5
6
7 – Constant nausea, frequent dry heaves and vomiting

### Paroxysmal Sweats
0 – No sweat visible
1 – Barely perceptible sweating, palms moist
2
3
4 – Beads of sweat obvious on forehead
5
6
7 – Drenching sweats

### Agitation
0 – Normal activity
1 – Somewhat more than normal activity
2
3
4 – Moderate fidgety and restless
5
6
7 – Paces back and forth during most of the interview or constantly thrashes about

### Visual Disturbances
0 – Not present
1 – Very mild photosensitivity
2 – Mild photosensitivity
3 – Moderate photosensitivity
4 – Moderately severe visual hallucinations
5 – Severe visual hallucinations
6 – Extreme severe visual hallucinations
7 – Continuous visual hallucinations

### Tremor
0 – No tremor
1 – Not visible, but can be felt at finger tips
2
3
4 – Moderate when patient's hands extended
5
6
7 – Severe, even with arms not extended

### Tactile Disturbances
0 – None
1 – Very mild paraesthesias
2 – Mild paraesthesias
3 – Moderate paraesthesias
4 – Moderately severe hallucinations
5 – Severe hallucinations
6 – Extremely severe hallucinations
7 – Continuous hallucinations

### Headache
0 – Not present
1 – Very mild
2 – Mild
3 – Moderate
4 – Moderately severe
5 – Severe
6 – Very severe
7 – Extremely severe

### Auditory Disturbances
0 – Not present
1 – Very mild harshness or ability to frighten
2 – Mild harshness or ability to frighten
3 – Moderate harshness or ability to frighten
4 – Moderately severe hallucinations
5 – Severe hallucinations
6 – Extremely severe hallucinations
7 – Continuous hallucinations

### Orientation and clouding of the Sensorium
0 – Oriented and can do serial additions
1 – Cannot do serial additions
2 – Disoriented for date but not more than 2 calendar days
3 – Disoriented for date by more than 2 calendar days
4 – Disoriented for place/person

### Cumulative scoring

| Cumulative scoring | Approach |
|---|---|
| 0 – 8 | No medication needed |
| 9 – 14 | Medication is optional |
| 15 – 20 | Definitely needs medication |
| >20 | Increased risk of complications |

**Fig. 39.1** CIWA-Ar scale.

**TABLE 39.3** ■ **Risk Factors for Admission into the Intensive Care Unit**

Age >40–45 years
Existing cardiac problems (heart failure, arrhythmia, MI, angina)
Hemodynamic instability
Marked acid-base disturbance
Severe electrolyte abnormality
Respiratory compromise (hypoxia, hypercapnia, pneumonia, asthma, COPD)
Serious infection (pneumonia, trauma, UTI, etc.)
GI distress/pathology (pancreatitis, GI bleed, liver failure)
Persistent hyperthermia
Rhabdomyolysis
Acute or chronic renal failure
Previously complicated alcohol withdrawal (seizures, DTs)
Requirement for high-dose sedatives to control symptoms

*COPD*, Chronic obstructive pulmonary disease; *DT*, delirum tremen; *GI*, gastrointestinal; *MI*, myocardial infarction; *UTI*, urinary tract infection.

*What is the next best step in his care?*

Severe alcohol withdrawal can lead to permanent brain damage and even death. The patient has severe withdrawal as evidenced by the delirium tremens as well as his high benzodiazepine requirement. It would be appropriate to transfer him to the intensive care unit (ICU) for closer monitoring and treatment. Generally speaking, the emergency room, ICU and postoperative acute care unit are the only places capable of fulfilling any hourly need a patient has, whether that involves suctioning for excessive secretions regularly or administering medication administration hourly. The patient currently requires hourly administration of medications and thus should be in an ICU for treatment of his alcohol withdrawal. Table 39.3 lists risk factors that would determine admission into the ICU.

*Are there other adjunctive treatments to consider?*

You have transferred the patient to the ICU. He continues to have CIWA scores >20 every 10 minutes after doses of IV benzodiazepines.

Phenobarbital, a barbiturate, is another common treatment. Similar to benzodiazepines, phenobarbital stimulates GABA receptors and affects α-amino-3-hydroxy-5-methyl-4-isoxazolepropionic acid (AMPA)-type glutamate receptors as well. Phenobarbital can have a synergistic effect when given simultaneously with benzodiazepines. Phenobarbital increases the duration of the GABA chloride channel opening, whereas benzodiazepines increase the frequency of the opening. Phenobarbital is often used as a first- or second-line agent for alcohol withdrawal, but unlike benzodiazepines, it has a more predictable dose-related effect. Presumably, this is related to variable GABA cross-tolerance to benzodiazepines and alcohol. A dose of 10 to 20 mg/kg of phenobarbital is generally effective for withdrawal. When dosing alone, phenobarbital should not lead to respiratory depression and thus may decrease the risk of intubation. This is also an attractive medication because it is an anti-epileptic, and thus may have additional preventive measures against withdrawal seizures. Many now are advocating for its use as monotherapy. Combination therapy with benzodiazepines is not additive and can lead to respiratory depression.

Additionally, many physicians are using dexmedetomidine, a highly selective α2-adrenergic agonist that works to increase the activity of GABA neurons. Although this is a non-FDA-approved use of the drug, it is being used more and more in conjunction with benzodiazepines or phenobarbital, because it does not lead to respiratory depression, even at high doses. It does not, however, decrease seizure risk. Many are now placing patients on a continuous dexmedetomidine IV drip, with additional doses of benzodiazepines or phenobarbital as needed according to symptoms per the CIWA-Ar scale. Adverse effects such as hypotension and bradycardia must be considered and monitored.

Propofol can also be an effective treatment with hypotension, with oversedation being the main adverse effect. If this medication is required, intubation is often, but not always, necessary and that decision should be based upon clinical evaluation.

---

You have ordered phenobarbital for the patient's continued severe withdrawal. He is NPO; however, despite close attention and good supportive care unfortunately he vomits and aspirates. He is now tachypneic to 38/min; desaturating to 79% on 3 liters of supplemental oxygen; and having continued tremors, diaphoresis, and adrenergic surge. His blood pressure and heart rate are very labile, and there is concern for his safety as he fights against the restraints aggressively whenever not heavily sedated. Control of his psychomotor agitation is very difficult, and during periods of rest he appears to have difficultly clearing his secretions and his breathing is becoming more labored.

---

### What should you do now?
No matter what the clinical situations, you should always default to your ABCs: airway, breathing and circulation. Currently, our patient does not have a secured airway, as he is vomiting and altered without airway protection. Thus he should be intubated for airway protection and hypoxic respiratory failure. Intubation will provide good airway protection from aspiration and significantly decreased work of breathing. This will also allow higher doses of medications to be given while ensuring greater safety as the treatment course progresses through the most danger.

---

The patient is intubated.

---

### Should you change your treatment plan for his alcohol withdrawal now that he is intubated?
Now that the patient has a secure airway, you should consider the addition of a benzodiazepine IV infusion. Given his high hourly requirement, this may lend to better symptom control. Remember, benzodiazepines work centrally to depress the respiratory drive, so now that the ventilator is in control of his breathing, a depressed respiratory drive is less concerning. Otherwise, you would continue supportive care and ventilator management.

### What is the normal time course for alcohol withdrawal resolution?
Symptoms of withdrawal generally last 5 to 7 days. It is important that patients who get admitted with alcohol withdrawal are given resources for alcohol cessation support groups upon discharge in the hopes of preventing relapse.

### BEYOND THE PEARLS:
- Plasma homocysteine levels are often elevated in alcoholic patients. Its is associated with high risk of first-onset alcohol withdrawal seizures.
- Cortical and cerebellar atrophy can have pathological features seen in patients with chronic alcohol abuse.
- Korsakoff syndrome is the advanced stage of Wernike's encephalopathy consisting of amnesia with confabulation and hallucinations.
- Mamillary bodies, part of the limbic system, are damaged in Wernike-Korsakoff syndrome.
- Majority of CIWA-Ar criteria are subjective and do not take into account objective data such as hypertension or tachycardia. Remember to also review objective information when assessing for alcohol withdrawal.

## References

American Psychiatric Association. (2013). *Diagnostic and statistical manual of mental disorders* (5th ed.). Washington, DC: Author.

Bayard, M., McIntyre, J., Hill, K. R., & Woodside, J. Jr. (2004). Alcohol withdrawal syndrome. *American Family Physician, 69*(6), 1443–1450.

Linn, D., & Loeser, K. (2015). Dexmedetomidine for alcohol withdrawal syndrome. *Annals of Pharmacotherapy, 49*(12), 1336–1342.

Puz, C. A., & Stokes, S. J. (2005). Alcohol withdrawal syndrome: Assessment and treatment with the use of the Clinical Institute Withdrawal Assessment for Alcohol-revised. *Critical Care Nursing Clinics of North America, 17*(3), 297–304.

Schmidt, K., Doshi, M. R., Holzhausen, J. M., Natavio, A., Cadiz, M., & Winegardner, J. E. (2016). Treatment of severe alcohol withdrawal. *Annals of Pharmacotherapy, 50*(5), 389–401.

Schuckit, M. (2014). Recognition and management of withdrawal delirium (delirium tremens). *New England Journal of Medicine, 371*, 2109–2113.

Sen, S., Grgurich, P., Tulolo, A., Smith-Freedman, A., Lei, Y., Gray, A., & Dargin, J. (2017). A symptom-triggered benzodiazepine protocol utilizing SAS and CIWA-Ar scoring for the treatment of alcohol withdrawal syndrome in the critically ill. *Annals of Pharmacotherapy, 51*(2), 101–110.

Note: Page numbers followed by "f" indicate figures, "t" indicate tables, and "b" indicate boxes.